Advanced Decision Making in Clinical Medicine

Advanced Decision Making in Clinical Medicine

Guest Editors

Kiril Tenekedjiev
Mike Calford

MDPI

Basel • Beijing • Wuhan • Barcelona • Belgrade • Novi Sad • Cluj • Manchester

Guest Editors
Kiril Tenekedjiev
Australian Maritime College
University of Tasmania
Launceston, TAS
Australia

Mike Calford
Hunter Medical Research
Institute
New Lambton, NSW
Australia

Editorial Office
MDPI AG
Grosspeteranlage 5
4052 Basel, Switzerland

This is a reprint of the Special Issue, published open access by the journal *Applied Sciences* (ISSN 2076-3417), freely accessible at: https://www.mdpi.com/journal/applsci/special_issues/advanced_decision_making_in_clinical_medicine.

For citation purposes, cite each article independently as indicated on the article page online and as indicated below:

Lastname, A.A.; Lastname, B.B. Article Title. *Journal Name* **Year**, *Volume Number*, Page Range.

ISBN 978-3-7258-6053-1 (Hbk)
ISBN 978-3-7258-6054-8 (PDF)
https://doi.org/10.3390/books978-3-7258-6054-8

Contents

About the Editors

Kiril Tenekedjiev

Kiril Tenekedjiev is an adjunct professor at the University of Tasmania, Australia. He is an established researcher in the areas of statistical decision sciences, machine learning, and systems engineering. He is a senior member of the IEEE, and a Fellow of Engineers Australia. He holds a PhD in statistical pattern recognition and a Doctorate of Sciences degree in decision support and data analysis. His career has seen him hold professorial appointments in Bulgaria and Australia, including Professor at the University of Tasmania and Professor in computer science with Varna Free University "Chernorizets Hrabar", Bulgaria. Kiril served as a Fulbright Scholar with the State University of New York (USA)—Binghamton and held a Visiting Scientist role at the European Union's Joint Research Centre in Ispra, Italy. His expertise is in intelligent systems, focusing on quantitative decision making, simulation modelling, risk analysis, technical diagnostics, and statistical pattern recognition. He has applied his expertise across reliability engineering, medical science, economic analyses, energy efficiency, transport management, and environmental modelling. He has been the CI on 55 grants in Europe and Southeast Asia and serves on eight Editorial boards of peer-reviewed journals. He reviews for over 20 reputable journals, serves as an expert for the Australian Academy of Sciences, and reviews proposals for the Australian Research Council and other funding programmes (Czech Science Foundation, Fulbright Commission, etc.). He has published over 260 works (book chapters, journal/conference papers) in five languages, with a total impact factor of 158, with over 2000 citations and an h-index of 19 (Google Scholar).

Mike Calford

Mike Calford has held the role of CEO of the Hunter Medical Research Institute. He has also held a number of other esteemed leadership roles at Australian universities, including Provost at the Australian National University, Provost at the University of Tasmania, Deputy Vice Chancellor (Research) and Pro Vice Chancellor (Health) at Newcastle, and Pro Vice Chancellor (Health and Medical Research) at Wollongong. He was also the CEO at the Illawarra Health and Medical Research Institute. He previously held research and teaching roles at the Universities of Queensland, Newcastle, and ANU. His eminent research is in the field of neuroscience, and he served as the Chief Investigator of an ARC Centre of Excellence and of an NHMRC Programme. He has been published in the highest impact journals, including two full papers in *Nature* and one in *Science* (this paper was the scientific basis for a clinical trial of stroke rehabilitation therapy run by the NIH Clinical Center at Bethesda (NCT00056706)). His research focus is neural plasticity and the premise that any hopes for therapy after major brain trauma depend ultimately on the capacity of the central nervous system to encode and integrate, into its working systems, a changed circuit. His experiments in this field, which began at the University of Queensland around 1985, were based firmly upon the need to understand the capacity for change in the adult brain and then to develop the tools necessary to manipulate that capacity. His approach was to develop appropriate animal models that allow this capacity to be studied in the intact brain.

Preface

In modern medical practice, patients are encouraged to actively participate in all decisions affecting their treatment, quality of life, and livelihood. However, patients are rarely qualified or confident enough to participate in all phases of decision-making about their treatment. Appropriate medical decision-making is at the heart of evidence-based medicine. It integrates the expertise of healthcare professionals with the patient's preferences and value system, as well as the best possible interpretation of medical information, to effectively guide medical decisions in clinical practice. Recent advances in artificial intelligence, data science and statistics can improve the quality of medical decisions and increase public confidence in the value of proposed medical solutions.

Our Special Issue features articles that explore how artificial intelligence, data science, and statistics come together to improve medical decision-making. We offer a collection of eleven research works that discuss advances in data analysis and risk management in medical treatment decisions, applications of artificial intelligence methods, modelling and simulation in medical decision-making, and policy development for better evidence-based practices and services. Each article addresses unique aspects of improving medical decision-making through intelligent methods and data analysis. Collectively, these works exemplify the translational potential of advanced decision methodologies to deliver safer, more equitable, and evidence-informed clinical care. The contributions of these works reflect the diversity and richness of current research, focusing on topics ranging from improving diagnostics using artificial intelligence, through fuzzy data analysis for better medical care, to exploring drug side effects and improving personalized healthcare cases and decision-making.

Kiril Tenekedjiev and Mike Calford
Guest Editors

applied sciences

MDPI

Editorial

Exploring Computational Methods to Advance Clinical Decision Making

Kiril Tenekedjiev [1,2,*] and Mike Calford [3,4]

1 Australian Maritime College (AMC), University of Tasmania (UTAS), Launceston, TAS 7248, Australia
2 School of Computer Science, Faculty of Social, Business and Computer Sciences, Varna Free University "Chernorizets Hrabar", Varna 9007, Bulgaria
3 Hunter Medical Research Institute, Locked Bag 1000, New Lambton Heights, NSW 2305, Australia; mike.calford@anu.edu.au
4 School of Medicine and Psychology, Australian National University, Canberra, ACT 2601, Australia
* Correspondence: kiril.tenekedjiev@fulbrightmail.org

The papers comprising our Special Issue on advanced decision making in clinical medicine (which is part of the series in applied bioscience and bioengineering) were conceived and written during a most challenging time for medical science and its delivery—the COVID-19 pandemic. Particularly in the pre-vaccine period, terms and concepts which are normally reserved for specialist journals were, for the first time, the parlance of the daily news. Public health officials and practitioners were called on to explain their technical frameworks and jargon to a wide audience. For most, it was a revelation to learn of the highly mathematical nature of modern medical practice. For many, this was reassuring, and for others, the message was foreign and fueled distrust.

Recent developments in artificial intelligence, data science, and statistics, however, have the potential to enhance the quality of medical decision making and bolster public confidence in the value of the offered solutions. There is a communication gap that is as much the responsibility of scientists and practitioners as it is of the media and politicians.

The landscape of clinical decision making is transforming, driven by the convergence of data science, systems engineering, cognitive analytics, and machine learning. As the complexity and volume of patient data expand thanks to genomic, imaging, sensor-derived, and electronic health record sources, the demand for robust, explicable, and adaptive decision-support tools has intensified. The challenge to combine, for the best effect, the knowledge of healthcare professionals (both frontline and their scientist and technical colleagues) with patient preferences, values and risk tolerance, has never been more pressing.

The role of decision theory and probabilistic reasoning has re-emerged in clinical contexts. Shared decision making frameworks, supported by Bayesian models and utilities elicited from patients, are facilitating more personalized and ethically grounded treatment choices [1]. Simulation-based methods have also gained traction. Studies apply agent-based models, system dynamics, and discrete-event simulations to optimize clinical pathways and resource allocation, especially in critical care and pandemic response scenarios [2].

Decision support also requires understanding causality. Advances in causal inference from observational data—through frameworks such as counterfactual reasoning [3], targeted maximum likelihood estimation (TMLE), and instrumental variable methods—enable clinicians to assess treatment effects more robustly in the absence of randomized trials [4].

Recent research has progressed to embed artificial intelligence (AI) in diagnostic and prognostic workflows. For example, ref. [5] demonstrated the potential of deep learning to match or exceed dermatologist-level accuracy in skin cancer classification. The study [6] advocated for a human-centered AI approach that enhances clinician judgment rather than replacing it. At the same time, explainable AI (XAI) approaches, as outlined in [7], have emerged as critical tools to improve transparency and trust in clinical environments, particularly in high-stakes decisions.

Another trend is the use of reinforcement learning (RL) as a decision-theoretic framework for sequential treatment planning, especially in chronic and critical care. The study referenced in [8] demonstrated how off-policy RL could recommend vasopressor and fluid management strategies for septic patients in the ICU, often aligning with expert decisions. Building on this, ref. [9] highlighted the challenges of implementing RL in healthcare, considering aspects of safety, fairness, and interpretability.

In this Special Issue we present state-of-the-art contributions that examine how artificial intelligence, data science, and statistics can improve and enhance effective medical decision making and evidence-based medicine. We curated a collection of studies that address innovative procedures in evidence-based medicine, data analytics advances and risk management in medical treatment decisions, applications of artificial intelligence methods, modeling and simulation in medical decision making, as well as policy development for better evidence-based practices and services. Collectively, these works exemplify the translational potential of advanced decision methodologies to deliver safer, more equitable, and evidence-informed clinical care. We strongly encouraged articles from interdisciplinary teams that include medical professionals, researchers, clinicians, data scientists, and AI experts.

There are eleven state-of-the-art research articles in this Special Issue that are pertinent to the issues covered. Each paper addresses unique aspects of the enhancement of medical decision making through intelligent methods and data analysis. The contributions made by these studies reflect the variety and richness of current research, focusing on topics ranging from improved diagnostics using AI, through fuzzy data analysis for improved medical treatment, to exploration of adverse drug reactions and improved personalized health case and decision making. In the following paragraphs, we shortly describe the articles included in this Special Issue.

Early or timely detection of serious medical conditions is an area where machine learning can considerably improve efficiency of medical care and patient outcomes. The work of Naeem Ullah, Javed Ali Khan, Mohammad Sohail Khan, Wahab Khan, Izaz Hassan, Marwa Obayya, Noha Negm and Ahmed S. Salama, titled *An Effective Approach to Detect and Identify Brain Tumors Using Transfer Learning* [10], explores the use of pre-trained deep transfer learning (TL) for the detection and recognition of the three types of brain tumors—gliomas, meningiomas, and pituitary tumors. The latter are among the most critical, widespread, and life-threatening illnesses worldwide. More specifically, they assess the performance of nine pre-trained TL classifiers by automatically identifying and classifying brain tumors using a detailed classification method. The TL algorithms are tested on a baseline brain tumor classification (MRI) dataset, which is freely accessible on Kaggle. The deep learning (DL) models are fine-tuned using their default parameters. The authors find that the inceptionresnetv2 TL algorithm yields the best performance and achieves the highest accuracy in detecting and classifying glioma, meningioma, and pituitary brain tumors, thereby ranking as the top classification algorithm, surpassing the other DL algorithms. The authors also verify their results through comparison with hybrid methods, where they employ convolutional neural networks (CNNs) for deep feature extraction and a support vector machine (SVM) for classification.

Another study that deals with improved detection of serious medical conditions is by Andressa C. M. da Silveira, Álvaro Sobrinho, Leandro Dias da Silva, Evandro de Barros Costa, Maria Eliete Pinheiro and Angelo Perkusich, titled *Exploring Early Predic-*

tion of Chronic Kidney Disease Using Machine Learning Algorithms for Small and Imbalanced Datasets [11]. The authors discuss chronic kidney disease (CKD), which is recognized as a global public health challenge, and is typically identified during the later stages of the condition due to imbalanced and small datasets. The work uses medical record data about Brazilians with and without a CKD diagnosis, which includes attributes such as hypertension, diabetes mellitus, creatinine levels, urea, albuminuria, age, gender, and glomerular filtration rate. They then apply oversampling methods with both manual and automated augmentation techniques, such as the synthetic minority oversampling technique (SMOTE), borderline-SMOTE, and borderline-SMOTE support vector machine (borderline-SMOTE SVM). Modeling is performed using decision trees (DTs), random forests, and multi-class AdaBoosted DT algorithms. The authors also apply methods for dynamic classifier selection, such as overall local accuracy and local class accuracy. For dynamic ensemble selection, they use k-nearest oracles-union, k-nearest oracles-eliminate, and META-DES. The performance of the models is assessed using hold-out validation, multiple stratified cross-validation (CV), and nested CV. The authors show superior accuracy for the decision tree model accuracy through manual augmentation and SMOTE. The outcomes of this work can contribute to the development of systems aimed at the early detection of CKD, particularly when dealing with imbalanced and limited datasets.

A third related work in this Special Issue addresses the use of artificial intelligence (AI) in the healthcare sector—the work of Saleem Ameen, Ming-Chao Wong, Kwang-Chien Yee and Paul Turner, titled *AI and Clinical Decision Making: The Limitations and Risks of Computational Reductionism in Bowel Cancer Screening* [12]. While AI techniques are often praised as enhancers of precision, safety, and quality of clinical decisions, treatments, and patient care, they depend on reductive reasoning and computational determinism that incorporate problematic assumptions regarding clinical decision making and practice. They tend to simplify the autonomy, expertise, and judgment of clinicians to inputs and outputs that are framed as binary or multi-class classification challenges measured against a clinician's ability to identify or predict disease conditions. The authors investigate this reductive reasoning within AI systems for colorectal cancer (CRC) to underscore their limitations and dangers. Those refer to the issues caused by intrinsic biases found in retrospective training datasets and the embedded assumptions present in fundamental AI architectures and algorithms. They also relate to the inadequate and limited evaluations performed on AI systems before their integration into clinical practice. Another limitation is the underrepresentation of socio-technical factors concerning the context-specific interactions between clinicians, their patients, and the wider healthcare system. As a result, the authors recommend that to maximize the advantages of AI systems and prevent adverse unintended effects on clinical decision making and patient care, it is essential to adopt more nuanced and balanced approaches to the deployment and evaluation of AI systems in CRC.

Two of the works in the Special Issue explore diagnostics techniques of adverse drug reactions.

The first work is by Jianxiang Wei, Lu Cheng, Pu Han, Yunxia Zhu and Weidong Huang, titled Decision Tree-Based Data Stratification Method for the Minimization of the Masking Effect in Adverse Drug Reaction Signal Detection [13]. They posit that data masking is an inherent flaw in the measures of disproportionality used for detecting signals in adverse drug reactions (ADRs). They introduce a decision tree stratification approach to reduce the masking effect by incorporating both patient- and drug-related factors. They utilize adverse drug reaction monitoring records from the Jiangsu Province in China from 2011 to 2018. The authors define the age divisions for antibiotic-related data and perform correlation analysis on the gender and age of patients in relation to the properties of drug categories. They then develop a decision tree using the J48 algorithm, which classified whether drugs were categorized as antibiotics based on age and gender. They also introduce performance evaluation metrics such as recall, precision, and F score (the harmonic mean of recall and precision). Using four experiments (based on the proportional reporting ratio methodology: non-stratification, gender-stratification, age-stratification, and decision tree stratification), the authors show that decision tree stratification outperformed the other three approaches, and the data-masking effect can be further reduced by thoroughly considering confounding factors related to both patients and drugs.

The second work is by Jianxiang Wei, Jimin Dai, Yingya Zhao, Pu Han, Yunxia Zhu and Weidong Huang, titled *Application of Association Rules Analysis in Mining Adverse Drug Reaction Signals* [14]. The authors emphasize the use of spontaneous reporting systems (SRSs) as a key method for tracking ADRs that occur during clinical drug use. To detect signals for ADRs, researchers often use disproportionality analysis (DPA) and do not incorporate data mining techniques. Here, the authors rely again on the spontaneous reports from Jiangsu Province, China for the period from 2011 to 2018 and apply association rules analysis (ARA) to extract signals. For their analysis, they define crucial metrics for ARA, e.g., confidence and lift, and develop performance evaluation indicators like precision, recall, and F1 as objective benchmarks. The results show improvement of the F1 score using the ARA method, representing a significant enhancement. To mitigate drug risks and support decision making regarding drug safety, it is essential to integrate and utilize more data mining techniques for ADR signal detection.

The study by Kiril Tenekedjiev, Daniela Panayotova, Mohamed Daboos, Snejana Ivanova, Mark Symes, Plamen Panayotov and Natalia Nikolova, titled *Quasi-Experimental Design for Medical Studies with the Method of the Fuzzy Pseudo-Control Group* [15], explores the effect of interventions over a given parameter representing the medical condition of patients. The authors propose a novel fuzzy quasi-experimental computational approach, called the method of the fuzzy pseudo-control group (MFPCG), which addresses the limitations of methods commonly used (e.g., the difference-in-differences (DID) method). The method uses four fuzzy samples as input and statistically compares the favorability of the differences in a continuous parameter before and after the intervention for the experimental and the pseudo-control groups. MFPCG applies four modifications of fuzzy Bootstrap procedures to perform each of the nine statistical tests. As a case study, the team explores a dataset related to the effect of annuloplasty that acts in conjunction with revascularization over two continuous parameters that characterize the condition of patients with ischemic heart disease complicated by moderate and moderate-to-severe ischemic mitral regurgitation. The statistical results proved the favorable effect of annuloplasty on two parameters, both for patients with a relatively preserved medical state and patients with a relatively deteriorated medical state. The results of the MFPCG are compared with those of a fuzzy DID. The work discusses the limitations and adaptability of MFPCG, indicating that it is not a technique competing with DID but instead should be used alongside it.

Artificial intelligence, machine learning, and data science are becoming commonplace in data analysis and statistics. However, a versatile software tool tailored to the interactions in small biomedical teams is often missing. Proprietary commercial software packages bear inherent risks of abandonment or unpredictable company policies. Open-source software libraries may require too much effort to use. In the work, titled *Anatomy of a Data Science Software Toolkit That Uses Machine Learning to Aid 'Bench-to-Bedside' Medical Research—With Essential Concepts of Data Mining and Analysis Explained*, the authors László Beinrohr, Eszter Kail, Péter Piros, Erzsébet Tóth, Rita Fleiner and Krasimir Kolev [16] describe a toolkit to address this problem. Their toolkit is designed from bottom to top with small teams in mind, which allows individuals with very different expertise to work together with only specific parts of the software dedicated to their expertise. The proposed approach is based on open-source components (existing modular Python platform libraries); thus, company policy risks are alleviated. This paper also summarizes basic concepts in data science that serve the structured data organization through a contemporary data analysis applied in the described toolkit. The authors also show examples from their laboratory using blood sample and blood clot data from thrombosis patients (suffering from stroke, heart and peripheral thrombosis disease) and how such tools can help to set realistic expectations and show caveats.

A different scope of exploration is offered by Andrzej Walczak, Paweł Moszczyński and Paweł Krzesiński, in their work titled *Evolution of Hemodynamic Parameters Simulated by Means of Diffusion Models* [17]. They explore the similarity between diffusion as a physical concept in particle movement, heat transfer, etc., and the behavior of medical data. They posit that changes in medical parameters recorded during patient treatment can also be described using diffusion models. They view a patient medical condition by a set of discrete values, and the progression of condition is represented as a transition of continuously changing, temporal attributes from one discrete parameter value to another, linked to given parameters. The capacity to forecast such diffusion-related characteristics provides invaluable support in diagnostic decision making. The authors assess several hundred patients to study how to stabilize their hemodynamic parameters and introduce a diffusion model based on the simulation of treatment outcomes. As a case study, they explore the time evolution of thoracic fluid content (TFC). They use the Fokker–Planck equation (FPE) to verify that the diffusion phenomenon effectively accounts for the changes observed in heart disease parameters.

The study by Joana Magalhães, Maria José Correia, Raquel M. Silva, Ana Cristina Esteves, Artur Alves and Ana Sofia Duarte, titled *Molecular Techniques and Target Selection for the Identification of Candida spp. in Oral Samples* [18], explores candidiasis and the ability to avoid overuse of antifungal medications. The use of high-throughput technologies for diagnosing yeast pathogens offers notable advantages in terms of sensitivity, precision, and rapidity. While molecular techniques are the subject of considerable investigation, their implementation in clinical practice faces significant obstacles. In their review, the authors explore the pros and cons of existing molecular techniques used for identifying Candida spp., particularly in the context of oral candidiasis. A discussion on their use for diagnosing oral infections seeks to pinpoint the most rapid, cost-effective, precise, and user-friendly molecular approaches suitable for point-of-care testing. The authors pay attention to the challenges healthcare professionals must overcome to ensure an accurate diagnosis.

Another review by Daniela Gifu, titled *Soft Sets Extensions: Innovating Healthcare Claims Analysis* [19], focuses on the development and use of soft sets and their various extensions and how they are used in the analysis of healthcare claims data. They offer adaptable frameworks for handling the uncertainty and indeterminacy that are characteristic of healthcare claims data. The review traces the evolution of these mathematical tools and how they have advanced healthcare research and improved data analysis techniques. Through real-world illustrations, the author highlights the impact of these tools, emphasizing their critical role in supporting informed decision making and facilitating knowledge discovery within the healthcare sector. The author discussed several case studies to demonstrate the practical usefulness of soft set extensions. The recommendations of this work are to suggest incorporating soft sets and their extensions as a way to enhance the accuracy and effectiveness of healthcare data analysis, leading to improved healthcare results.

In our Special Issue, we were able to accommodate a perspectives paper by Franco Musio, titled The Critical Link in the Successful Application of Advanced Clinical Decision Making—Revisiting the Physician–Patient Relationship from a Practical and Pragmatic Perspective [20]. The author explores the rapidly growing field of advanced clinical decision making influenced by healthcare technologies and the new dimensions of how physicians and patients interact to support medical treatment and shared decision making. The discussion examines the models being researched and utilized in clinical decision making, as well as the connections between physicians and patients, highlighting their complex interactions. Moreover, both clinical decision making and the physician–patient relationship exhibit dynamic, reciprocal relationships that work together in a synergistic manner. The author presents innovative frameworks to clarify these intricate processes, alongside real-life clinical examples. The author widely discusses that the physician–patient relationship serves as a "filter" through which decision-making processes must navigate in order to be executed.

We express our appreciation to the authors for their significant contributions and to the reviewers for their thorough feedback, which allowed us to prepare a Special Issue of such quality. We hope that this Special Issue will motivate future research and findings in innovative data analytics for improved medical decision making, medical diagnostics, and healthcare.

Author Contributions: Conceptualization, K.T. and M.C.; methodology, K.T. and M.C.; resources, K.T. and M.C.; writing—original draft preparation, K.T. and M.C.; writing—review and editing, K.T. and M.C.; supervision, K.T. and M.C.; project administration, K.T. and M.C. All authors have read and agreed to the published version of the manuscript.

Conflicts of Interest: The authors declare no conflict of interest.

References

1. Elwyn, G.; Durand, M.A.; Song, J.; Aarts, J.; Thomas, V. A three-talk model for shared decision making: Multistage consultation process. *BMJ* **2020**, *359*, j4891. [CrossRef] [PubMed]
2. Currie, C.S.; Fowler, J.W.; Kotiadis, K.; Monks, T.; Onggo, B.S.; Robertson, D.A.; Tako, A.A. How simulation modelling can help reduce the impact of COVID-19. *J. Simul.* **2020**, *14*, 83–97. [CrossRef]
3. Pearl, J. *Causality: Models, Reasoning and Inference*, 2nd ed.; Cambridge University Press: Cambridge, UK, 2009.
4. Schwab, P.; Linhardt, L.; Karlen, W. Granger-causal attentive mixtures of experts: Learning important features with neural networks. *Proc. AAAI 2020* **2020**, *34*, 4712–4719. [CrossRef]
5. Esteva, A.; Robicquet, A.; Ramsundar, B.; Kuleshov, V.; DePristo, M.; Chou, K.; Cui, C.; Corrado, G.; Thrun, S.; Dean, J. A guide to deep learning in healthcare. *Nat. Med.* **2021**, *25*, 24–29. [CrossRef] [PubMed]
6. Topol, E. *Deep Medicine: How Artificial Intelligence Can Make Healthcare Human Again*; Basic Books: New York, NY, USA, 2019.
7. Tjoa, E.; Guan, C. A survey on explainable artificial intelligence (XAI): Toward medical XAI. *IEEE Trans. Neural Netw. Learn. Syst.* **2021**, *32*, 4793–4813. [CrossRef] [PubMed]
8. Komorowski, M.; Celi, L.A.; Badawi, O.; Gordon, A.C.; Faisal, A.A. The artificial intelligence clinician learns optimal treatment strategies for sepsis in intensive care. *Nat. Med.* **2018**, *24*, 1716–1720. [CrossRef] [PubMed]
9. Gottesman, O.; Johansson, F.; Komorowski, M.; Faisal, A.A.; Sontag, D.; Doshi-Velez, F.; Celi, L.A. Guidelines for reinforcement learning in healthcare. *Nat. Med.* **2019**, *25*, 16–18. [CrossRef] [PubMed]
10. Ullah, N.; Khan, J.A.; Khan, M.S.; Khan, W.; Hassan, I.; Obayya, M.; Negm, N.; Salama, A.S. An effective approach to detect and identify brain tumors using transfer learning. *Appl. Sci.* **2022**, *12*, 5645. [CrossRef]
11. da Silveira, A.C.M.; Sobrinho, A.; da Silva, L.D.; de Barros Costa, E.; Pinheiro, M.E.; Perkusich, A. Exploring early prediction of chronic kidney disease using machine learning algorithms for small and imbalanced datasets. *Appl. Sci.* **2022**, *12*, 3673. [CrossRef]
12. Ameen, S.; Wong, M.-C.; Yee, K.-C.; Turner, P. AI and clinical decision making: The limitations and risks of computational reductionism in bowel cancer screening. *Appl. Sci.* **2022**, *12*, 3341. [CrossRef]
13. Wei, J.; Cheng, L.; Han, P.; Zhu, Y.; Huang, W. Decision tree-based data stratification method for the minimization of the masking effect in adverse drug reaction signal detection. *Appl. Sci.* **2021**, *11*, 11380. [CrossRef]
14. Wei, J.; Dai, J.; Zhao, Y.; Han, P.; Zhu, Y.; Huang, W. Application of association rules analysis in mining adverse drug reaction signals. *Appl. Sci.* **2021**, *11*, 10828. [CrossRef]
15. Tenekedjiev, K.; Panayotova, D.; Daboos, M.; Ivanova, S.; Symes, M.; Panayotov, P.; Nikolova, N. Quasi-experimental design for medical studies with the method of the fuzzy pseudo-control group. *Appl. Sci.* **2025**, *15*, 1370. [CrossRef]

16. Beinrohr, L.; Kail, E.; Piros, P.; Tóth, E.; Fleiner, R.; Kolev, K. Anatomy of a data science software toolkit that uses machine learning to aid 'bench-to-bedside' medical research—With essential concepts of data mining and analysis explained. *Appl. Sci.* **2021**, *11*, 12135. [CrossRef]
17. Walczak, A.; Moszczyński, P.; Krzesiński, P. Evolution of hemodynamic parameters simulated by means of diffusion models. *Appl. Sci.* **2021**, *11*, 11412. [CrossRef]
18. Magalhães, J.; José Correia, M.; Silva, R.M.; Esteves, A.C.; Alves, A.; Duarte, A.S. Molecular techniques and target selection for the identification of candida spp. in oral samples. *Appl. Sci.* **2022**, *12*, 9204. [CrossRef]
19. Gifu, D. Soft sets extensions: Innovating healthcare claims analysis. *Appl. Sci.* **2024**, *14*, 8799. [CrossRef]
20. Musio, F. The critical link in the successful application of advanced clinical decision making—Revisiting the physician–patient relationship from a practical and pragmatic perspective. *Appl. Sci.* **2025**, *15*, 2446. [CrossRef]

applied sciences

MDPI

Article

Application of Association Rules Analysis in Mining Adverse Drug Reaction Signals

Jianxiang Wei [1,2,*], Jimin Dai [3], Yingya Zhao [3], Pu Han [1], Yunxia Zhu [3] and Weidong Huang [1,2]

1 School of Management, Nanjing University of Posts and Telecommunications, Nanjing 210003, China; hanpu@njupt.edu.cn (P.H.); huangwd@njupt.edu.cn (W.H.)
2 Key Research Base of Philosophy and Social Sciences in Jiangsu-Information Industry Integration Innovation and Emergency Management Research Center, Nanjing 210003, China
3 School of Internet of Things, Nanjing University of Posts and Telecommunications, Nanjing 210003, China; b19060238@njupt.edu.cn (J.D.); b19060208@njupt.edu.cn (Y.Z.); zhuyx@njupt.edu.cn (Y.Z.)
* Correspondence: jxwei@njupt.edu.cn

Abstract: Adverse drug reactions (ADRs) are increasingly becoming a serious public health problem. Spontaneous reporting systems (SRSs) are an important way for many countries to monitor ADRs produced in the clinical use of drugs, and they are the main data source for ADR signal detection. The traditional signal detection methods are based on disproportionality analysis (DPA) and lack the application of data mining technology. In this paper, we selected the spontaneous reports from 2011 to 2018 in Jiangsu Province of China as the research data and used association rules analysis (ARA) to mine signals. We defined some important metrics of the ARA according to the two-dimensional contingency table of ADRs, such as Confidence and Lift, and constructed performance evaluation indicators such as Precision, Recall, and F1 as objective standards. We used experimental methods based on data to objectively determine the optimal thresholds of the corresponding metrics, which, in the best case, are Confidence = 0.007 and Lift = 1. We obtained the average performance of the method through 10-fold cross-validation. The experimental results showed that F1 increased from 31.43% in the MHRA method to 40.38% in the ARA method; this was a significant improvement. To reduce drug risk and provide decision making for drug safety, more data mining methods need to be introduced and applied to ADR signal detection.

Keywords: association rule; data mining; adverse drug reaction; signal detection

1. Introduction

Adverse drug reaction (ADR) refers to an appreciably harmful or unpleasant reaction, resulting from an intervention related to the use of a medicinal product, which predicts hazards from future administration and warrants prevention, specific treatment, alteration of the dosage regimen, or withdrawal of the product [1]. ADR is a common clinical manifestation, and we must pay attention to the frequency of this potential injury. Because it is related to morbidity and mortality, it may cause unnecessary economic loss, and, to a certain extent, it harms the doctor–patient relationship [2]. Under normal circumstances, it is difficult to detect all possible ADRs before the drug is marketed. After the drug is marketed and put into use, we can detect more comprehensive ADRs through long-term observation. To ensure the safety of medication for each patient and reduce ADRs, all countries have established a spontaneous reporting system (SRS) to collect adverse drug events (ADEs) as an essential data source for ADR signal detection. SRS has been defined as an unsolicited communication by a healthcare professional or consumer to a company, regulatory authority, or other organizations (e.g., the WHO, Regional Centre, Poison Control Centre) that describe one or more ADRs in a patient who was given one or more medicinal products and that does not derive from a study or any organized data collection scheme.

The traditional ADR signal detection method is mainly based on disproportionality analysis (DPA). The proportional reporting ratio (PRR) method is the most basic signal detection algorithm in the early stage [3–5]. On this basis, the British Medicines and Healthcare Products Regulatory Agency (MHRA) combined the value of PRR with the target drug, the target ADR report number, and the Pearson Chi-square value as a more stable signal detection method, called the MHRA method [6]. At present, this method has been widely used by the Pharmacovigilance Center in the Netherlands, the Drug ADR Monitoring System in the United Kingdom, the Uppsala Monitoring Center of the World Health Organization (WHO, UMC), and the Drug ADR Spontaneous Reporting System in the United States [7]. However, the results of the MHRA method are easily affected by spontaneous reports. Although the MHRA method is determined by three metrics and the results are relatively stable and accurate, as the number of spontaneous reports increases, the value calculated by the formula of the index will inevitably decrease as the base increases due to the limitations of the metrics themselves. When the specified thresholds remain unchanged, the sensitivity of the MHRA method will decrease.

As an important data mining method, association rules analysis (ARA) has been introduced into signal detection to solve the problems of drug safety. Through research on relevant papers, we found that (1) most of the researchers applied the ARA method to specific drugs and performed personalized analysis of the ADRs of some drugs. That is to say, researchers rarely used SRS for many drugs and a larger range of studies to detect ADR signals. (2) Most researchers used ARA as a preliminary screening tool for the detection of ADR signals. By calculating the Support, Confidence, or other metrics of each ADR combination, they filtered out the combinations that were not in the ideal range and used other algorithms to further detect the ADR signals in the selected high-quality combinations. This approach failed to tap the maximum potential of ARA, increased the research cost of data mining, and complicated the experiment. (3) When using ARA to filter data, only Support, Confidence, or other metrics were used as the screening criteria, and the performance of the criteria were not evaluated. Therefore, it was difficult to confirm whether the experimental results were the optimum.

In response to the above situation, we put forward our research hypothesis: firstly, we tried to introduce SRS in ARA for a larger range of ADR signal detection. Secondly, we believed that ARA cannot only be used as a preliminary screening tool for data; it has the ability to do more work. Thus, we proposed using ARA to complete the whole process of ADR signal detection, using Confidence and lift to finalize the ADR signals, and using F1 and other indicators to objectively describe the detection performance of ARA to ensure the best results. In order to verify that our research does make the ability to mine ADR signals with ARA stronger than other methods, we also compared the ARA method with the MHRA method to prove the reliability of the ARA.

This paper aims to fully utilize ARA to mine ADR signals, improve the accuracy of ADR signal detection at a minimum cost, provide more reliable decision support for drug safety, and strive to minimize the side effects of drugs used to improve health services and health practices.

The remainder of this paper is organized as follows: related works are given in Section 2. The process of the experiment and the explanation of the relevant theory are formulated in Section 3. In Section 4, the experimental results are presented and compared with other methods. The discussion about the advantages and limitations of the ARA method proposed in this paper is in Section 5. Finally, the concluding remarks are provided in Section 6.

2. Related Works

Based on the concept of strong rules, Rakesh Agrawal, Tomasz Imieliński, and Arun Swami introduced association rules [8]. They used them to mine the rules between products in large-scale transaction data recorded by supermarket point-of-sale systems. Today, many ARA algorithms have been proposed. Apriori uses a breadth-first search strategy to count the Support of item sets and uses a candidate generation function that exploits the downward closure property of Support [9]. Eclat (alt. ECLAT, stands for Equivalence Class Transformation) is a depth-first search algorithm based on set intersection. It is suitable for both sequential as well as parallel execution with locality-enhancing properties [10–12]. The ASSOC procedure is a GUHA method that mines for generalized association rules using fast bit string operations [13]. The association rules mined by this method are more general than those output by Apriori, for example "items" can be connected both with conjunction and disjunctions, and the relation between the antecedent and consequent of the rule is not restricted to setting minimum Support and Confidence as in Apriori: an arbitrary combination of supported interest measures can be used.

ARA has a wide range of applications in many aspects, such as Web usage mining, intrusion detection, continuous production, and bioinformatics. The research in this paper applies ARA to the field of biomedicine. In this field, many researchers have used ARA for research. Jenna M. Reps et al. proposed a proof-of-concept method that learned common associations and used this knowledge to automatically refine side effect signals (i.e., exposure–outcome associations) by removing instances of the exposure–outcome associations that are caused by confounding [14]. They then calculated a novel measure termed the confounding-adjusted risk value, a more accurate absolute risk value of a patient experiencing the outcome within 60 days of the exposure. Tentative results suggested that the method works. Sharma D extracted useful information from the quarterly tables produced, synthesized the information to obtain the rules using Apriori algorithm to vary the Confidence and other measure levels. Interactions of Patients' demographic characteristics (such as age, gender, etc.), length of therapy, and dosages of the drugs taken were also explored to determine if such factors play a role in driving the reactions [15].

In this paper, we proposed an ARA method based on Confidence and Lift and used simulation experiments to objectively find their optimal thresholds. Under our performance evaluation system, this ARA method performed well.

3. Methods

3.1. Date Source

The data source was monitoring reports of ADRs in Jiangsu Province, China, from 2011 to 2018. The reference dataset contains known ADR combinations extracted from drug package inserts, and it is used as an objective standard for performance evaluation of signal detection.

3.2. MHRA

The MHRA is a signal detection method adopted by the British Medicines and Healthcare Products Regulatory Agency, also known as the comprehensive standard method or MHRA method. It bases on the PRR method and comprehensively considers the chi-square value x^2 and the absolute number of reports a. Only when the three conditions of $a \geq 3$, $PRR \geq 2$, and $x^2 \geq 4$ are met simultaneously can the signal be considered to exist, indicating that there is a relationship between a specific drug and a specific ADR.

The PRR method was first applied to the ADR monitoring system in the United Kingdom. It is a method used to quantitatively analyze the data of ADR records collected by the SRS [16]. The three metrics mentioned above are all based on two-dimensional contingency tables of ADRs. In Table 1, a represents the number of the target ADR caused by the target drug, b represents the number of all other ADRs caused by the target drug, c represents the number of the target ADR caused by other drugs other than the target drug, and d represents the number of all other ADRs caused by other drugs other than the target drug. The MHRA method is more rigorous than the PRR method; it guarantees the minimum number of combination cases, and the result is relatively more stable.

$$PRR = \frac{a/(a+b)}{c/(c+d)}, \tag{1}$$

$$\chi^2 = \frac{\left(|ad-bc| - \frac{n}{2}\right)^2 \cdot n}{(a+b)(c+d)(a+c)(b+d)}, \; n = a+b+c+d, \tag{2}$$

Table 1. Two-dimensional contingency table of ADRs.

Signal	Suspected ADE	All Other ADEs
Suspected drug	a	b
All other drugs	c	d

3.3. Association Rules Analysis

ARA is a commonly used data mining method used to discover the interrelationships between data in large datasets [17]. ARA is defined as the implicit expression of X→Y, where X and Y are sets of items that originate from the same dataset but do not intersect [8]. Furthermore, X is called the antecedent or left-hand side (LHS) and Y the consequent or right-hand side (RHS). In this paper, X means "drug" in spontaneous reports, and Y means "adverse reaction". In order to filter the signals that meet the requirements, researchers have designed many different functional metrics, of which the most commonly used are Support, Confidence, and Lift. According to Table 1, we defined the calculation formulas of these three metrics as follows:

$$Support = \frac{a}{a+b+c+d}, \tag{3}$$

$$Confidence = \frac{a}{a+b}, \tag{4}$$

$$Lift = \frac{confidence}{a+c/a+b+c+d}, \tag{5}$$

Support indicates the proportion of the data combination that contains both X and Y to the total data volume. From Formula (3), it can be seen that the denominator in the expression of Support is the number of records in the entire dataset, and the numerator only contains the number of records in which the target ADR caused by the target drug "a". The base of the denominator is too large, and the numerator is relatively too small, which causes the value of Support to infinitely approach to 0. If Support were used as the metric of signal detection in this experiment, the accuracy and sensitivity of the detection result would be greatly reduced. Thus, we deprecated Support.

Confidence indicates the proportion of data containing X that also contain Y. It can also be interpreted as an estimate of the conditional probability P(Y | X), the probability of finding the RHS of the rule in transactions under the condition that these transactions also contain the LHS [18,19].

Lift indicates the ratio of "the proportion of data containing X that also contain Y" and "the proportion of data containing Y in the population". Lift reflects the correlation between X and Y in the ARA. If Lift = 1, it means that X and Y are not correlated. If Lift > 1, the higher the Lift, and the higher the positive correlation between X and Y. If Lift < 1, the lower the Lift, and the higher the negative correlation between X and Y [18].

3.4. Performance Evaluation

When the metrics for the detection of ADR signals were determined to be Confidence and Lift, our core task was to determine the best thresholds for Confidence and Lift.

In order to better compare the performance of different methods for detecting ADR signals, we defined three indicators to describe the performance of detecting ADR signals, namely: Precision, Recall [20], and F1 [21,22]. The expressions of these three indicators depend on Table 2.

Table 2. Performance evaluation metrics of MHRA/ARA method.

Signal	MHRA/ARA Method Tested Positive	MHRA/ARA Method Tested Negative
Known as positive in the ADR dataset	TP	FN
Known as negative in the ADR dataset	FP	TN

Our dataset contains known ADR combinations extracted from package inserts. We used them as an objective standard for performance evaluation. In Table 2, "Known as positive in the ADR dataset" means the ADR combination has been recorded in the dataset as a known ADR combination. "Known as negative in the ADR dataset" means the ADR combination was not been recorded in the dataset, so we temporarily denied that it was an objective ADR combination. "MHRA/ARA method tested positive" means the ADR combination was detected as an ADR signal by MHRA/ARA method. "MHRA/ARA method tested negative" means the ADR combination was not been detected as an ADR signal by MHRA/ARA method.

As shown in the Table 2, TP (True Positive) represents the number of known positive ADR combinations in the ADR dataset that can be detected as positive by the MHRA/ARA method. FN (False Negative) represents the number of known positive ADR combinations in the ADR dataset that can be detected as negative by the MHRA/ARA method. FP (False Positive) represents the number of known negative ADR combinations in the ADR dataset that can be detected as positive by the MHRA/ARA method. TN (True Negative) represents the number of known negative ADR combinations in the ADR dataset that can be detected as negative by the MHRA/ARA method [23].

$$Precision = \frac{TP}{TP + FP} \times 100\%, \tag{6}$$

$$Recall = \frac{TP}{TP + FN} \times 100\%, \tag{7}$$

$$F1 = \frac{2 \times Precision \times Recall}{Precision + Recall} \times 100\%, \tag{8}$$

Precision represents the proportion of the number of true ADR signals predicted by a method to the number of all ADR signals predicted by the method, and it considers the accuracy of the detection. Recall represents the proportion of the number of true ADR signals to the number of actual ADR signals in the prediction of a certain method. It considers integrity20. The value of F1 is the harmonic average of Precision and Recall21,22. The higher the value of F1, the better the performance of the method.

3.5. Method of Determining the Thresholds

We imported the data in the dataset into Microsoft Visual FoxPro and used Microsoft Visual FoxPro for simulation experiments. Through the existing research data of Confidence and Lift, the approximate range of the thresholds of the two metrics was determined, and through continuous precision and refinement, the ideal thresholds were obtained. Due to the limitation of the definition of performance indicators, when the value of Precision becomes larger, the value of Recall will inevitably become smaller, so we used F1 (the harmonic average of Precision and Recall) as the final indicator to reflect the performance of the ARA.

3.6. Method Comparison

In order to analyze the advantages of the ARA method more objectively, we used 10-fold cross-validation on the ARA method to obtain the average performance level of the ARA method and compared it with the performance of the MHRA method. In addition, we compared the two methods from the perspective of formulation, and used specific drug event examples to concretely present the performance of the two methods.

4. Results

4.1. Study Dataset

A total of 751,606 reports were selected as the study dataset, and all experiments were conducted based on this dataset. We first processed the data through the above formulas to obtain the values of all indicators such as PRR, Confidence, and Lift, and further obtained our experimental results through these data.

4.2. Optimal Threshold

According to the method described above, we determined appropriate thresholds for the Confidence and Lift to maximize the effectiveness. The specific results are shown in Tables 3 and 4.

Table 3. The value of F1(Preliminary).

F1	Lift = 1	Lift = 1.5	Lift = 2	Lift = 2.5	Lift = 3
Confidence = 0.005	39.91%	36.85%	34.40%	32.04%	30.38%
Confidence = 0.010	40.30%	36.77%	33.74%	30.94%	29.03%
Confidence = 0.015	39.50%	35.73%	32.70%	29.70%	27.72%
Confidence = 0.02	38.29%	34.51%	31.36%	28.47%	26.56%
Confidence = 0.025	37.22%	33.27%	30.10%	27.07%	25.23%

Table 4. The value of F1(Finally).

F1	Lift = 1	Lift = 1.1	Lift = 1.2	Lift = 1.3	Lift = 1.4	Lift = 1.5
Confidence = 0.006	40.28%	39.50%	38.83%	38.17%	37.65%	37.07%
Confidence = 0.007	40.51%	39.71%	38.98%	38.27%	37.71%	37.15%
Confidence = 0.008	40.49%	39.66%	38.93%	38.21%	37.62%	37.01%
Confidence = 0.009	40.35%	39.52%	38.76%	38.07%	37.45%	36.82%

Starting from the definition of Confidence and Lift, we first selected some reasonable thresholds for them and observed the value of F1 obtained from that place. As shown in Table 3, the effective threshold of the Lift should start from 1. We selected five values of 1, 1.5, 2, 2.5, and 3 and found that the value of F1 decreases with the increase in Lift. Additionally, we chose 0.005, 0.01, 0.015, 0.02, and 0.025 as the Confidence's threshold and found that when the Confidence's threshold is 0.01, the ARA performs best.

On this basis, we analyzed the adjacent values of the current optimal thresholds and reasonably suspected that the optimal thresholds would appear between Confidence $\in [0.005,0.01]$ and Lift $\in [1,1.5]$. Thus, we used more exact values for the simulation experiments. It can be seen from Table 4 that when confidence = 0.007 and lift = 1, F1 achieves a maximum value of 40.51%. Thus, we finally determined that Confidence = 0.007 and Lift = 1 are the optimal thresholds.

4.3. Comparison of the MHRA Method and the ARA Method at the Performance Level

However, the best thresholds obtained from the overall sample and the performance they exhibited were the best results that the ARA method could achieve. In order to obtain the average performance level of the ARA method, we used 10-fold cross-validation to evaluate the performance of our method. We divided the dataset into 10 subsets on average, selected 9 of them as the training set and the other as the test set, and performed

10 experiments without repeating them. In the training set, we used the ARA method to obtain the optimal thresholds, then used them as the optimal thresholds in the test set, and evaluated the performance indicators of the thresholds which we obtained from training set in the test set. When we determined the thresholds of the metrics used in the training set, we could divide each piece of data in the test set into four categories: TP, TN, FP, and FN based on the threshold, and then we used Formulas (6)–(8) to obtain the performance of the ARA method to detect ADR signals through the simulation experiments and found the average performance of ten experiments. We used the three average performance indicators obtained from ten experiments as the final result of the threshold determination, respectively: Precision = 36.28%, Recall = 45.65%, and F1 = 40.38%. Figure 1 is a comparison of the performance of the ARA method and the MHRA method.

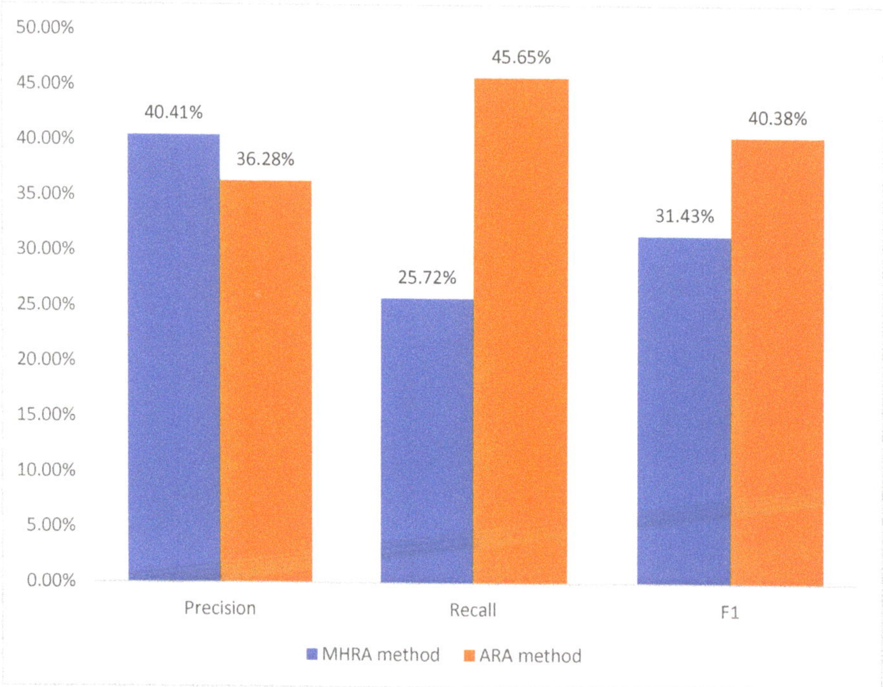

Figure 1. Comparison of the performance of the MHRA method and the ARA method.

As shown in Figure 1, Precision was reduced from 40.41% in the MHRA method to 36.28% in the ARA method; Recall increased from 25.72% in the MHRA method to 45.65% in the ARA method; F1 increased from 31.43% in the MHRA method to 40.38% in the ARA method. As can be seen from Section 3.4, we used F1 as the main indicator to judge the performance of ADR signal detection, and the F1 of the ARA method was increased by 28.48% compared to the F1 of the MHRA method. These results showed that the performance of the ARA method was much better than that of the MHRA method.

We used the data of levofloxacin in the dataset to concretely characterize the superior performance of ARA. We screened the top ten potential ADRs that may be caused by levofloxacin from the dataset and reported the results in Table 5 (the frequency of adverse symptoms is in descending order). "Has been identified as a positive signal" means the ADR was determined as the drug's ADR. "Detected as a positive signal by MHRA method" means that the ADR was detected as an ADR signal by the MHRA method. "Detected as a positive signal by ARA method" means that the ADR was detected as an ADR signal by the ARA method.

Table 5. ADRs of levofloxacin and related detection signals.

Adverse Drug Reaction	Has Been Identified as a Positive Signal	Detected as Positive Signal by MHRA Method	Detected as Positive Signal by ARA Method
Pruritus	Yes	Yes	Yes
Rash	Yes	No	Yes
Nausea	Yes	No	Yes
Vomiting	Yes	No	Yes
Allergy	Yes	No	Yes
Phlebitis	Yes	Yes	Yes
Dizziness	Yes	No	No
Chest distress	No	No	No
Anaphylactoid reaction	No	No	Yes
Abdominal pain	Yes	No	No

In this dataset, the number of rashes caused by levofloxacin was 7088, accounting for about 15.60% of the ADRs caused by the drug. Moreover, a rash was determined as levofloxacin's ADR, but the MHRA method did not detect this as an ADR signal, while the ARA method detected it as an ADR signal. Similarly, 4226 people had nausea after using levofloxacin, 2967 people vomited after using levofloxacin, and 2644 people had allergies after using levofloxacin. These were all determined as levofloxacin's ADRs, but were only detected as ADR signals by the ARA method. Moreover, pruritus and phlebitis were detected as ADR signals in the three situations.

In conclusion, the ARA mined six kinds of ADRs that were determined as ADRs before. This was enough to illustrate the effectiveness of the method. Furthermore, the anaphylactoid reaction was not previously determined as an ADR signal, but it was detected as an ADR signal by the ARA method, and relevant medical research has confirmed our conjecture [24]. This showed that the ARA method's accuracy and performance are higher than those of the MHRA method.

4.4. Comparison of the MHRA Method and the ARA Method at the Formula Level

We used the controlled variable method to analyze and compared the formulas of the MHRA method and the ARA method to study the influence of the formulas on the detection of ADR signals. We took levonorgestrel ethinyl estradiol and etimicin as examples for analysis, and the specific results are shown in Tables 6 and 7.

Table 6. Levonorgestrel ethinyl estradiol test results.

	MHRA Method Tested Positive	ARA Method Tested Positive
a Not up to standard, other formulas are up to standard	0	6
All formulas are up to standard	1	13
Recorded in the package inserts	0	4

Number of reports: 17; number of ADR combinations: 13; total amount of data: 751,606.

Table 7. Etimicin test results.

	MHRA Method Tested Positive	ARA Method Tested Positive
PRR Not up to standard, other formulas are up to standard	0	8
All formulas are up to standard	26	16
Recorded in the package inserts	3	6

Number of reports: 3710; number of ADR combinations: 209; total amount of data: 751,606.

In Table 6, levonorgestrel ethinyl estradiol is a long-acting contraceptive that affects the endocrine. Only 17 cases of its ADRs have been reported in the entire dataset. The amount of data is minimal. Even when the PRR and x^2 met the standard, six ADR combinations appeared negative under the

MHRA method and appeared positive under the ARA method because the value 'a' did not meet the standard. For example, the ADR of uterine bleeding caused by levonorgestrel ethinyl estradiol focused on a = 1, b = 16, c = 14, and d = 751,575; the ADR of menstrual disorders caused by levonorgestrel ethinyl estradiol focused on a = 1, b = 16, c = 227, and d = 751,362. The drug reported a total of 13 ADR combinations, of which 1 group was detected positive by the MHRA method, and 13 groups were detected positive by the ARA method. That is, because the number of cases of target ADRs caused by the target drug is not up to the standard of MHRA, the detection difference between the MHRA method and the ARA method reached 50%. If the ADRs recorded in the package inserts are used as the reference standard, then under the dataset, the detection accuracy rate of the drug by the MHRA method is 0, and the detection accuracy rate of the ARA method is 30.77%.

In Table 7, etimicin is an aminoglycoside antibiotic drug. There are 3710 ADRs that have been reported in this dataset, accounting for 0.49% of the data in this dataset. In the reported case of this drug, because it did not meet the criteria of the PRR formula, the number of ADR combinations that tested negative under the MHRA method and tested positive under the ARA method reached eight groups. For example, the ADR of palpitations caused by etimicin focused on a = 105, b = 3605, c = 11,104, and d = 736,792; the ADR of rash caused by etimicin focused on a = 641, b = 3069, c = 114,059, and d = 633,837. A total of 209 ADR combinations were reported for the drug, among which the detection difference between the MHRA method and the ARA method due to the PRR formula was 3.83%. If the ADRs recorded in the package inserts are used as the reference standard, then under the dataset, the detection accuracy rate of the drug by the MHRA method is 11.54%, and the detection accuracy rate of the ARA method is 37.5%.

In conclusion, the ARA method has better universality, and it can handle smaller or larger datasets more calmly while maintaining high accuracy. This also means that when we want to process data in other datasets, we only need to execute the methods provided in this paper step by step, and we can obtain each dataset's own optimal threshold.

5. Discussion

5.1. Progress in the ARA Field

ARA has become a common method in the field of data mining. Kai Guo et al. used ARA as a data screening tool combined with embedded models to detect ADR signals and proved that this method could effectively detect potential ADRs through specific studies on rofecoxib and gadoversetamide [25]. Heba Ibrahim et al. used an optimized tailored mining algorithm called "hybrid Apriori". The results showed that the proposed method could extract signals of serious ADRs, and various association patterns could be identified based on the relationships among the elements which composed a pattern [26]. Dan Zhang et al. used ARA to analyze the characteristics and regularities of cardiac ADRs induced by Chinese materia medica. They found that the cardiac ADRs had strong correlations with the ADRs of the nervous system and digestive system, and the aconitum species and other toxic Chinese materia medica were intimately associated with the ADRs of the nervous system and digestive system [27]. Through the critical research of the above papers and other papers, we proposed the research provided in this paper on the use of ARA to mine ADR signals and achieved good results. The specific manifestations are as follows: 1. We introduced SRS, which greatly expanded the scope of ARA to detect ADR signals and demonstrated the powerful potential of ARA. 2. We used ARA as the only tool to mine ADR signals, which fully demonstrated the powerful capabilities of ARA. 3. Because there was no need to use more tools, the economic cost was greatly saved, which has important practical significance. 4. We added a performance evaluation mechanism, which ensured the accuracy of the results to a greater extent. These are also the advantages of our research results.

5.2. Advantages over the Traditional MHRA

Compared with the traditional DPA method, (1) the advantage of ARA lies in the higher adaptability to datasets with different characteristics. Taking the MHRA method as an example, this method has fixed index combination thresholds. If the data for the dataset were increased, the sensitivity would decrease. While the ARA method's index thresholds change dynamically, the thresholds can be determined by simulation experiments based on the specific characteristics of the dataset. Similarly, due to the limitation of the combination of metrics of the MHRA method, the amount of data in the dataset using this method cannot be too small. Otherwise, it will cause few positive signals to be detected, which leads to no research values. All metrics of the ARA method are expressed in the form of proportions, so the result is relatively more stable even if the amount of data is small. (2) The ARA method has better detection performance for rare ADR signals. We have verified this in the above experiment. At the theoretical level, due to the different data characteristics of each dataset and some unavoidable interference factors, such as individual selective reporting of ADRs and over-reporting of ADRs, these may cause some real and rare ADRs to be masked. If we used the MHRA method, the positive ADR signal might be ignored due to the fact that the number of records of specific ADRs is small, or the frequency of ADRs caused by specific drugs is relatively lower in the same ADR range. The ARA method is more accurate and stable for detecting ADR signals because of its metrics' proportional representation and dynamics.

From the perspective of formulas, The MHRA method requires that the ADR combination completely meets $a \geq 3$, $PRR \geq 2$, and $x^2 \geq 4$, then it is determined as an ADR signal. The ARA method requires that the ADR combination completely meets $Confidence \geq 0.007$ and $Lift \geq 1$, then it is determined as an ADR signal.

The three formulas of MHRA method can be explained as

(1) The number of target ADR caused by the target drug $\geq$3;
(2) The probability of target ADR caused by the target drug $\geq$ the probability of target ADR caused by all other drugs $\times$2;
(3) The Chi-square value of the ADR $\geq$4, which means the drug is related to the ADR.

The two formulas of the ARA method can be explained as:

(1) The number of cases of target drug producing target ADR accounted for the number of cases of target drug producing all ADRs $\geq$ 0.007 (the probability of target ADR occurring when the target drug is used $\geq$ 0.007);
(2) When using the target drug, the probability of the target ADR is greater than the probability of using all the drugs to produce the target ADR. At the same time, Lift also reflects the correlation between the drug and the ADR.

By analyzing the definitions of the formulas of the two methods and their meaning of expressions, we divided the variable 'a' in the MHRA method and Formula (4) in the ARA method into a group for comparison, at the same time, we divided Formulas (1) and (2) in the MHRA method and Formula (5) in the ARA method into a group for comparison.

Formula (5) in the ARA method is more comprehensive Formulas (1) and (2) in the MHRA method. The function of Lift's formula expression is similar to that of the PRR's formula expression in MHRA, but because it also has the implication of "correlation", the Chi-square value is added to MHRA to compensate for the implication of "correlation". For the PRR's expression in the MHRA method and the Lift's expression in the ARA method, the values of their denominators $c/c + d$ and $a + c/a + b + c + d$ tend to behave in the same way when the amount of data in the dataset is large enough, so the requirements needed to achieve the PRR's formula are more stringent, but this also reduces the ability of the MHRA method to capture rare ADR signals. When the amount of data in the dataset is moderate or small, the requirements for reaching the PRR's formula are similar to those for reaching the Lift's formula.

In practical applications, if the amount of data reported for a drug is small or the drug produces rare ADRs, the value of 'a' in the MHRA method may not meet the standard, and the ratio is used in the ARA method to determine whether the number of cases that the target drug producing target ADR meets the standard; thus, the ARA method has better stability and can capture rare ADR signals more accurately, and it also makes the ARA method fairer and more accurate in processing different levels of data.

It can be seen from the formula that the MHRA method is more suitable for data analysis in a dataset with a moderate amount of data and the number of ADR reports for each independent drug in the dataset is sufficient, while the ARA method has better general applicability. Additionally, the ARA method is more capable of capturing rare ADR signals.

5.3. Limitations of the ARA

However, in the course of the experiment, we still found some limitations. In the dataset we used, we used the two variables of Confidence and Lift as metrics to mark the ADR signals according to the characteristics of this dataset and performed simulation experiments based on the data in this dataset to obtain the best thresholds of the two metrics. Nevertheless, if we need to update the dataset or apply it to a new dataset, the performance of these two metrics might fluctuate greatly. Because the data characteristics of different datasets are different, we may need to replace or add new metrics, such as the Support mentioned above. Moreover, because of the change of data, the metric threshold has to be reconfirmed through simulation experiments. That is to say, we have not been able to find a universal indicator combination and an objective method that can be used to confirm the metric threshold directly.

From the perspective of data, the unbalanced distribution of the ADR spontaneous report data means that the frequency of using different tablets may vary greatly, and the frequency of ADRs caused by drugs may also vary greatly. Therefore, when we use the same index to detect the dataset, it will produce unfairness, which will lead to inaccuracy of detection. In subsequent improvements, we will consider using data stratification methods to separate different characteristic data according to a certain method and, respectively, confirm more effective index thresholds to detect ADR signals. We are committed to further improving the universality and performance of ARA for mining ADR spontaneous report datasets.

6. Conclusions

In this paper, we analyzed the current research related to ARA and found some shortcomings in the process of using ARA. On this basis, we put forward our own research hypothesis: we introduced SRS and tried to use only ARA as a tool to mine ADR signals because this could better utilize the capabilities of ARA and save costs to a certain extent. According to the actual situation of the dataset used, we chose Confidence and Lift as metrics for detecting ADR signals. We used 10-fold cross-validation. Through the three indicators of Precision, Recall, and F1, we compared the results of the ARA method with the results of the MHRA method and proved that the ARA method is effective. Furthermore, at the performance level, we took the drug levofloxacin and its ADRs as an example to further prove the reliability of the ARA method. At the formula level, by analyzing the mathematical and physical meanings of the formulas, we have confirmed that the ARA method has better universal applicability to various datasets.

Finally, we summarized the progress of the ARA method proposed in this paper in ARA-related fields, and its advantages over other traditional data mining methods. At the same time, we also reflect on the limitations of the ARA and consider continuing to improve on this basis to make them more universal and reliable.

Author Contributions: J.W. conceived of the study. J.D. participated in data processing and experimental simulation. J.W. and J.D. participated in data analysis, and drafting of the manuscript. Y.Z. (Yingya Zhao), P.H., Y.Z. (Yunxia Zhu), and W.H. were involved in critically revising the manuscript and reviewing experiment results. All authors have read and agreed to the published version of the manuscript.

Funding: This study was funded by the National Social Science Foundation of China (No. 17CTQ022) and the Major Project of Philosophy and Social Science Research in Jiangsu Universities (2020SJZDA102).

Institutional Review Board Statement: Not applicable.

Informed Consent Statement: Not applicable.

Data Availability Statement: The data are not publicly available due to the policy of confidentiality of the CFDA but are available from the corresponding author on reasonable request and with permission of the CFDA.

Conflicts of Interest: The authors declare no conflict of interest.

References

1. Edwards, I.R.; Aronson, J.K. Adverse drug reactions: Definitions, diagnosis, and management. *Lancet* **2000**, *356*, 1255–1259. [CrossRef]
2. Coleman, J.J.; Pontefract, S.K. Adverse drug reactions. *Clin. Med.* **2016**, *16*, 481–485. [CrossRef]

3. Banks, D.; Woo, E.J.; Burwen, D.R.; Perucci, P.; Braun, M.M.; Ball, R. Comparing data mining methods on the VAERS database. *Pharmacoepidemiol. Drug Safe* **2005**, *14*, 601–609. [CrossRef] [PubMed]
4. Matsushita, Y.; Kuroda, Y.; Niwa, S.; Sonehara, S.; Hamada, C.; Yoshimura, I. Criteria revision and performance comparison of three methods of signal detection applied to the spontaneous reporting database of a pharmaceutical manufacturer. *Drug Saf.* **2007**, *30*, 715–726. [CrossRef]
5. Hauben, M. Early postmarketing drug safety surveillance: Data mining points to consider. *Ann. Pharm.* **2004**, *38*, 1625–1630. [CrossRef]
6. Singh, S.; Loke, Y.K.; Furberg, C.D. Long-term Risk of Cardiovascular Events with Rosiglitazone: A Meta-analysis. *JAMA J. Am. Med. Assoc.* **2007**, *298*, 1189–1195. [CrossRef] [PubMed]
7. Hauben, M.; Zhou, X.F. Quantitative Methods in Pharmacovigilance: Focus on Signal Detection. *Drug Saf.* **2003**, *26*, 159–186. [CrossRef] [PubMed]
8. Agrawal, R.; Imieliński, T.; Swami, A. Mining association rules between sets of items in large databases. *SIGMOD Rec.* **1993**, *22*, 207–216. [CrossRef]
9. Agrawal, R.; Srikant, R. Fast algorithms for mining association rules in large databases. In Proceedings of the 20th International Conference on Very Large Data Bases (VLDB), Santiago de, Chile, Chile, 12–15 September 1994; pp. 487–499.
10. Zaki, M.J. Scalable algorithms for association mining. *IEEE Trans. Knowl. Data Eng.* **2000**, *12*, 372–390. [CrossRef]
11. Zaki, M.J.; Parthasarathy, S.; Ogihara, M.; Li, W. New Algorithms for Fast Discovery of Association Rules. In Proceedings of the 3rd International Conference on Knowledge Discovery and Data Mining, Newport Beach, CA, USA, 14–17 August 1997; pp. 283–286.
12. Zaki, M.J.; Parthasarathy, S.; Ogihara, M.; Li, W. Parallel Algorithms for Discovery of Association Rules. *Data Min. Knowl. Discov.* **1997**, *1*, 343–373. [CrossRef]
13. Hájek, P.; Havránek, T. *Mechanizing Hypothesis Formation: Mathematical Foundations for a General Theory*; Springer: Berlin/Heidelberg, Germany, 1978.
14. Reps, J.M.; Aickelin, U.; Ma, J.; Zhang, Y. Refining Adverse Drug Reactions Using Association Rule Mining for Electronic Healthcare Data. In Proceedings of the 2014 IEEE International Conference on Data Mining Workshop, Shenzhen, China, 14 December 2014; pp. 763–770.
15. Sharma, D. Application of Association Rules in Clinical Data Mining: A Case Study for Identifying Adverse Drug Reactions. *Value Health* **2016**, *19*, 101. [CrossRef]
16. Evans, S.J.W.; Waller, P.C.; Davis, S. Use of proportional reporting ratios (PRRs) for signal generation from spontaneous adverse drug reaction reports. *Pharm. Drug Saf.* **2001**, *10*, 483–486. [CrossRef] [PubMed]
17. Frawley, W.J.; Piatetsky-Shapiro, G.; Matheus, C.J. Knowledge Discovery in Databases: An Overview. *AI Mag.* **1992**, *13*, 57–70.
18. Hahsler, M.; Grün, B.; Hornik, K. Arules—A Computational Environment for Mining Association Rules and Frequent Item Sets. *J. Stat. Softw.* **2005**, *14*, 1–25. [CrossRef]
19. Hipp, J.; Güntzer, U.; Nakhaeizadeh, G. Algorithms for association rule mining—A general survey and comparison. *SIGKDD Explor. Newsl.* **2000**, *2*, 58–64. [CrossRef]
20. Olson, D.L.; Delen, D. *Advanced Data Mining Techniques*, 1st ed.; Springer: Berlin/Heidelberg, Germany, 2008; p. 138.
21. Sasaki, Y. The truth of the F-measure. *Teach Tutor Mater.* **2007**, *1*, 1–5.
22. Perruchet, P.; Peereman, R. The exploitation of distributional information in syllable processing. *J. Neurolinguist.* **2004**, *17*, 97–119. [CrossRef]
23. Powers, D.M. Evaluation: From Precision, Recall and F-Measure to ROC, Informedness, Markedness & Correlation. *J. Mach. Learn. Technol.* **2011**, *2*, 37–63.
24. Lee, J.-H.; Lee, W.-Y.; Yong, S.J.; Shin, K.C.; Lee, M.K.; Kim, C.W.; Kim, S.-H. A case of levofloxacin-induced anaphylaxis with elevated serum tryptase levels. *Allergy Asthma Immunol. Res.* **2013**, *5*, 113–115. [CrossRef] [PubMed]
25. Guo, K.; Lin, H.; Xu, B.; Yang, Z.; Wang, J.; Sun, Y.; Xu, K.; Cai, Z.; Daescu, O.; Li, M. Detecting Potential Adverse Drug Reactions Using Association Rules and Embedding Models. *Lect. Notes Comput. Sci.* **2017**, *10330*, 373–378.
26. Ibrahim, H.; Saad, A.; Abdo, A.; Eldin, A.S. Mining association patterns of drug-interactions using post marketing FDA's spontaneous reporting data. *J. Biomed. Inf.* **2016**, *60*, 294–308. [CrossRef] [PubMed]
27. Zhang, D.; Lv, J.; Zhang, B.; Zhang, X.; Jiang, H.; Lin, Z. The characteristics and regularities of cardiac adverse drug reactions induced by Chinese materia medica: A bibliometric research and association rules analysis. *J. Ethnopharmacol.* **2020**, *252*, 112582. Available online: https://pubmed.ncbi.nlm.nih.gov/31972324/ (accessed on 21 October 2021). [CrossRef] [PubMed]

applied sciences

MDPI

Article

Decision Tree-Based Data Stratification Method for the Minimization of the Masking Effect in Adverse Drug Reaction Signal Detection

Jianxiang Wei [1,2,*], Lu Cheng [3], Pu Han [1], Yunxia Zhu [3] and Weidong Huang [1,2]

1 School of Management, Nanjing University of Posts and Telecommunications, Nanjing 210003, China; hanpu0725@163.com (P.H.); huangwd@njupt.edu.cn (W.H.)
2 Key Research Base of Philosophy and Social Sciences in Jiangsu-Information Industry Integration Innovation and Emergency Management Research Center, Nanjing 210003, China
3 School of Internet of Things, Nanjing University of Posts and Telecommunications, Nanjing 210003, China; 1020072104@njupt.edu.cn (L.C.); zhuyunxia2005@163.com (Y.Z.)
* Correspondence: jxwei@njupt.edu.cn

Abstract: Data masking is an inborn defect of measures of disproportionality in adverse drug reactions signal detection. Some improved methods which used gender and age for data stratification only considered the patient-related confounding factors, ignoring the drug-related influencing factors. Due to a large number of reports and the high proportion of antibiotics in the Chinese spontaneous reporting database, this paper proposes a decision tree-stratification method for the minimization of the masking effect by integrating the relevant factors of patients and drugs. The adverse drug reaction monitoring reports of Jiangsu Province in China from 2011 to 2018 were selected for this study. First, the age division interval was determined based on the statistical analysis of antibiotic-related data. Secondly, correlation analysis was conducted based on the patient's gender and age respectively with the drug category attributes. Thirdly, the decision tree based on age and gender was constructed by the J48 algorithm, which was used to determine if drugs belonged to antibiotics as a classification label. Fourthly, some performance evaluation indicators were constructed based on the data of drug package inserts as a standard signal library: recall, precision, and F (the arithmetic harmonic mean of recall and precision). Finally, four experiments were carried out by means of the proportional reporting ratio method: non-stratification (total data), gender-stratification, age-stratification and decision tree-stratification, and the performance of the signal detection results was compared. The experimental results showed that the decision tree-stratification was superior to the other three methods. Therefore, the data-masking effect can be further minimized by comprehensively considering the patient and drug-related confounding factors.

Keywords: decision tree; data masking effect; adverse drug reaction; signal detection; data stratification

1. Introduction

Adverse drug reaction (ADR) refers to the harmful effects and negative reactions of qualified drugs without any relation to the purpose of the drug under normal usage and normal dosage, that is, discomfort symptoms or pathogenic reactions [1]. Spontaneous reporting system (SRS) is the main data source of risk reassessment of post-marketing drugs in various countries. ADR signal detection is the main work of pharmacovigilance, which is to explore the relationship between drug and adverse event (AE) by using statistical analysis or data-mining methods. The current methods of signal detection used in many countries are based on disproportionality analysis (DPA). These methods are mainly used to calculate whether the reported frequency of adverse reactions of a certain drug in the database is higher than the expected reported frequency of all drugs, and to qualitatively measure the correlation between drugs and adverse reactions. Methods include proportional reporting ratio (PRR) [2], reporting odds ratio (ROR) [3], information component (IC) [4], multi-item gamma passion shrinker (MGPS) [5], empirical Bayesian geometric mean (EBGM) [6], and so on.

DPA has been widely used in various countries, and plays a positive role in the pharmacovigilance of post-marketing drugs. However, DPA has an inherent defect, the masking effect, which can be caused by data deviation, competition deviation, confounding factors, low data quality and so on [7]. The most common masking effect is due to overreporting. That is, assuming that there is a large number of reports of drug A and adverse reaction B in the data, the ADR combination may reduce the contact strength generated by the combination of drug A and other adverse reactions, or the contact strength generated by the combination of other drugs and adverse reaction B, so that a part of the valuable signals will be masked and the detection efficiency will be reduced. Many scholars have proposed methods to address this issue. The commonly used method for the minimization of the masking effect is to adopt a data stratification strategy, which is to stratify the data according to the different classifications of certain variables that need to be controlled, and then estimate the relationship between a certain exposure factor and a certain AE. Dodd et al. [8] investigated the impact of age stratification and age adjustment on the performance of PRR and EBGM based on pediatric data from the US FDA adverse event reporting system. They thought that stratification could reveal new associations, and therefore suggest recommendations as to when drug use is age-specific or when an age-specific risk is suspected. Zeinoun et al. [9] evaluated the impact of stratification, the comparator dataset and the potential for masking, and conducted a semi-quantitative assessment by comparing the changes in the disproportionality scores and the number of vaccine-event pairs that exceeded an arbitrary threshold as a measure of the impact of any of these choices. The results showed that stratification by age and region has a significant impact. Hopstadius et al. [10] studied the impact of potential confounding factors based on stratification—such as gender, age, reporting quarter—and compared the changes in IC values before and after stratification. Mickael et al. [11] combined the method of removing the masking factor and the stratification of the confounding factor, and proposed a method based on the competition index (ComIn) to identify the disproportionate strength of competitors. They compared the competition factor with the masking factor (MF) and the masking ratio (MR), and found that the ComIn can minimize the competition bias. However, when stratifying confounding factors, these researchers only considered the two major confounding factors, age and gender, and ignored the influence of drug category. Therefore, the improvement effect of stratification was not obvious in the results.

Classification is an important subject in data mining. In recent years, researchers have begun to use the decision tree model to classify datasets. In order to verify the performances of data mining methodology in the evaluation of cardiovascular risk in athletes, and whether the results may be used to support clinical decision making, Barbieri et al. [12] used resampling to balance positive/negative class ratios, and used a decision tree and logistic regression to classify individuals according to risk, so as to improve balance in the classification of medical datasets. The results showed that resampling by decision tree can be effectively applied to biomedical data in order to optimize clinical decision making, and—at the same time—minimize the amount of unnecessary examinations.

Since the mass production and use of penicillin by American pharmaceutical companies in 1942, hundreds of antibiotics have been synthesized. Antibiotic resistance affects the development of the world economy and threatens public health. Antibiotic-induced reactions account for half of spontaneous reports of adverse events in China [13]. Due to the high proportion of antibiotics in the Chinese spontaneous reporting database (CSRD), this paper proposes a decision tree-stratification method for the minimization of the masking effect in ADR signal detection by integrating the relevant factors of patients (age, gender) and drug category (whether or not antibiotics).

2. Methods

2.1. Data Source

The ADR monitoring reports of Jiangsu Province in China between January 1, 2011 and 31 December 2018 were selected for this study, including 754,882 reports. The original dataset includes the fields of drug category, drug name, ADR name, gender and age. The object to be predicted in this study is the combination of drugs and adverse reactions. Due to the lack of age, gender and other information in some reports, a study dataset is obtained after deleting the records with missing information and standardizing the terms of drug name and ADR name. The study dataset contains a total of 751,606 ADR records, which included 1252 drugs, 1262 ADRs and 64,846 drug-event combinations (DECs).

A reference database was established to evaluate the performance of signal detection, including 53,774 kinds of DECs collected from the package insert of drugs.

2.2. Stratification Strategy

The traditional method based on data stratification selects only a single confounding factor, such as age or gender. The reason gender can become a confounding factor is that men and women have many differences in physiological organs and body structures, such as height and weight, hormone secretion, fat distribution, etc., which can change the efficacy of drugs and affect the adverse reactions to drugs. The same is true for age. Due to the large proportion of antibiotic-related reports in CSRD and the complex relationship between age, gender and antibiotics (for example, metronidazole is mainly used for female gynecological diseases, and quinolone is mainly used for the elderly), this paper proposes a stratification method based on a decision tree by integrating the relevant factors of patients and drugs. The specific steps include:

(1) Determining the age division intervals by using the cumulative distribution of antibiotic-related reports based on the patient's age;
(2) χ^2 was used to analyze the correlation between age and drug category ("Antibiotics" or "Non-antibiotics"), as well as gender and drug category;
(3) Data stratification was conducted by a classification algorithm, based on a decision tree by using drug category as the class label, and the two confounding factors of "gender" and "age" as the stratification conditions;
(4) DPA was performed on the multiple datasets generated by the decision tree;
(5) The performance of this method is compared with that of non-stratification, gender-stratification and age-stratification. Classification performances were assessed by means of precision, recall and F-measure.

The overall research framework is shown in Figure 1.

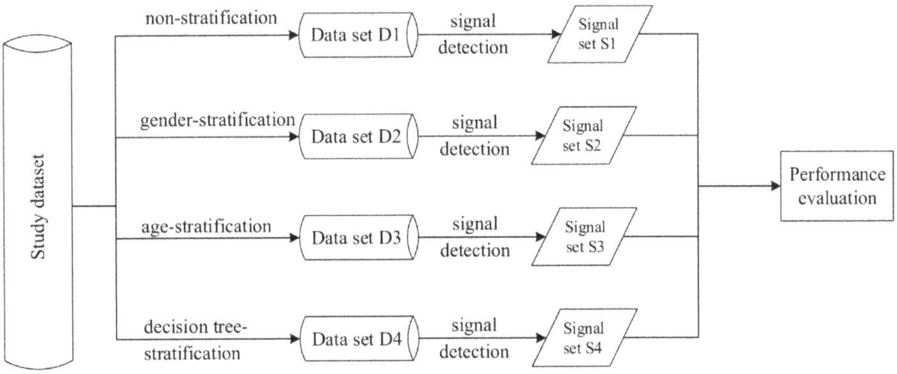

Figure 1. Overall research framework.

2.3. Decision Tree

The decision tree is a widely used technology in classification algorithms. Compared with other algorithms, the classification accuracy of the decision tree is competitive, and the efficiency is also very high. The classification model representation obtained by this algorithm is in the form of a tree. Among them, the more commonly used algorithm is the C4.5 [14]. The J48 algorithm is the application of the C4.5 algorithm in Waikato Environment for Knowledge Analysis (WEKA) [15]. Based on the recursive strategy from top to bottom, the algorithm uses information-gain ratio as attribute separation [16], searches for a property field with a maximum amount of information, establishes a decision tree root node, and then generates a branch for each possible attribute value, dividing instances into multiple subsets, where each subset corresponds to a branch of the root node. The process repeats recursively on each branch. Recursion stops when all instances have the same classification or when the Gini value is less than a certain point with no new leaf nodes generated.

In the design of the algorithm, a good pruning process is considered and added, making it easy for users to understand the classification rules and which has good accuracy in data processing. It has attracted the attention of data mining researchers and solved many practical application problems.

2.4. Signal Detection Method

The calculation of DPA is based on the 2 × 2 contingency table shown in Table 1. If a specific DEC in the database is significantly higher than the background frequency in the entire database and reaches a certain threshold, it is considered a positive signal.

Table 1. Two-by-two contingency table.

	The Target ADR	The Other ADRs
the target drug	A	B
the other drugs	C	D

A represents the number of reports caused by the target drug and the target ADR, B represents the number of reports of the other ADRs caused by the target drug, C represents the number of reports of the target ADR caused by the other drugs, and D Represents the number of reports of the other ADRs caused by the other drugs.

The PRR method is adopted for ADR signal detection. Based on Table 1, the calculation formula is as follows:

$$\text{PRR} = \frac{A/(A+B)}{C/(C+D)} \tag{1}$$

A positive signal is an output if PRR ≥ 2.

2.5. Performance Evaluation

As an objective standard, the reference database is used for performance evaluation. If the signal result is positive and appears in the reference database, it is denoted as a true positive (*TP*), otherwise it is a false positive (*FP*). If the signal result is negative and appears in the reference database, it is denoted as a false negative (*FN*). Precision (*P*) is the proportion of true positive in all predicted positives, and can be defined as follows:

$$P = \frac{TP}{TP + FP} \tag{2}$$

Recall (*R*), the proportion of true positive in all actual positives, is defined as follows:

$$R = \frac{TP}{TP + FN} \tag{3}$$

F-Measure (*F*) is the arithmetic harmonic mean of Precision and Recall, is defined as follows:

$$F = \frac{2 \bullet P \bullet R}{P + R} \tag{4}$$

The larger the *F* value, the higher the performance overall, and the more ideal the effect of minimizing data masking.

3. Results

3.1. Data Analysis

Due to the high proportion of antibiotics-related reports in CSRD, this paper analyzes the correlation between age and drug category, and gender and drug category. The proportion of ADR reports for Antibiotics and Non-antibiotics in the study dataset is given in Table 2.

Table 2. The proportion of reports for antibiotics and non-antibiotics.

Drug Category	Number of Reports (Proportion)
Non-antibiotics	392,113 (52.17%)
Antibiotics	359,493 (47.83%)
Total	751,606

From Table 2, we can see that the proportion of reports for antibiotics accounted for 47.83% of the total reports.

Previous related literature does not have a unified division for the confounding factor of age, they are all subjective individual divisions [17]. Therefore, this paper uses cumulative distribution graphs of the antibiotics-related ADR reports for division of age range, where the length of the age interval is set to five years. The resulting cumulative distribution diagram is shown in Figure 2.

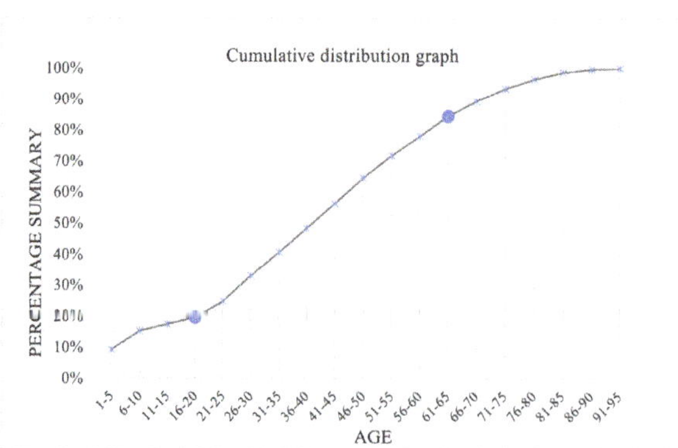

Figure 2. Age cumulative distribution of spontaneous reporting of antibiotics.

It can be seen from Figure 2 that the reported number of antibiotics before and after the age of 60 tends to be flat, while the reported number between 20 and 60 years old has increased significantly. Therefore the age of patients in the data set was discretized into three values: younger than 20 years old is "Young"; 20–60 years old is "Middle"; and older than 60 years is "Senior".

Correlation analysis between gender and drug category was conducted based on Chi-square. The χ^2 value is 343.42, which is far greater than the critical value 3.84 when the degree of freedom is 1 and the significance level is 95%. In the same way, the χ^2 value between age and drug category based on Chi-square is 36,435.81, which is much larger than the critical value of 5.99 when the degree of freedom is 2 and the significance level is 95%. Therefore, the drug category is closely related to gender and age. The contingency table of drug category with gender and age is shown in Table 3.

Table 3. The contingency table of drug category with gender and age.

	Male	Female	Young (≤20)	Middle (21~60)	Senior (≥61)
Antibiotics	170,739	188,754	25,979	225,676	140,458
Non-antibiotics	194,618	197,495	70,145	209,886	79,462
χ^2	343.42			36,435.81	

3.2. Decision Tree

The J48 classification algorithm in WEKA software is used to construct the decision tree (Figure 3).

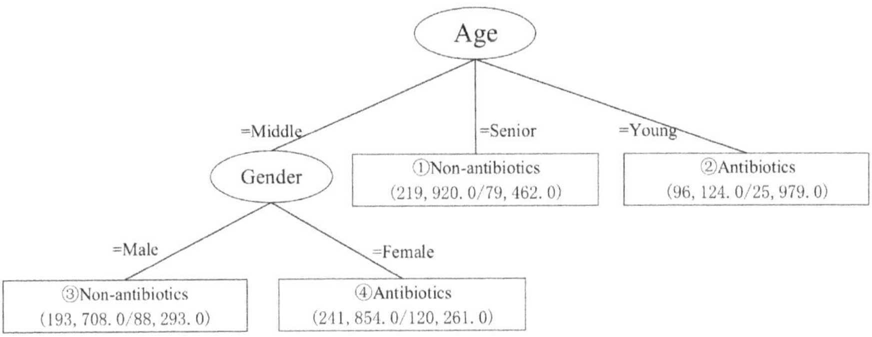

Figure 3. Decision tree.

This decision tree realizes the optimal division of data by using age and gender as conditions and drug category as a class label. The study data set is divided into four data sets:

(1) The data meeting the condition "Age = Senior" are classified into "Non-antibiotics class", including 219,920 reports. The accuracy rate is 63.87%.
(2) The data meeting the condition "Age = Young" are classified into "Antibiotics class", including 96,124 reports. The accuracy rate is 72.97%.
(3) The data meeting the condition "Age = Middle" and "Gender = Male" are classified into "Non-antibiotics class", including 193,708 reports. The accuracy rate is 54.42%.
(4) The data meeting the condition "Age = Middle" and "Gender = Female" are classified into "Antibiotics class", including 241,854 reports. The accuracy rate is 50.28%.

3.3. Performance Evaluation

PRR was used to detect signals in datasets (D1, D2, D3, D4) generated by non-stratification, gender-stratification, age-stratification and decision tree-stratification. Signal sets (S1, S2, S3, S4) were generated (See Figure 1). The comparison results are shown in Table 4.

Table 4. Comparison of detection results of different stratification methods.

Method	TP	FP	FN	R	P	F
non-stratification	7293	28,781	6661	52.26%	20.22%	29.16%
gender-stratification	8369	34,236	5585	59.98%	19.64%	29.59%
age-stratification	8977	35,591	4977	64.33%	20.14%	30.68%
decision tree-stratification	9605	38,225	4349	68.83%	20.08%	31.09%

As can be seen from Table 4, *F* of the three stratification methods has been improved. Among them, the *F* value obtained by decision tree-stratification is the largest, and the *F* value of decision tree-stratification is 1.93% higher than that of non-stratification. In addition, the *R* obtained by decision tree-stratification is significantly improved, which is 16.57% higher than that of non-stratification.

4. Discussion

4.1. Discussion of Methods

Unlike other countries, China has a large population and is one of the largest manufacturers and users of antibiotics. The more kinds of antibiotics that are used, the more ADRs are produced [18]. In this study dataset, antibiotic-related reports accounted for 47.83% of the total reports. Of all 1262 different ADRs, 969 were caused by antibiotics, accounting for 77% of the total. The essence of the signal masking effect is that when a group of DECs are reported too frequently, other DECs associated with these drugs will produce signal delay or direct masking phenomenon [19]. Therefore, drug category is considered an important confounding factor in CSRD, which could cause the data masking effect. The method based on a decision tree is to minimize the signal masking effect by separating antibiotics from other drugs.

In the study data set, among the adverse reaction reports of Epirubicin, 1143 were female and 317 were male, as Epirubicin was mainly used in the treatment of female breast cancer. For Cefpiramide, there are 1851 cases for the young, 1299 cases for the middle, and only 380 cases for the senior. Chi-square analysis revealed a strong correlation between drug category and gender, as well as drug category and age. Therefore, previous studies were also used for reference in our method, and gender and age were considered as two confounding factors. The proposed method integrated the information of patients and drug categories, so it showed advantages in signal detection performance.

In addition, the age interval division in previous studies was subjective and there was no unified standard. An objective method was proposed to discretize age data based on the cumulative distribution of antibiotic-related reports with age.

4.2. Discussion of Results

In this study, four performance comparison experiments are conducted on the same dataset: non-stratification, gender-stratification, age-stratification and decision tree-stratification. The first three are previous methods and the last one is proposed in this study. Experimental results show that the proposed method improves the performance of signal detection in different degrees compared with the previous three methods. Specifically, compared with non-stratification, the R obtained by decision tree-stratification increased greatly from 52.26% to 68.83%, an increase of 16.57%, when the P remains basically unchanged. In addition, the value of *F*-measure increased from 29.16% to 31.09%, an increase of 1.93%. Moreover, the F-measure of our method was higher than that of age-stratification and gender-stratification, which proved the effectiveness of our method.

4.3. Limitations

First of all, the accuracy of the decision tree algorithm adopted in this paper is only 58.22%. If higher classification accuracy is needed, more classification attributes need to be added. However, this will also lead to excessive stratification, which is not good for minimizing the masking signal [20]. Therefore, optimizing the algorithm to improve the accuracy of classification without adding more attributes is what we need to do in the future.

Secondly, while the signal detection method adopted in this paper was PRR, some other methods, such as ROR, IC and MHRA, also need further tested.

5. Conclusions

Data stratification can effectively reduce the data masking effect. The traditional methods were based on the patient's age and gender and other confounding factors, ignoring the drug information. Because there were a large number of reports related to antibiotics in CSRD, we proposed a decision tree-stratification method for the minimization of the masking effect by integrating the relevant information of patients and drug categories, and achieved better performance in ADR signal detection.

Author Contributions: J.W. conceived of the study. L.C. participated in data processing and experimental simulation. J.W. and L.C. participated in data analysis, and drafting of the manuscript. P.H., Y.Z. and W.H. were involved in critically revising the manuscript and reviewing experiment results. All authors have read and agreed to the published version of the manuscript.

Funding: This study was funded by the Major Project of Philosophy and Social Science Research in Jiangsu Universities (2020SJZDA102).

Institutional Review Board Statement: Not applicable.

Informed Consent Statement: Not applicable.

Data Availability Statement: All ADR spontaneous reporting data in this study is licensed by the CFDA. The datasets are not publicly available due to the policy of confidentiality of the CFDA but are available from the corresponding author on reasonable request and with permission of the CFDA.

Conflicts of Interest: The authors declare no conflict of interest.

References

1. Edwards, I.R.; Aronson, J.K. Adverse drug reactions: Definitions, diagnosis, and management. *Lancet* **2000**, *356*, 1255–1259. [CrossRef]
2. Slattery, J.; Alvarez, Y.; Hidalgo, A. Choosing thresholds for statistical signal detection with the proportional reporting ratio. *Drug Saf.* **2013**, *36*, 687–692. [CrossRef] [PubMed]
3. Bate, A.; Leufkens, H.G.M.; Lindquist, M.; Orre, R.; Egberts, T. A comparison of measures of disproportionality for signal detection in spontaneous reporting systems for adverse drug reactions. *Pharmacoepidemiol. Drug Saf.* **2002**, *11*, 3–10. [CrossRef]
4. Bate, A.; Lindquist, M.; Edwards, I.R.; Orre, R. A data mining approach for signal detection and analysis. *Drug Saf.* **2002**, *25*, 393–397. [CrossRef] [PubMed]
5. Hauben, M.; Bate, A. Decision support methods for the detection of adverse events in post-marketing data. *Drug Discov. Today* **2009**, *14*, 343–357. [CrossRef] [PubMed]
6. Martin, D.; Menschik, D.; Bryant-Genevier, M.; Ball, R. Data mining for prospective early detection of safety signals in the vaccine adverse event reporting system (VAERS): A case study of febrile seizures after a 2010–2011 seasonal influenza virus vaccine. *Drug Saf.* **2013**, *36*, 547–556. [CrossRef] [PubMed]
7. Almenoff, J.; Tonning, J.M.; Gould, A.L.; Szarfman, A.; Hauben, M.; Ouellet-Hellstrom, R.; Ball, R.; Hornbuckle, K.; Walsh, L.; Yee, C.; et al. Perspectives on the use of data mining in pharmacovigilance. *Drug Saf.* **2005**, *28*, 981–1007. [CrossRef] [PubMed]
8. Caster, O.; Norén, G.N.; Madigan, D.; Bate, A. Large-scale regression-based pattern discovery: The example of screening the WHO global drug safety database. *Stat. Anal. Data Min. ASA Data Sci. J.* **2010**, *3*, 197–208. [CrossRef]
9. Zeinoun, Z.; Seifert, H.; Verstraeten, T. Quantitative signal detection for vaccines: Effects of stratification, background and masking on GlaxoSmithKline's spontaneous reports database. *Hum. Vaccines* **2009**, *5*, 599–607. [CrossRef] [PubMed]
10. Hopstadius, J.; Norén, G.N.; Bate, A.; Edwards, I.R. Impact of stratification on adverse drug reaction surveillance. *Drug Saf.* **2008**, *31*, 1035–1048. [CrossRef] [PubMed]
11. Mickael, A.; Francesco, S.; Ismaïl, A.; Philip, R.; Nicholas, M.; Bernard, M.; Tubert-Bitter, P.; Pariente, A. A method for the minimization of competition bias in signal detection from spontaneous reporting databases. *Drug Saf.* **2016**, *39*, 251–260.
12. Barbieri, D.; Chawla, N.; Zaccagni, L.; Grgurinović, T.; Šarac, J.; Čoklo, M.; Missoni, S. Predicting cardiovascular risk in Athletes: Resampling improves classification performance. *Int. J. Environ. Res. Public Health* **2020**, *17*, 7923. [CrossRef] [PubMed]
13. Li, Y.; Xu, J.; Wang, F.; Wang, B.; Liu, L.; Hou, W.; Fan, H.; Tong, Y.; Zhang, J.; Lu, Z. Overprescribing in China, driven by financial incentives, results in very high use of antibiotics, injections, and corticosteroids. *Health Aff.* **2012**, *31*, 1075–1082. [CrossRef] [PubMed]
14. Quinlan, J.R. *C4.5: Programs for Machine Learning*; Morgan Kaufmann Publishers: San Francisco, CA, USA, 1993.
15. Garner, S.R. *WEKA: The Waikato Environment for Knowledge Analysis*; Department of Computer Science, University of Waikato: Hamilton, OH, USA, 1995.

16. Li, C.B.; Li, S.J. *Data Warehouse and Data Mining Practice and Application*; Publishing House of Electronics Industry: Beijing, China, 2014; pp. 328–330.
17. Zhao, L.; Ye, X.; Wang, C.; Qian, W.; Du, W.; He, J. Application of stratification analysis in adverse drug reaction signal detection. *Chin. J. Pharmacovigil.* **2011**, *8*, 158–160.
18. Walley, J.D.; Zhang, Z.; Wei, X. Antibiotic overuse in China: Call for consolidated efforts to develop antibiotic stewardship programmes. *Lancet Infect. Dis.* **2021**, *21*, 597. [CrossRef]
19. Wang, H.-W.; Hochberg, A.M.; Pearson, R.K.; Hauben, M. An experimental investigation of masking in the US FDA adverse event reporting system database. *Drug Saf.* **2010**, *33*, 1117–1133. [CrossRef] [PubMed]
20. Hopstadius, J.; Norén, G.N.; Bate, A.; Edwards, I.R. Stratification for spontaneous report databases. *Drug Saf.* **2008**, *31*, 1145–1147. [CrossRef] [PubMed]

applied sciences

MDPI

Article

Evolution of Hemodynamic Parameters Simulated by Means of Diffusion Models

Andrzej Walczak [1,*], Paweł Moszczyński [1] and Paweł Krzesiński [2]

1 Institute of Computer and Information Systems, Military University of Technology, ul. gen. Kaliskiego 2, 00-908 Warsaw, Poland; pawel.moszczynski@wat.edu.pl
2 Department of Cardiology and Internal Diseases, Military Institute of Medicine, ul. Szaserów 128, 04-141 Warsaw, Poland; pkrzesinski@wim.mil.pl
* Correspondence: andrzej.walczak@wat.edu.pl

Abstract: Diffusion is a well-known physical phenomenon governing such processes as movement of particles or transportation of heat. In this paper, we prove that a close analogy to those processes exists in medical data behavior, and that changes in the values of medical parameters measured while treating patients may be described using diffusion models as well. The medical condition of a patient is usually described by a set of discrete values. The evolution of that condition and, consequently, of the disease has the form of a transition of that set of discrete values, which correspond to specific parameters. This is a typical medical diagnosis scheme. However, disease evolution is a phenomenon that is characterized by continuously varying, temporal characteristics. A mathematical disease evolution model is, in fact, a continuous diffusion process from one discrete slot of the diagnosed parameter value to another inside the mentioned set. The ability to predict such diffusion-related properties offer precious support in diagnostic decision-making. We have examined several hundred patients while conducting a medical research project. All patients were under treatment to stabilize their hemodynamic parameters. A diffusion model relied upon simulating the results of treatment is proposed here. Time evolution of thoraric fluid content (TFC) has been used as the illustrative example. The objective is to prove that diffusion models are a proper and convenient solution for predicting disease evolution processes. We applied the Fokker-Planck equation (FPE), considering it to be most adequate for examining the treatment results by means of diffusion. We confirmed that the phenomenon of diffusion explains the evolution of the heart disease parameters observed. The evolution of TFC has been chosen as an example of a hemodynamic parameter.

Keywords: Fokker-Planck equation; diffusion; heart failure; impedance cardiography; thoracic fluid content

1. Introduction

The current state of the art in predicting disease evolution may be summarized in the following manner. Hemodynamic assessment procedures are widely described in the literature, primarily by means of biological models for flow or response functions [1–4]. Numerous investigations aimed to estimate the risk of heart failure by relying on common statistical data processing tools and regression models [5–7]. Highly illustrative investigations were proposed by Lassnig at al. [8]. Other clinical prediction models (CPMs), also known as clinical prediction scores or rules, are used to estimate the risk of an existing disease (diagnostic prediction model) or future outcomes (prognostic prediction model) for a given individual and consist of analyzing the values of numerous predictors (prognostic or risk factors), such as age, sex, and biomarkers [9–12]. Generic prediction models are widely used in adult intensive care medicine. These include, for instance, acute physiology and chronic health evaluation (APACHE) II, APACHE III, APACHE IV, simplified acute physiology score (SAPS) II, SAPS 3, and mortality probability model

III [13]. So, different predictive approaches are present in the literature. The results presented in there are organized in accordance with risk analysis, and such an approach does not allow us to simulate disease evolution. The following question arises: are we able to simulate the evolution of hemodynamic parameters during medical treatment? In this paper, we propose a model explaining the rules of hemodynamic parameter evolution in patients with heart failure. Simulation of the disease evolution seems to be possible with the presented approach.

The activities undertaken may be divided into experimental and theoretical phases. In the experimental phase of the project, a multicenter, prospective, randomized, open-label, and controlled, parallel group trial was conducted (ClinicalTrials.gov Identifier: NCT03476590). Here, 605 patients suffering from heart failure were recruited to participate in the project. In the theoretical phase, we propose to describe the behavior of the hemodynamic parameters measured by relying on diffusion models.

In Section 2, experimental observations and analyses are presented. Section 3 presents theoretical models describing the diffusion phenomena. Section 3 contains the results of confrontation theoretical models with experimental data. Finally, Section 4 contains a summary and a discussion.

The achieved aim is the creation of a continuous, differential model for disease evolution.

2. Experimental Data

The experimental data used in this study were sourced from the AMULET research project [14], under which a multicenter, prospective, randomized, open-label and controlled, parallel group trial was conducted (ClinicalTrials.gov Identifier: NCT03476590) at nine locations throughout Poland. In total, 605 patients with heart failure were recruited. To our study, we examined electrocardiogram (ECG—electrocardiogram) and impedance (ICG—impedance cardiogram) curves recorded with the use of an ICG device (Cardioscreen 2000, Medis, Illmenau, Germany). This non-invasive diagnostic method allows one to collect a set of specific hemodynamic parameters, such as: heart rate (HR—heart rate), diastolic and systolic blood pressure (DBP—diastolic blood pressure, SBP—systolic blood pressure), stroke volume (SV—stroke volume), and thoracic fluid content (TFC—thoraric fluid content). In our analysis, TFC has been used as an illustrative example. The value of TFC is the inverse of chest impedance with unit (1/Ohm).

TFC values were measured during a clinical examination of 605 patients, performed in a relaxed, seated position [14]. The total number of measurements made is 2860, with the number of individual patient observations differing for each patient within the measurement set. The results registered are illustrated in Figure 1. At least half of the patients were investigated several times, with the observation period lasting for up to 12 months per patient.

All intervals of the investigated TFC value have been divided arbitrarily into 15 discrete value slots, as shown in Figure 1. The assumed number of slots must be greater than five to allow statistical analysis (especially χ^2 tests) but not too high to avoid complexity of calculations. With computer calculation, we estimate that 15 slots allow an acceptable accuracy of calculations. The time series was registered as follows: due to the irregular flow of the measured data, we adopted a registration period that was 31 days long for each slot. The result of the measurement was placed inside a given slot if number of days between the sequenced examination of the patient remained within the $k \pm 0.5$ range, with k being the duration of the registration period between measurements. Each slot includes hits counted during measurements registered over a five-month period. Hits registered during each single measurement period are illustrated below.

One can observe that, for the increasing Δt, the total number of TFC hits registered tends to have the same stationary distribution of TFC, as shown in Figure 1. We assumed that the period of 5 months during which the measurements were made (see Figure 2 and comments to Figure 1) is sufficient for proper estimation of stationary distribution.

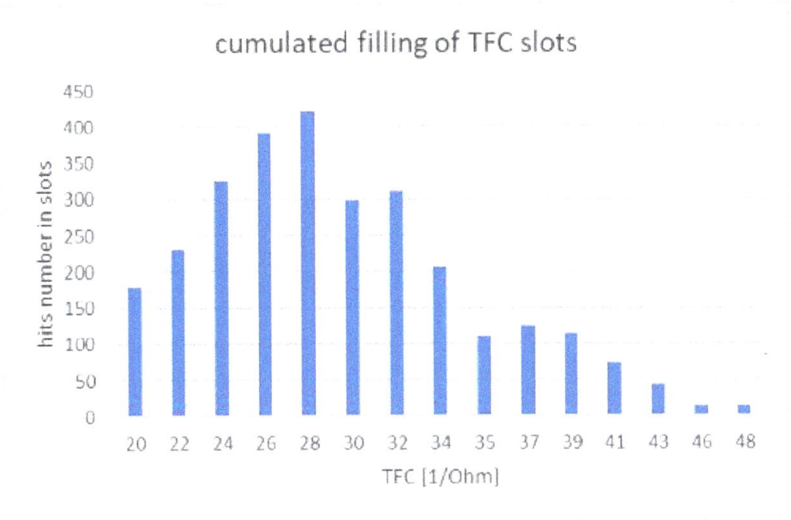

Figure 1. Values of TFC slots filled with the number of measurements.

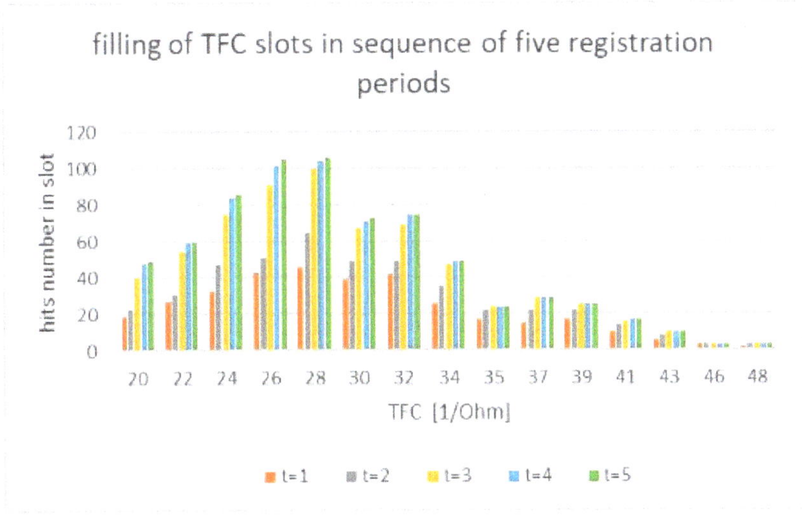

Figure 2. Stepped registration of TFC values in measurement intervals denoted as t in the figure.

3. Theoretical Model and Calculation

The Fokker-Planck equation with one variable (here, variable x denotes the TFC value) has the following form [15]:

$$\frac{\partial P}{\partial t} = \left[-\frac{\partial}{\partial x} D^{(1)}(x) + \frac{\partial^2}{\partial x^2} D^{(2)}(x) \right] P \tag{1}$$

In this equation, $D^{(2)}(x) > 1$ is the diffusion coefficient, and $D^{(1)}(x)$ is called the drift coefficient. In general, both coefficients may also depend on time. The equation describes behavior $P(x, t)$, i.e., the $P(x, t)$ is distribution of probability. We assumed stochastic process characterizes the linear drift coefficient, and the diffusion coefficient is constant.

$$\frac{\partial P}{\partial t} = \gamma \frac{\partial (xP)}{\partial x} + D\frac{\partial^2}{\partial x^2} P \tag{2}$$

In our experiment, drift γx is present due to therapy data registration, so drift presence is necessary. Diffusion describes the transition between slots of parameter values measured. A solution of Equation (2) is of the form [15]:

$$P(x, t|x', t\prime) = \sqrt{\frac{\gamma}{2\pi D\left(1 - e^{-2\gamma(t-t')}\right)}}\, exp\left(-\frac{\gamma\left(x - x' e^{-\gamma(t-t')}\right)^2}{2D\left(1 - e^{-2\gamma(t-t')}\right)}\right) \tag{3}$$

Green function (3) of Equation (2) is one of the basic ways for system dynamic description [15,16]. The stationary solution for $\gamma > 0$ and a sufficiently long-period $\gamma(t - t') >> 1$ takes the following form:

$$W(x) = \sqrt{\frac{\gamma}{2\pi D}} exp\left(\frac{-\gamma x^2}{2D}\right) \tag{4}$$

For $\gamma \leq 0$, no stationary solutions exist. Formal mathematical procedures enable us to find coefficients γ and D with a normalization condition and a boundary condition. Due to the existence of a stationary shape of $W(x)$ distribution obtained in the experiment, we can assume that the boundary conditions are properly fulfilled despite not being fully established in the formal way. In such a situation, the assumption that coefficients γ and D are well-matched by means of conjugated gradient algorithm and, simultaneously, to minimize root mean square error (RMSE) between the experiment data and the theoretical model (4) is permissible.

The set of solutions for $W(x)$ is placed in Table 1, where local and global minima have been shown for the illustrative subset of γ and D. The shape for stationary distribution with γ and D for the global minimum is presented in Figure 3.

Table 1. Illustrative values of RMSE, with the global minimum highlighted in bold print obtained by means of conjugated gradient algorithm.

RMSE	γ	D
0.09810952	0.4	11.99
0.09838436	0.06	1.75
0.09811257	0.2	5.99
0.09811050	0.3	8.99

The results obtained with the conjugated gradient solution are placed in Table 1. The global minimum is placed in the first row of Table 1.

The green function of FPE with adjusted γ and D values, and stationary distribution $W(x')$ is applied to determine $P(x, t)$ distribution in accordance with:

$$P(x, t) = \int P(x, t|x' - x_0) W(x' - x_0) dx' \tag{5}$$

Distribution $P(x, t)$ allows us to verify if the calculated and measured evolution of TFC values is statistically convergent by conducting an χ^2 test. Item x_0 is commonly the maximum observed value of $W(x')$ or may also be the boundary point. A comparison of the theoretical $P(x, t)$ with the experiment's results is presented in Table 2, and the outcomes of statistical tests are shown in Table 3.

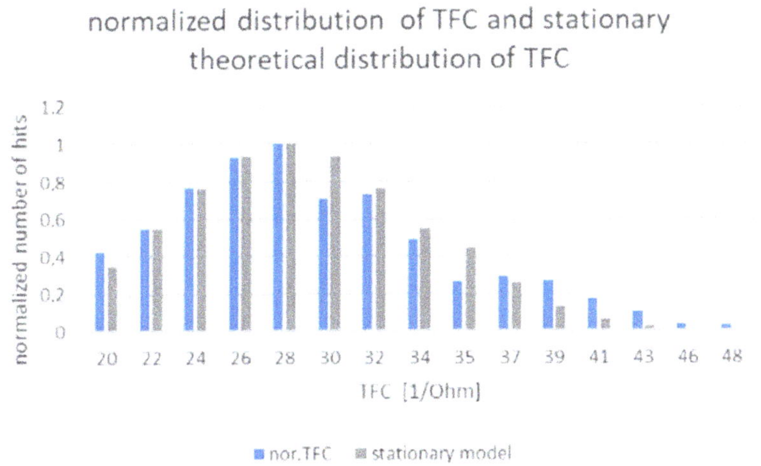

Figure 3. Result of minimization of RMSE between experimental TFC distribution data and the stationary distribution model $W(x)$.

Table 2. The TFC slots filling obtained during measurements (see also Figure 2) and values predicted with $P(x, t)$.

TFC Slot Number	Observation Period t2–t1		Observation Period t3–t2		Observation Period t4–t3		Observation Period t5–t4	
	Registered hits of TFC	Predicted TFC hits	Registered hits of TFC	Predicted TFC hits	Registered hits of TFC	Predicted TFC hits	Registered hits of TFC	Predicted TFC hits
1	19	18.9475	23	22.8236	40	29.9024	48	28.6218
2	27	31.5513	31	39.8768	55	55.6347	59	55.9634
3	33	40.8633	47	53.8865	75	79.7512	84	84.2399
4	43	39.6876	51	55.9473	91	87.9519	102	97.5805
5	46	37.5247	65	54.1467	100	86.493	104	97.1694
6	39	39.6876	49	55.7919	67	83.7667	71	89.5681
7	42	40.8643	49	44.0522	69	62.3851	75	63.5276
8	26	31.5513	35	15.541	47	20.981	49	20.549
9	17	10.9594	22	19.0808	24	24.5837	24	23.2358
10	15	13.509	22	7.9594	29	9.5469	29	8.5716
11	17	5.8755	22	2.5746	25	2.8579	25	2.4346
12	10	0.7917	14	0.7780	16	0.6587	17	0.5322
13	6	0.5562	8	0.6613	10	0.1285	10	0.0982
14	3	0.1235	3	0	3	0	3	0

Table 3. Calculations of χ^2 test for sequence of period of measurement.

Time Period in Experiment	χ^2 Test Value	Number of Independent Variables	Significance Level (Critical Value α)
t2–t1	314,375	14	$\alpha = 0.005$
t3–t2	570,858	14	$\alpha < 0.001$
t4–t3	811,461	14	$\alpha < 0.001$
t5–t4	922,901	14	$\alpha < 0.001$

4. Discussion and Conclusions

Claiming that hemodynamic parameter values measured in a population of patients behave in accordance with the rules of drifted diffusion, we have identified a step-by-step procedure allowing to verify such a statement. From the green function of FPE, we obtained stationary distribution $W(x)$ of the thoracic fluid content (TFC) parameter observed, and by minimizing RMSE between the theoretical model and the experimental observations of stationary distribution, we adjusted the parameters of the stochastic process with the use of conjugated gradient algorithms. It turned out that the resulting form of the stochastic process is the Ornstein–Uhlenbeck process. So, we found the Ornstein–Uhlenbeck diffusion process as a model for medical treatment of heart failures. From the analytical form of the FPE solution (green function of FPE), we determined the "ex definition" distribution $P(x, t)$ for the observed hemodynamic parameters and determined dynamics of TFC evolution. The last step had the form of a statistical χ^2 test, aiming to accept or to reject the proposed theoretical model. The χ^2 test confirms the accepted level of efficiency of the theoretical model of the Ornstein–Uhlenbeck process, describing TFC evolution.

Finally, we may conclude that the diffusion processes have turned out to be useful tools for predicting disease evolution. We have also proved that:

1. The Ornstein–Uhlenbeck process, including the linear drift component, seems to be a precise tool for simulating the evolution of TFC and, supposedly, other hemodynamic parameters, also during medical treatment.
2. We obtained the distribution $P(x, t)$, allowing us to predict and simulate TFC evolution.
3. Parameter γ describes the effectiveness of medical treatment in the population of patients, thus being a mathematical measure of such treatment effectiveness that is worth being analyzed in a more thorough manner, e.g., by focusing on variations depending on sex, occupation, age, severity of heart failure in accordance with the NYHA standard, etc.

The idea of diffusion occurring inside a potential force field is deeply exploited in solid state physics and quantum electronics [16–22], but its successful application in medical diagnostics seems to be a new approach that suggests, to some extent, the existence of a "hidden general symmetry" between physics and biology as well. Diffusion theory is relevant not only for microscopic observations made in physics, but also for much larger scale phenomena, e.g., in medicine. In medicine, fluctuations take place due to multiple and multilevel interactions occurring in the patient's system. Such fluctuations are hard to describe in a precise manner, although their presence seems to be obvious.

The results presented herein are based on data processed during a medical experiment and, to the best of the authors' knowledge, form the first model of its type proposed in medical diagnostics. The results we obtained allows us to predict the time evolution of TFC. Simultaneously, we have confirmed that the fluctuation theory, reflected here by means of FPE, is an inherent element of medical diagnostic processes.

It must be underlined that prospective validation of the model is continued now in collaborative clinics under Amulet project. We do suppose that limitations of the model will be analyzed during further validation. An evident strength of the model is its continuous, differential model of disease evolution. As far as authors know, it seems to be a new approach.

Author Contributions: Conceptualization, methodology, software, formal analysis—A.W.; validation and statistics—P.M.; investigation, resources—P.K. All authors have read and agreed to the published version of the manuscript.

Funding: This work was supported by the National Centre for Research and Development under the program 'Prevention and treatment of lifestyle diseases'—STRATEGMED III STRATEGMED3/305274/8/NCBR/2017).

Institutional Review Board Statement: The study was conducted according to the guidelines of the Declaration of Helsinki, and approved by the Institutional Ethics Committee of Military Institute of Medicine (No. 70/WIM/2016).

Informed Consent Statement: Informed consent was obtained from all subjects involved in the study.

Data Availability Statement: The data used to support the findings of this study are available from the corresponding author upon request.

Acknowledgments: The authors would like to thank the medical staff of their centers for the nursing care and data collection.

Conflicts of Interest: The authors declare that there are no conflict of interest regarding the publication of this paper.

References

1. Chen, X.; Schwarz, K.Q.; Phillips, D.; Steinmetz, S.D.; Schlief, R. A Mathematical Model for the Assessment of Hemodynamic Parameters Using Quantitative Contrast Echocardiography. *IEEE Trans. Biomed. Eng.* **1998**, *45*, 754–765. [CrossRef] [PubMed]
2. Aquinoab, K.M.; Robinsonab, P.A.; Drysdaleab, P.M. Spatiotemporal hemodynamic response functions derived from physiology. *J. Theor. Biol.* **2014**, *347*, 118–136. [CrossRef] [PubMed]
3. Mukkamala, R.; Gao, M. A Comparative Analysis of Reduced Arterial Models for Hemodynamic Monitoring. In Proceedings of the 2013 35th Annual International Conference of the IEEE Engineering in Medicine and Biology Society (EMBC), Osaka, Japan, 3–7 July 2013; pp. 225–228. [CrossRef]
4. Morris, P.; Ryan, D.; Morton, A.; Lycett, R.; Lawford, P.; Hose, D.R.; Gunn, J. Virtual Fractional Flow Reserve from Coronary Angiography: Modeling the significance of coronary lesions. *JACC Cardiovasc. Interv.* **2013**, *6*, 149–157. [CrossRef] [PubMed]
5. Priyanka, H.; Vivek, R. Multi Model Data Mining Approach for Heart Failure Prediction. *Int. J. Data Min. Knowl. Manag. Process* **2016**, *6*, 31–37.
6. Bouvy, M.L.; Heerdink, E.R.; Leufkens, H.G.M.; Hoes, A.W. Predicting mortality in patients with heart failure: A pragmatic approach. *Heart* **2003**, *89*, 605–609. [CrossRef] [PubMed]
7. Jiang, W.; Siddiqui, S.; Barnes, S.; Barouch, L.A.; Korley, F.; Martinez, D.; Toerper, M.; Cabral, S.; Hamrock, E.; Levin, S. Readmission Risk Trajectories for Patients with Heart Failure Using a Dynamic Prediction Approach: Retrospective Study. *JMIR Med. Inf.* **2019**, *7*, e14756. [CrossRef] [PubMed]
8. Lassnig, A.; Rienmueller, T.; Kramer, D.; Leodolter, W.; Baumgartner, C.; Schroettner, J. A novel hybrid modeling approach for the evaluation of integrated care and economic outcome in heart failure treatment. *BMC Med. Inform. Decis. Mak.* **2019**, *19*, 229. [CrossRef] [PubMed]
9. Steyerberg, E.; Moons, K.; Van der Windt, D.; Hayden, J.; Perel, P.; Schroter, S.; Riley, R.D.; Hemingway, H.; Altman, D.G.; PROGRESS Group. Prognosis Research Strategy (PROGRESS) 3: Prognostic Model Research. *PLoS Med.* **2013**, *10*, e1001381. [CrossRef] [PubMed]
10. Labarère, J.; Bertran, R.; Fine, M.J. How to derive and validate clinical prediction models for use in intensive care medicine. *Intens. Care Med.* **2014**, *40*, 513–527. [CrossRef] [PubMed]
11. Laupacis, N.; Sekar, N.; Stiell, I. Clinical prediction rules. A review and suggested modifications of methodological standards. *JAMA* **1997**, *277*, 488–494. [CrossRef] [PubMed]
12. Moons, K.; Altman, D.; Vergouwe, Y.; Royston, P. Prognosis, and prognostic research: Application and impact of prognostic models in clinical practice. *BMJ* **2009**, *338*, b606. [CrossRef] [PubMed]
13. Vincent, J.; Moreno, R. Clinical review: Scoring systems in the critically ill. *Crit. Care* **2010**, *14*, 207. [CrossRef] [PubMed]
14. Krzesiński, P.; Siebert, J.; Jankowska, A.E.; Galas, A.; Piotrowicz, K.; Stańczyk, A.; Siwołowski, P.; Gutknecht, P.; Chrom, P.; Murawski, P.; et al. Nurse-led ambulatory care supported by non-invasive haemodynamic assessment improves the functional state and well-being of patients suffering from acute heart failure decompensation—A pilot study. *ESC Heart Fail.* **2021**, *8*, 1018–1026. [CrossRef] [PubMed]
15. Risken, H. The Fokker-Planck equation. In *Method of Solution and Applications*; Springer: Berlin/Heidelberg, Germany, 1989.
16. Gardiner, C.W. *Handbook of Stochastic Methods for Physics, Chemistry and Natural Sciences*; Springer: Berlin/Heidelberg, Germany, 1990.
17. Peliti, L.; Vulpiani, A. (Eds.) *Measures of Complexity*; Springer: Berlin/Heidelberg, Germany, 1988.
18. Takayama, H. (Ed.) *Cooperative Dynamics in Complex Systems*; Springer: Berlin/Heidelberg, Germany, 1989.
19. Carslaw, H.S.; Jaegher, J.C. *Conduction of Heat in Solids*; Clarendon Press: Oxford, UK, 1959.
20. Nelson, E. *Dynamical Theories of Brownian Motion*; Princeton University Press: Princeton, NJ, USA, 1967.

21. de Groot, S.R.; Mazur, P. *Non-Equilibrium Thermodynamics*; North-Holland: Amsterdam, The Netherlands, 1969.
22. Coley, W.T.; Kalmykov, Y.P.; Waldron, J.T. *The Langevin Equation*; World Scientific: Singapore, 1996.

applied sciences

MDPI

Communication

Anatomy of a Data Science Software Toolkit That Uses Machine Learning to Aid 'Bench-to-Bedside' Medical Research—With Essential Concepts of Data Mining and Analysis Explained

László Beinrohr [1,*], Eszter Kail [2], Péter Piros [2], Erzsébet Tóth [1], Rita Fleiner [2] and Krasimir Kolev [1]

1 Department of Biochemistry, Semmelweis University, Tűzoltó utca 37–47, 1094 Budapest, Hungary; toth.erzsebet@med.semmelweis-univ.hu (E.T.); Krasimir.Kolev@eok.sote.hu (K.K.)
2 John von Neumann Faculty of Informatics, Óbuda University, Bécsi út 96/b, 1034 Budapest, Hungary; kail.eszter@nik.uni-obuda.hu (E.K.); piros.peter@nik.uni-obuda.hu (P.P.); fleiner.rita@nik.uni-obuda.hu (R.F.)
* Correspondence: beinrohr.laszlo@med.semmelweis-univ.hu

Abstract: Data science and machine learning are buzzwords of the early 21st century. Now pervasive through human civilization, how do these concepts translate to use by researchers and clinicians in the life-science and medical field? Here, we describe a software toolkit, just large enough in scale, so that it can be maintained and extended by a small team, optimised for problems that arise in small/medium laboratories. In particular, this system may be managed from data ingestion statistics preparation predictions by a single person. At the system's core is a graph type database, so that it is flexible in terms of irregular, constantly changing data types, as such data types are common during explorative research. At the system's outermost shell, the concept of 'user stories' is introduced to help the end-user researchers perform various tasks separated by their expertise: these range from simple data input, data curation, statistics, and finally to predictions via machine learning algorithms. We compiled a sizable list of already existing, modular Python platform libraries usable for data analysis that may be used as a reference in the field and may be incorporated into this software. We also provide an insight into basic concepts, such as labelled-unlabelled data, supervised vs. unsupervised learning, regression vs. classification, evaluation by different error metrics, and an advanced concept of cross-validation. Finally, we show some examples from our laboratory using our blood sample and blood clot data from thrombosis patients (sufferers from stroke, heart and peripheral thrombosis disease) and how such tools can help to set up realistic expectations and show caveats.

Keywords: thrombosis; stroke; data science; machine learning; graph database; python; PyTanito; user story; classification; cross-validation

1. Introduction

Coronary artery disease (CAD), acute ischemic stroke (AIS), peripheral artery disease (PAD) are cardiovascular diseases and represent the leading morbidity and mortality causes globally [1]. The acute tissue damage is mostly due to thrombi occluding the supplying arteries [2]. The lysis susceptibility and stability of these thrombi ultimately determines the fate of the patient [3]. Can we tell more from their structure and from common blood test data of patients? Can we predict the diseases from this data? Even better, can we predict it before disease onset? These are questions that we address with the help of the data analysis approach described in this paper.

2. Data Science Project Organisation—Industry 'Best Practices'

As with any project, the question arises: where to begin? This is especially so with complex, data-driven projects, such as the 'bench-to-bedside' projects often seen in the medical and life science field. Fortunately, this problem has been seen before and some solutions, or rather, guidelines were devised. Industrial Micro Machines (IBM) researchers and automotive engineers (Daimler-Chrysler) did indeed face the same problem in the 1990s. The resultant guidelines were standardized in the CRISP-DM standard which stands for Cross Industry Standard Process for Data Mining [4]. The model, illustrated in Figure 1, consists of six steps [5].

1. Business understanding. In the medical field, we would need to determine if the project is for research purposes only. Do we have obvious clinical implications (with rigorous safety, regulatory and legal requirements)? Do we eye business potential—which in turn may need strict documentation and reporting?
2. Data understanding. In the medical and life science field, we often have to gather data via experiments ourselves, and the quality of this data will be crucial. (In the era of big data, many projects may rely on published open data sources.) What data can we gather and in what amount? Can we collect enough in a realistic timeframe? Will the data be sufficient for the questions asked? Do we have good recipes so that the data is reproducible over large timespans, with changing personnel?
3. Data preparation. We must gather data from handwritten notes or other sources, collect them in machine-readable form, and normalize or otherwise standardize them. Watch out for reproducibility issues often encountered with difficult experiments. Can our data be quantified and compared across different investigators and with human subjects involved? Even standard laboratory tests may differ in testing methodology. With human subjects, legal issues also arise privacy rights need to be respected, and data anonymized.
4. Modelling. We need to use our data—somehow. Do we have continuous variables or categorical ones? Do we have an initial hypothesis to test, or do we need methods that are suitable for 'walking in the dark'?
5. Evaluation. We need to use metrics by which we quantify 'successes. Do we have concise research questions so that an answer to them can be made? Are we descriptive or do we have new hypotheses as a result? Without clear questions, no metrics will be satisfactory, as metrics are often meaningless themselves. Can we compare our work to that of others via the metrics?
6. Deployment. Pure research may result in scientific outputs, such as presentations or scientific papers or openly published datasets. However, does our research yield tangible results such as new scientific hypotheses? Does our research have clinical implications?

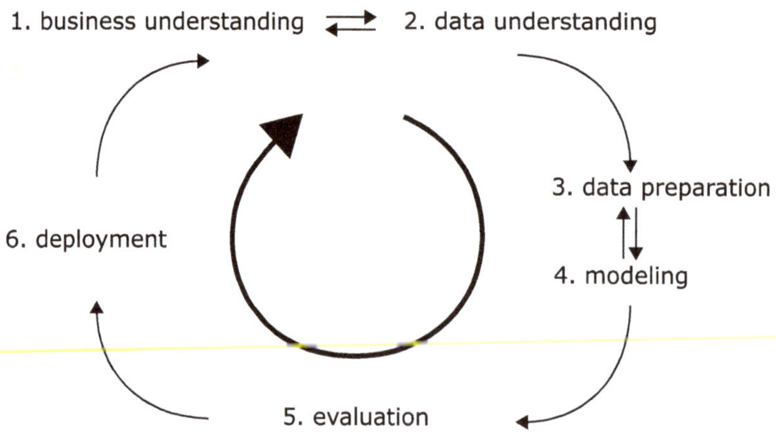

Figure 1. The six elementary steps in a data science project as outlined in the CRISP-DM standard.

This is the model we will follow and around which we build our homemade software, which will be described in more detail in the next sections.

2.1. Software Architecture—Incorporation of 'Best Practices' for User-Friendliness

The software we are developing is an aid for a small-scale medical research team. To borrow from the beforementioned concepts, we are developing software that helps with steps 2–5, with 3–4 essential parts of it. The focus is deliberately limited, it does not want to do more: it is simply a framework by which a team can gather all their research data, test various hypotheses and models with it, and report it automatically in a user-readable form. We feel that this scope fits with a few developers and new functions may be added as needed; in contrast with large software frameworks, where such incorporation may take a long time or workarounds.

However, the CRISP-DM standard deliberately does not provide a guideline, how to actually implement the functionality required. This problem is as old as software development itself. Fortunately, industry 'best practices' are available. One of these is the widely popular 'Agile' methodology [6]. The 'Agile Manifesto' of software developers describes essential concepts and introduced the concept of 'user stories' [7]. With Agile and with 'user stories', the system is approached from outside, from the perspective of the users. Everything else is developed around the needs of the users, every user has a 'story' with the software piece.

In a small research project, we usually have four types of participants:

1. Assistants, who usually have a narrow, well-defined scope of work.
2. Junior researchers (e.g., undergraduate students) and other personnel, who are strongly dependent on input in their work.
3. Senior researchers (e.g., postdocs), who are able to work independently with minimal input.
4. Principal investigator, who oversees the whole project and sets goals.

To meet the requirements of data processing in such teams, we have devised a software toolkit, a data learning framework we named 'PyTanito'. The Py stands for 'Python', an increasingly popular, open-source, machine programming language [8], with a large following in the science field as of 2021. We have deliberately made this choice, so that our software may be extended by future researchers without 'strings attached' or without potential large costs that come with proprietary systems managed by large corporations. A secondary benefit of this adoption is that an increasingly large amount of 'libraries' are available for it. These 'libraries' are pieces of independent programs performing specific tasks so that one can rely on the work of others. We do not need to program every function, especially data analysis or machine learning tasks, which are usually difficult to code.

Illustrated in Figure 2, the system builds around the needs of four types of users. The respective four 'user stories' are as follows, roughly corresponding to the natural composition of a small medical research team:

1. Software/database manager, who manages the software; may not need to be a research person; sets up environment and checks database and software function.
2. Data curator, the role of assistants and junior researchers; collects and inputs data into the system.
3. Simple data analyser, the role of more senior researchers; may perform simple analyses on certain selected data.
4. Complex model builder and analysis, the role of the most senior researchers; sets up different machine learning models.

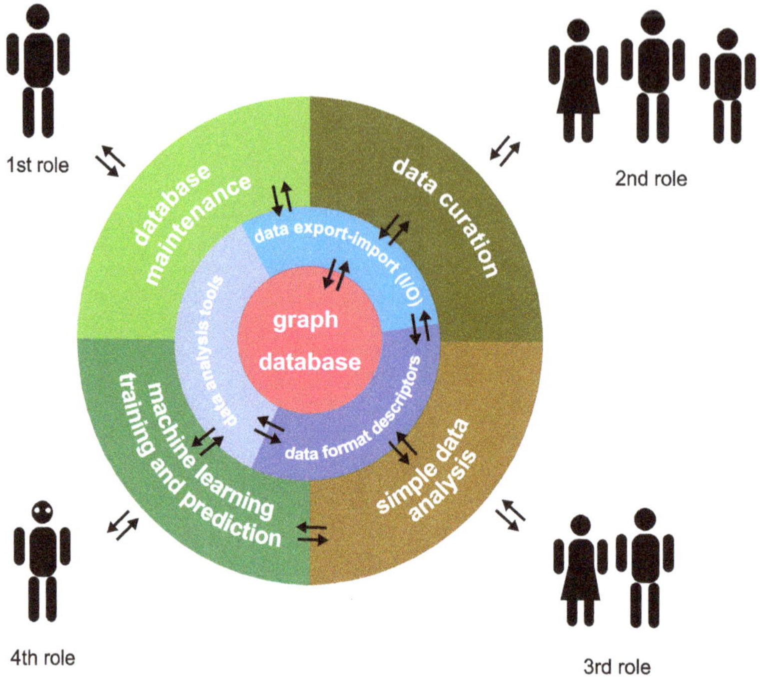

Figure 2. Architecture of 'PyTanito', organised into three layers. The outermost shell is the user-interactable components, corresponding to the four roles in a small research team. The middle layer is the part corresponding to data input-output, managing data formats, and the data analysis tools themselves. A database is placed at the core, serving as the 'single point of truth'. The arrows denote flow of information.

'PyTanito' incorporates another software development 'best practice': the layers only interact with the single layer below their level—or, at maximum, at their level. This key part is illustrated in Figure 2, which shows the direction of information flow. For example, it is not possible and not desirable for any user to interact directly with the database sitting in the centre. Simply use the 2nd role functions that read and input data into it. Another advantage is that 3rd and 4th role users do not need to know where the data comes from, as they work with the database, where all data is unified.

2.2. Data Storage and Organisation—An Up-to-Date Solution Using a Graph Database

At the core of the system is a database. It is a central, 'single point of truth' type organisation so that all data we work with will be consistent. We do not have to worry about differently formatted spreadsheet files or other nonstandard sources. We have chosen a graph-type database [9], instead of a traditional, relational type (such as SQL types, like Oracle SQL or MySQL [10]). Traditional relational type databases are organised into columns and rows, and usually need to have clearly defined data types/fields/tables [11]. That is, we need to have a clear concept beforehand of what we will store. Unfortunately, we found out that our exploratory research is not kind to this type of organisation. New variables emerge constantly as a result of research. In our case, not all parameters are measured for all patients, and new parameters are added routinely to certain patients. Patients do not have all their parameters measured—some patients have extra parameters. From a traditional relational database viewpoint, it is untidy and would require constantly changing its tables and columns, thus rebuilding the entire database structure.

A graph database does not rely on such assumptions. A graph, as a mathematical principle, consists of only 'nodes' and 'links. The nodes may be connected with links to each other, describing their relation. We illustrate the use of this graph-type organisation on our dataset in Figure 3 [12], which consists of ~200 thrombosis patients along with their blood and blood clot parameters. Illustrated in Figure 3a, our minimal graph database consists of a 'patient' node and a 'measurement' node. That is, the minimal sensible unit is a single patient with a single laboratory parameter value.

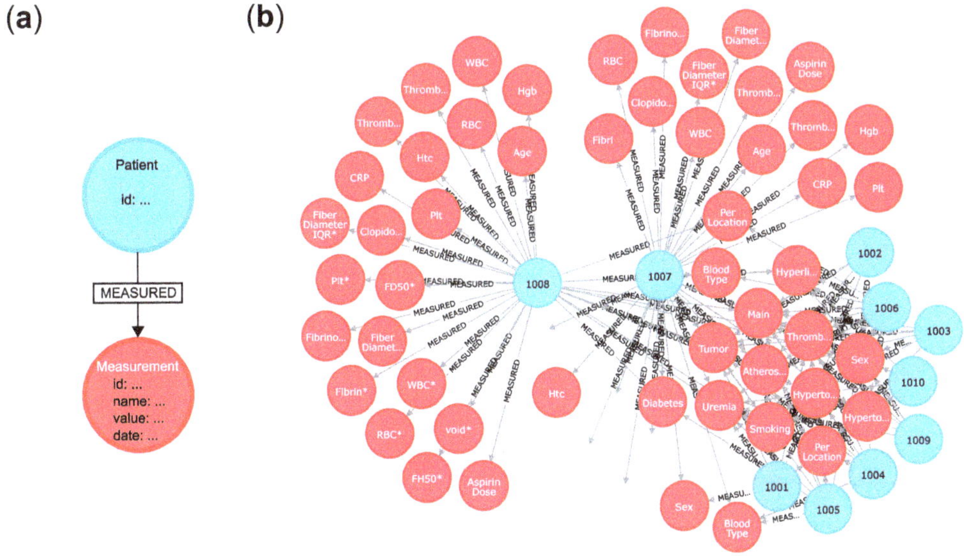

Figure 3. The organisation of our graph-type database using Neo4j [13] on our actual blood and blood clot data [12]. (**a**) The minimal unit of the database consist of a 'patient' node (blue) and an attached 'measurement' node (red). The two elements are linked together with a link named 'measured'. (**b**) A part of the actual database as viewed with the built-in Neo4j browser by opening the address http://localhost:7474 in any web browser. The patient nodes are connected to many red nodes. The patient IDs are shown (e.g., '1008'), just as the names of the measured parameters on the nodes (e.g., 'Sex' for sex, 'Hgb' for haemoglobin, 'WBC*' for white blood cell count, etc.).

Patients have an ID as a property of the node. The ID we added is a four-letter number and is anonymized; it cannot be used to reveal the identity of the patients. The laboratory measurements are of course nodes themselves. Patients are linked to their laboratory parameter(s) with a 'measured' relation link. The 'measurement' nodes have the value of the measured parameter as property, but others may be added, such as the name of the parameter, the method by which it was measured, the date, etc.). This arrangement gives extreme flexibility: patients may be added without much data, new data types may be added as simple new nodes with different labels, and this does not need database rework, just an additional operation to an already existing database. The question arises, that with such advantages, why graph databases are not more widespread? The answer is that the background processes driving graph databases are more computationally intensive than those driving SQL databases, but this is not a concern when using relatively small datasets with contemporary hardware.

Our actual implementation uses the Neo4j Community Edition database, which is open source, and was chosen on grounds discussed before. We note that many more types of graphs exist, such as hypergraphs, where links (the edges) may link to any number of nodes. The more commonly encountered 'property graphs' described in this paper and software are a subset of such hypergraphs since a particular link 'only' connects two nodes. The universality of hypergraphs makes them more difficult to comprehend and use computationally, nevertheless, see [14].

2.3. Data Analysis—Typical Tasks, Terms and Algorithms

In the next sections, now that we have data on hand, we need to specify, what we do with it [15,16]. For the sake of simplicity, we will provide examples using our actual patient dataset with blood parameters. In broad terms, we usually have three different types of analysis. Let us also have two types of variables, X and Y.

- Regression/classification analysis. We would like to predict Y from given X. X is the independent variable and Y is the dependent variable ($X \rightarrow Y$).
- Hypothesis testing. If, e.g., given two patient populations (Y_A and Y_B), is the so-called null hypothesis true? The 'null hypothesis' usually is that the two populations are different ($Y_A \rightarrow X$ is not equal to $Y_B \rightarrow X$). The 'alternative hypothesis' is the opposite, exclusive hypothesis: the two populations are identical.
- Clustering/dimensionality reducing algorithms. Sometimes we do not even have labelled data (here denoted Y), only raw data X. We need algorithms that work when we want to reduce the complexity somehow. In effect, can we cluster/label/group/classify the data based on X alone?

To put these analysis possibilities in context, taken our clotting disorder data [12], usually the Y dependent variable is a fundamental, clinically relevant label: what disease did our patients suffer from? Stroke, myocardial infarction or peripheral thrombosis? The Xs, the independent variables are usually the measured blood/blood clot parameters, such as cell counts, molecular marker (e.g., CRP) levels, etc. Please note that in a 'regression analysis', the Y is a continuous, quantifiable variable, while in a 'classification analysis' the Ys are discrete, non-quantifiable labels.

It is also useful to know that when we talk about 'labelled data', we mean data, which was appropriately tagged with useful (in the medical field this means clinically relevant) properties using discrete, non-quantifiable variables. This is, e.g., the disease type mentioned before. Unlabelled data are usually less worthy, as the number of analysis tools available are reduced. Here, using our dataset as an example, raw data would be, e.g., blood test numbers. If we add disease type and other clinically relevant labels, our data becomes labelled. This labelling task can be a hard problem, and often requires human intervention.

Supervised vs. unsupervised learning are additional terms encountered. In supervised learning, we have some expectations about the data, we have labels on the data, and we direct the analysis using this expectation. The analysis tools mentioned before Types 1 and 2 are supervised types. Type 3 is of the unsupervised type.

We provide two tables: one lists the common machine learning algorithms Table 1. The second table lists the evaluation metrics that may be used to determine how successful we were by using the beforementioned algorithms Table 2.

Table 1. Machine learning algorithms. This table provides an overview of algorithms that may be used in a Python language environment. The list may be extended significantly as new algorithms emerge and get incorporated into the Python environment. Of course, discussions on these methods fall beyond the scope of this paper, so the interested readers are directed to the excellent books of Hastie and Landau [15,16] for more information.

Name of Method	Recommended Use	Method Type	Input Variables	Output	Reference to Python Implementation
Decision tree	To visualize and break down complex decision making processes. It also provides an explainable output.	Supervised learning (in its basic form it is used for classification, but can be extended for regression)	Discrete and continuous data	Trained model (tree, in the case of CART it is a binary tree), cllassified points, (predicted values in the case of regression)	From sklearn.tree import DecisionTreeClassifier, from sklearn.tree import DecisionTreeRegressor
Random forest	It performs well on large datasets and reduces overfitting compared to decision trees. Random Forest is faster than Bagging	Supervised learning (both Classification and Regression)	Discrete and continuous data	trained model (trees for decision making) and classified points or predicted values (in the case of regression)	From sklearn.ensemble import RandomForest-Classifier, from sklearn.ensemble import RandomFore-stRegressor

Table 1. *Cont.*

Name of Method	Recommended Use	Method Type	Input Variables	Output	Reference to Python Implementation
SVM (support vector machine)	It is often used for text classification tasks such as category assignment, image recognition, and performs especially well in aspect-based recognition. It can be used in linearly separable and non-separable cases as well.	Supervised learning (both Classification and Regression) In basic form it supports binary classification, but it can be extended for multiclass classification problems and for regression (support vector regression, SVR) as well.	Discrete and continuous data	Trained model, classified points or predicted values (in the case of regression)	From sklearn.svm import SVC
KNN (K-nearest neighbour)	It is a very simple algorithm, which performs much better if all of the data have the same scale, and works well with a small number of input variables, but struggles when the number of inputs is very large. It is also needed, that the training is continuous and it only works when new data is coming.	Supervised learning (classification)	Discrete and continuous data	Classified points or predicted values (in the case of regression)	From sklearn.neighbors import KNeighborsClassifier
Linear Regression	One of the most frequently used regression methods, when a linear relationship is assumed between the input and output variables.	Supervised learning (Regression)	Continuous data	Regression line (predicted points)	From sklearn.neighbors import KNeighborsClassifier
Logistic regression	It is a commonly used algorithm for solving binary classification problems.	Supervised learning (Binary Classification with Softmax extension it can solve multiclass classification problems)	Discrete and continuous data	Classified points-binary (discrete) value	From sklearn.linear_model import LogisticRegression
ANN (artificial neural network)	State of the art. It performs well on a large and multi-dimensional dataset, and should be applied when there is no explicit mathematical equation for solving the problem. it is especially useful in image analysis, text classification, voice processing tasks. The results are not explainable.	Supervised learning (both classification and regression). It can be used also for unsupervised learning tasks, but it is not so widespread.	Discrete and continuous data	Trained model, classified points or predicted values (in the case of regression)	From sklearn.neural_network import MLPClassifier, from sklearn.neural_network import MLPRegressor

Table 1. *Cont.*

Name of Method	Recommended Use	Method Type	Input Variables	Output	Reference to Python Implementation
k-means	Clustering is used when we want to divide our datapoints into groups according to smilarity. The k-means algorithm can find spherical clusters easily, while DBSCAN can find clusters of any shape as long as the dataset has balanced density. Moreover, there are algorithms which are also good at the clustering of datasets with unbalanced density, such as mean-shift.	Unsupervised learning (clustering)	Discrete and Continuous data	Trained model, clusters	From sklearn.cluster import KMeans
DBSCAN					From sklearn.cluster import DBSCAN
Gaussian mixture model					From sklearn.mixture import GaussianMixture
Mean-shift					From sklearn.cluster import MeanShift
Others					From sklearn.cluster import AffinityPropagation, from sklearn.cluster import AgglomerativeClustering, from sklearn.cluster import Birch
PCA (principal component analysis)	Dimensionality reduction can serve as data preparation, as the machine learning algortihms work better on low-dimension data. However, the reduction can be the main exercise too.	Unsupervised learning (dimensionality reduction)	Discrete and continuous data	Data with reduced dimensionality (less features), where as much information as possible about the original data is preserved.	From sklearn.decomposition import PCA
LDA (linear discriminant analysis)					From sklearn.discriminant_analysis import LinearDiscriminantAnalysis
Others					From sklearn.decomposition import TruncatedSVD, from sklearn.manifold import Isomap, from sklearn.manifold import LocallyLinearEmbedding
Association	One uses Association when the aim is to study the connection between the datapoints, and make recommendation for new datapoints.	Unsupervised learning (association)	Discrete and continuous data	Association rules, associations	From mlxtend.frequent_patterns import apriori, association_rules
T-test	To compare the means of 2 groups. It assumes that the samples are (approximately) normally distributed and are independent, and have a similar amount of variance within each group.	Hypothesis testing	Continuous data, normally distributed, small sample with unknown variance	t-value, p-value, degrees of freedom	From scipy.stats import ttest_ind

Table 1. *Cont.*

Name of Method	Recommended Use	Method Type	Input Variables	Output	Reference to Python Implementation
F-test	The hypothesis that the means of a given set of normally distributed populations, all having the same standard deviation, are equal. The hypothesis that a proposed regression model fits the data well. (lack-of-fit sum of squares). The hypothesis that a data set in a regression analysis follows the simpler of two proposed linear models that are nested within each other.	Hypothesis testing	Independent and normally distributed data with a common variance.	F-value, *p*-value, degrees of freedom	From scipy.stats import f_oneway
Z-test	One can use Z-test when the sample size is greater than 30, the data points are independent from each other, the data is (approximately) normally distributed, sample sizes are equal. To check whethet sample mean of the two groups are equal or not.	Hypothesis testing	Independent and normally distributed data with large (>50) sample size or the variance is known	Z-value, *p*-value, degrees of freedom	From statsmodels.stats.weightstats import ztest
Chi-cquare Test	Chi-squared test is used to determine whether there is a statistically significant difference between the expected frequencies and the observed frequencies in one or more categories.	Hypothesis testing	Random sample that are classified into k mutually exclusive classes	*p*-value	From scipy.stats import chisquare

Table 2. Metrics used for evaluation of machine learning models. In this table, we provide a list of useful metrics used when quantifying success in a data analysis experiment, be it a regression or classification problem. As with Table 1, the list is not exhaustive, and interested users are directed to [17–19] for more information.

Name of Error Metrics	Recommended Use	Typical Drawback	Input Variable	Output Type and Range	Reference to Python Implementation
Mean absolute error/MAE	Regression. Gives an absolute measure; can be used to compare regression models on the same dataset.	Specific for the given model and dataset.	Continuous	Continuous value, $[0; \infty]$	From sklearn.metrics import mean_absolute_error
Mean square error/MSE					From sklearn.metrics import mean_squared_error
Root mean square error/RMSE					From sklearn.metrics import mean_squared_error
Standard error/residual standard error					From scipy.stats import sem

Table 2. *Cont.*

Name of Error Metrics	Recommended Use	Typical Drawback	Input Variable	Output Type and Range	Reference to Python Implementation
R2-value/R squared	Regression. A basic metric to evaluate regression models.	Does not take into account the number of independent variables.	Continuous	Continuous value, [0; 1]	From sklearn.metrics import r2_score
Adjusted R2/adjusted R square	Regression. Useful to compare models with differing numbers of independent variables.		Continuous	Continuous value, [0; 1]	Import statsmodels.api
Confusion matrix	Classification. Can be used to calculate other classification metrics.	The simple quantities of true positives (TP)/true negatives (TN)/false positives (FP)/false negatives (FN) refer only to the given model and dataset.	Discrete	Matrix for each classes values [0; ∞]	From sklearn.metrics import confusion_matrix
True positive rate/TPR/recall/ sensitivity/probability of detection	Classification. Recommended when the costs of FN is high (such as sick patient detection).	Not recommeded to use alone.	Discrete	Continuous value, [0; 1]	From sklearn.metrics import recall_score
True negative rate/TNR/specificity	Classification				From sklearn.metrics import confusion_matrix
False positive rate/FPR/type I error	Classification				From sklearn.metrics import confusion_matrix
False negative rate/FNR/type II error	Classification				From sklearn.metrics import confusion_matrix
Accuracy	Classification. Useful to compare classification models on the same dataset. Recommended when every class is equally important.	Can be largely contributed by a large number of TN. Not recommended when the costs of having a mis-classified actual positive is high (ex. virus carrier). Not recommeded to use alone.	Discrete	Continuous value, [0; 1]	From sklearn.metrics import accuracy_score
Misclassification rate/classification error	Classification. Since it is = 1-Accuracy, all properties are the same				
Precision	Classification. Recommended when the costs of FP is high (such as email spam detection).	Not recommeded to use alone.	Discrete	Continuous value, [0; 1]	From sklearn.metrics import precision_score
F1 score/F-score/F-measure	Classification. To have a balance between Precision and Recall and there is an uneven class distribution (large number of actual negatives)		Discrete	Continuous value, [0; 1]	From sklearn.metrics import f1_score
F2 score	Classification. The same as F1 score, but we nominate twice importance to recall over precision.				From sklearn.metrics import fbeta_score

Table 2. *Cont.*

Name of Error Metrics	Recommended Use	Typical Drawback	Input Variable	Output Type and Range	Reference to Python Implementation
Micro F1, macro F1, weighted F1	Multi-class classification. Advanced versions of F1 score where the difference (micro, macro, weighted) is the type of averaging performed on the data. Micro precision, micro recall weighted precision, macro precision, etc., also exist.		Discrete	Continuous value, [0; 1]	From sklearn.metrics import f1_score
ROC (receiver operating characteristics)	Classification. Visualizes the tradeoff between TPR and FPR.	In some cases, can be difficult to compare more curves *2	Discrete	Curve, X axis = FPR, Y axis = TPR	From sklearn.metrics import roc_curve
ROC AUC (area under ROC)	Classification. A quantity to describe the ROC curve.	Not recommended when the data is heavily imbalanced *3	Discrete	Continuous value, [0; 1]	From sklearn.metrics import roc_auc_score
PR curve (precision–recall curve)	Classification. Combines precision and recall in a single visualization.		Discrete	Curve, X axis = Recall, Y axis = Precision	From scikitplot.metrics import plot_precision_recall
PR AUC (area under PR curve)	Classification. A quantity to describe the PR curve.		Discrete	Continuous value, [0; 1]	From sklearn.metrics import aver-age_precision_score

2.4. A Machine Learning Workflow—Common Processes Explained with Examples

In a traditional scientific project, we are convinced of our models and hypotheses when these are repeated and verified by independent researchers. A single team collects data, and then 'trains' their model/algorithm on a part (or whole) of the available data [16]. Thus, this data is called 'training data'. Training a model/algorithm means the setting of the model's parameters so that the model from Table 1 describes the data 'best', according to selected metrics seen in Table 2. Training often involves other kinds of parameters (hidden variables) during the construction of the model ('hyperparameters') that refine/restrict the behaviour of an otherwise complex model. The model's ordinary parameters are, e.g., the two coefficients of a simple linear regression, and in this case, the training may be called 'linear fitting'. Linear regression is simple, and it has not hidden 'hyperparameters', but more complex models, such as a 'decision tree' may have more parameters and several hyperparameters that describe it.

However, it is possible that the model is not optimal for the problem, for example, a linear regression does not capture the phenomena studied, and so does not make sense from a medical/physical/chemical standpoint. To see that the fitted model is reasonable (and does not depend on cherry-picked 'training' datapoints), it is good practice to have a 'validation set' of data. This 'validation dataset' is data totally separated from the 'training data'. It is not used for the training (e.g., linear regression fitting), and so is 'unseen' by the model-building procedure. The trained model's error on this 'validation dataset' is more indicative of the model's appropriateness.

However, even this train-validation procedure may be less than optimal in real life. For example, because of inherent systematic errors during the experiments or if it just happens that the particular picking of data into train/validation sets skew results. Figure 4 illustrates how independent observations by different researchers solve the problem. However, in the medical field, this is often not possible, because the experiments may be too costly or there is simply not enough interest or resources to reproduce results.

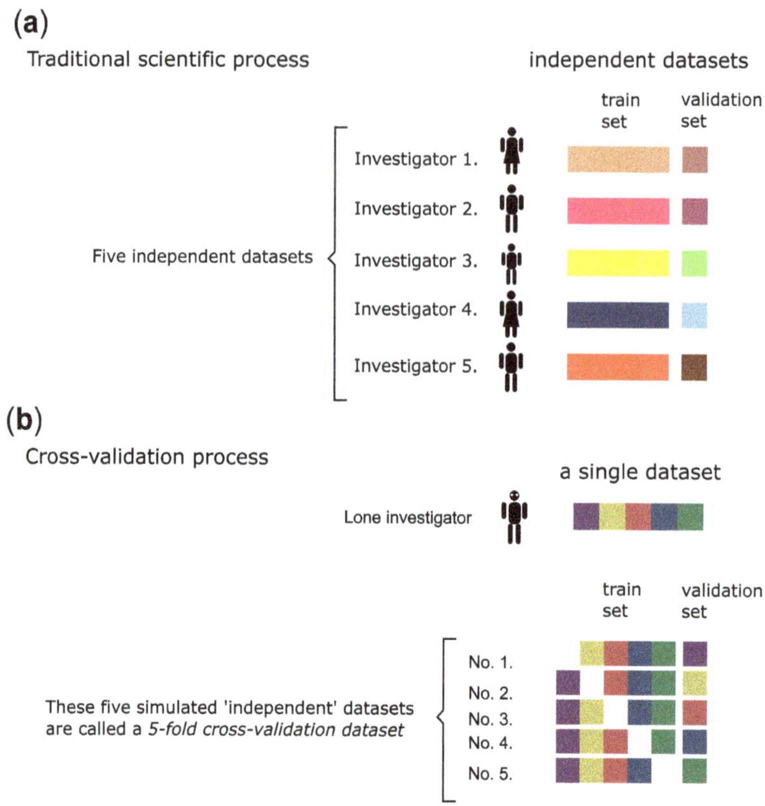

Figure 4. The scientific process and the cross-validation process compared. (**a**) In an ideal world, experiments can be repeated many times, and the results are reproducible. (**b**) In the real world, relatively few experiments can be executed (e.g., expensive and time-consuming medical types with human subjects). In our case, ex vivo examination of blood clots from thrombosis patients is a costly and time-consuming endeavour. Therefore, a cross-validation type procedure is used to evaluate the data analysis results. A k-fold cross-validation procedure produces 'k' number of simulated 'identical' and 'random' datasets. The original dataset is split into 'k' number of equal parts, then each part is used for validation only once—while the rest is used for training.

A so-called cross-validation procedure Figure 4b may solve this problem with caveats [20,21]. In a cross-validation procedure, we produce simulated 'independent' datasets randomly. A k-fold cross-validation procedure produces 'k' number of simulated datasets. This procedure minimizes at least the 'cherrypicking' problem of the train-validation dataset split. Still, the problem of systematic errors remains, therefore, this procedure produces only a hint on the minimum error, and the real error is certainly larger than that. Still, the procedure will prevent over-optimistic error estimations by setting a minimum error expectation and is best used to compare the appropriateness of different machine learning model types (e.g., linear regression vs. polynomial regression, etc.). Another advantage is that this procedure may be used 'on top' of other error metrics, because any error metrics may be used with these 'independent' datasets.

In the last part of this paper, we show the actual outputs of the software. Figure 5 depicts the use of the software to check the data and available measurements for further analysis (a simple 'data curator' user role). Figure 5 displays the command-line interface which is always available for Python programming. The output is also always available as a command-line type. Although not as wieldy or 'nice' as graphical user interfaces (GUIs), command-line interfaces and outputs serve an important purpose: they are read and parsed easily by machines, e.g., by other parts of the same program or even third-party software. For this reason, efficient software implements both the command-line interface and the GUI.

(a)

```
print ("Data curation demo...")

print("We are connecting to the database:")

ourdatabase=exportimport.Neo4jImport("bolt://localhost:7687", "neo4j", "password")

print("Let's see what we have in the database:")

ourdatabase.Stat()
```

(b)

```
Data curation demo...

We are connecting to the database:
Neo4j Connector: database connection established.
Let's see what we have in the database:

-------------------
Database statistics
-------------------
Patients total: 209    Measurements total: 6997

Measurement types: 43

================
 List of labels
================
(1) Age    (2) Aspirin Dose    (3) Atherosclerosis    (4) Blood Type    (5) CRP

(6) Cer Location    (7) Clopidogrel Dose    (8) Cor Location    (9) Diabetes    (10) ECG

(11) ECG Location    (12) Etiology    (13) FD50*    (14) FH50*    (15) FN50*

(16) FW50*    (17) Fiber Diameter IQR*    (18) Fiber Diameter*    (19) Fibrin*    (20) Fibrinogen

(21) Glucose    (22) Hgb    (23) Htc    (24) Hyperlipid    (25) Hypertonia

(26) INR    (27) Main    (28) Per Location    (29) Plt    (30) Plt*

(31) RBC    (32) RBC*    (33) Sex    (34) Smoking    (35) Thrombophilia

(36) Thrombus Age    (37) Thrombus Diameter    (38) Tumor    (39) Uremia    (40) WBC

(41) WBC*    (42) rTPA    (43) void*
```

Figure 5. 'PyTanito' software in actual use—example of a 'data curation' role use. (**a**) The input: these are code lines in Python for database import and for printing database statistics. (**b**) The output of the software in response to the commands in (**a**) lists the number of patients in our dataset [12] (209 total), as well as the number of measurements collected (6997 total), and as a bonus, it lists the type of measurements available for further analysis (43 different types). The asterisk (*) after a parameter name indicates that the parameter was measured using a pathological blood clot, unlike the rest, which are from ordinary blood samples.

In Figure 6, we show an actual example of decision making with the help of machine learning. The figure shows a pair of plots for two different, but related prediction problems using common 'Decision Tree' algorithm implementation. In each of the plots, we compare several 'tree' models and decide which 'tree' is the best if there is such a model. The provided example is realistic in the sense that it also displays commonly encountered, relatively unsuccessful models. A major takeaway is that relying on a single metric on a single training run is guaranteed to be flawed: even when it seems to be better, it is not when many random combinations of data are also validated. Extensive use of cross-validation helped in our case to set realistic expectations. For this particular example, the conclusion is that the decision trees are better than random guesses, but not by very much. It is an open question as to whether robust, clinically relevant predictions can be made. More data, more types of variables and more types of algorithms need to be tested. Thus, from this data only, the prediction of disease before onset is not practical.

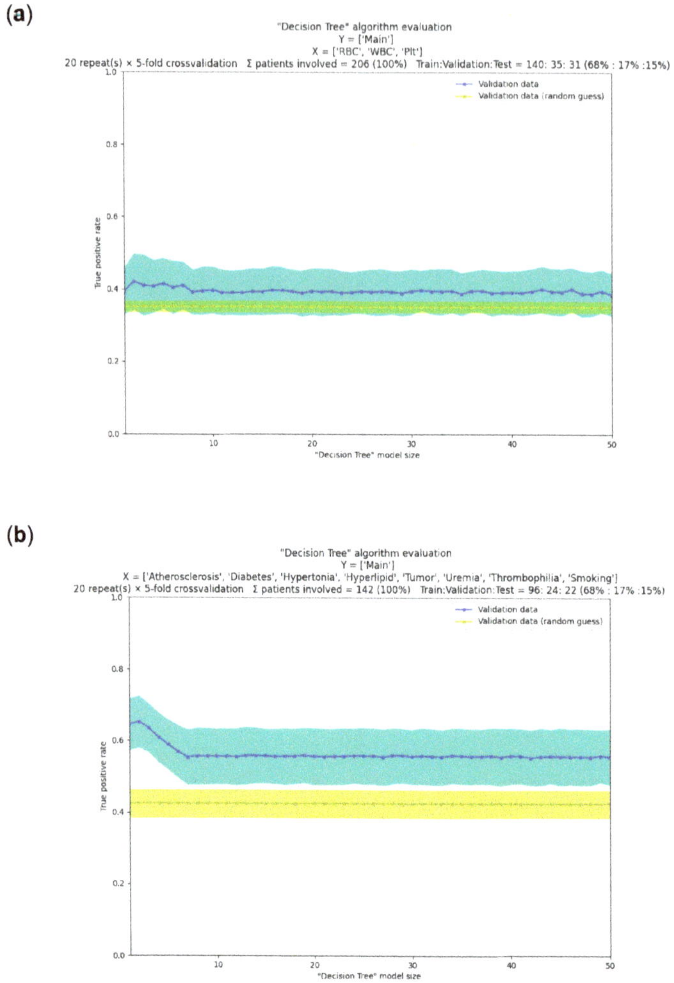

Figure 6. 'PyTanito' software in actual use—example use of the most advanced training and evaluation functions. (**a**) Decision tree models and their evaluation on our dataset [12]. Can we tell from mere blood cell counts (X independent variables are red 'RBC', white 'WBC' and platelet 'Plt' cell counts) what kind of thrombi were present (Y dependent variable is the 'Main' label, which has values 'stroke', 'myocardial' or 'peripheral')? We chose 'true positive' rate as error metrics (depicted on y scale) for a classification problem, 5-fold cross-validation was used with repeats. On the x scale are the different decision tree models, numbered 1–50. They are mostly identical in performance (on average they are ~40% correct, blue line) and not much better than random guessing (yellow line, 35% correct on average). (**b**) In a second problem, we used the same dataset and the same goal as before, but now X independent variables are clinically relevant labels (such as, do the patients have diabetes, atherosclerosis, etc.). Now, the results are better; all trained decision tree models (No. 1–50) seem better than random guessing. Models 1–8 appear better than the rest, with model 2 seemingly the best of all, with average success rate of ~65%, compared to the average success rate of ~45% of random guessing.

3. Conclusions and Remarks

We have seen that modern workflow (CRISP-DM standard) with modern software 'best practices' ('Agile' and software layering) can produce useful tools in medical research. We also provide a glimpse into how data may be stored in a humanly reasonable way using a graph database. We also provided lists of the incredible amount of contemporary machine learning methods and metrics for their evaluation.

We consider two kinds of readers and have conclusions for each.

- First, from the perspective of the software developer involved in a 'decision making' project, it is notable that software specification is a bottleneck during the initial steps. This often stems from a lack of clarity and vision during the initial stages of the project. Going forward in the project, the tuning of the machine learning models ('hyperparameter tuning') becomes the bottleneck and this remains so until the end. Curiously, the choice of algorithms does not appear critical now. Computational capacities are larger than ever, and several highly advanced machine learning methods are available (in fact, often more than needed in a project). Projects, however, may fail easily because of data quality issues, and this brings us to the second set of conclusions below.
- Second, from the perspective of the medical professional, the bottleneck is usually a lack of understanding between them and software specialists during the initial stages of the project. Going forward, the single but often critical bottleneck is the quality of their data. Experiments may span years and may be performed by different personnel over time. This may lead to inconsistent procedures, even if for mundane reasons, e.g., because of no longer available reagents or altered cell lines. These can introduce large systematic errors that make even advanced machine learning algorithms ineffective. Other kinds of experiments are inherently difficult to perform consistently for physical, economical or legal reasons. For example, in our case, the blood clots of ex vivo human origin pose a significant problem, since the number of experiments is severely limited. In summary, medical professionals must do everything to ensure reproducibility and consistency of their experiments and data over long timespans in sufficient quantity.

Author Contributions: L.B. developed software, conceptualization, wrote paper; E.K. wrote paper; P.P. wrote paper; E.T. data collection; R.F. wrote paper; K.K. funding, conceptualization, wrote paper. All authors have read and agreed to the published version of the manuscript.

Funding: K.K. This work was supported by the Hungarian National Research, Development and Innovation Office (NKFIH) #137563. K.K., E.T. and L.B.—Thematic Institutional Excellence Programme of the Ministry of Human Capacities in Hungary for the Molecular Biology thematic programme of Semmelweis University (TKP2021-EGA-24).

Institutional Review Board Statement: The study was approved by the Semmelweis University and regional ethical board (Ref.#2014/18.09.2014). The research also conforms to the principles outlined in the Declaration of Helsinki.

Informed Consent Statement: Informed written consent was obtained from all participants or their legal guardians.

Data Availability Statement: The software described in this paper is under development and is in a pre-release state. Only for information purposes—it is not suitable for public use. Code reuse, distribution and third-party use are restricted. With these limitations, it is available upon request from L.B. (laszlo@beinrohr.com). The blood clot data may be provided by K.K. (Krasimir.Kolev@eok.sote.hu) upon reasonable request.

Conflicts of Interest: The authors declare no conflict of interest.

References

1. The top 10 Causes of Death. Available online: https://www.who.int/news-room/fact-sheets/detail/the-top-10-causes-of-death (accessed on 11 November 2021).
2. Santos-Gallego, C.G.; Bayón, J.; Badimón, J.J. Thrombi of Different Pathologies: Implications for Diagnosis and Treatment. *Curr. Treat. Options Cardiovasc. Med.* **2010**, *12*, 274–291. [CrossRef] [PubMed]
3. Undas, A.; Ariëns, R.A.S. Fibrin Clot Structure and Function. *Arterioscler. Thromb. Vasc. Biol.* **2011**, *31*, e88–e99. [CrossRef] [PubMed]
4. Shearer, C. The CRISP-DM Model: The New Blueprint for Data Mining. *J. Data Warehous.* **2000**, *5*, 13–22.

5. Chapman, P.; Clinton, J.; Kerber, R.; Khabaza, T.; Reinartz, T.; Shearer, C.; Wirth, R. Step-by-Step Data Mining Guide. Available online: https://the-modeling-agency.com/crisp-dm.pdf (accessed on 11 November 2021).
6. Manifesto for Agile Software Development. Available online: https://agilemanifesto.org/ (accessed on 11 November 2021).
7. Dalpiaz, F.; Brinkkemper, S. Agile Requirements Engineering with User Stories. In Proceedings of the 2018 IEEE 26th International Requirements Engineering Conference (RE), Banff, AB, Canada, 20–24 August 2018; pp. 506–507. [CrossRef]
8. Welcome to Python.org. Available online: https://www.python.org/ (accessed on 11 November 2021).
9. Angles, R. A Comparison of Current Graph Database Models. In Proceedings of the 2012 IEEE 28th International Conference on Data Engineering Workshops, Arlington, VA, USA, 1–5 April 2012; pp. 171–177. [CrossRef]
10. MySQL. Available online: https://www.mysql.com/ (accessed on 11 November 2021).
11. Sahatqija, K.; Ajdari, J.; Zenuni, X.; Raufi, B.; Ismaili, F. Comparison between Relational and NOSQL Databases. In Proceedings of the 2018 41st International Convention on Information and Communication Technology, Electronics and Microelectronics (MIPRO), Opatija, Croatia, 21–25 May 2018; pp. 0216–0221. [CrossRef]
12. Farkas, Á.Z.; Farkas, V.J.; Gubucz, I.; Szabó, L.; Bálint, K.; Tenekedjiev, K.; Nagy, A.I.; Sótonyi, P.; Hidi, L.; Nagy, Z.; et al. Neutrophil Extracellular Traps in Thrombi Retrieved during Interventional Treatment of Ischemic Arterial Diseases. *Thromb. Res.* **2019**, *175*, 46–52. [CrossRef] [PubMed]
13. Neo4j Graph Data Platform—The Leader in Graph Databases. Available online: https://neo4j.com/ (accessed on 11 November 2021).
14. Alam, M.T.; Ahmed, C.F.; Samiullah, M.; Leung, C.K. Mining Frequent Patterns from Hypergraph Databases. In Proceedings of the Advances in Knowledge Discovery and Data Mining; Karlapalem, k., Cheng, h., Ramakrishnan, N., Agrawal, R.K., Reddy, P.K., Srivastava, J., Chakrabortya, T., Eds.; Springer International Publishing: Cham, Switzerland, 2021; pp. 3–15.
15. Landau, S.; Everitt, B. *A Handbook of Statistical Analyses Using SPSS*; Chapman & Hall/CRC: Boca Raton, FL, USA, 2004.
16. Hastie, T.; Tibshirani, R.; Friedman, J. *The Elements of Statistical Learning: Data Mining, Inference, and Prediction, Edition*, 2nd ed.; Springer Series in Statistics; Springer: New York, NY, USA, 2009. [CrossRef]
17. Hossin, M.; Sulaiman, M.N. A Review on Evaluation Metrics for Data Classification Evaluations. *Int. J. Data Min. Knowl. Manag. Process* **2015**, *5*, 1. [CrossRef]
18. Fawcett, T. ROC graphs: Notes and practical considerations for researchers. *Mach. Learn.* **2004**, *31*, 1–38.
19. Saito, T.; Rehmsmeier, M. The Precision-Recall Plot Is More Informative than the ROC Plot When Evaluating Binary Classifiers on Imbalanced Datasets. *PLoS ONE* **2015**, *10*, e0118432. [CrossRef]
20. Yadav, S.; Shukla, S. Analysis of K-Fold Cross-Validation over Hold-Out Validation on Colossal Datasets for Quality Classification. In Proceedings of the 2016 IEEE 6th International Conference on Advanced Computing (IACC), Bhimavaram, India, 27–28 February 2016; pp. 78–83. [CrossRef]
21. Wong, T.-T.; Yeh, P.-Y. Reliable Accuracy Estimates from K-Fold Cross Validation. *IEEE Trans. Knowl. Data Eng.* **2020**, *32*, 1586–1594. [CrossRef]

applied sciences

MDPI

Article

AI and Clinical Decision Making: The Limitations and Risks of Computational Reductionism in Bowel Cancer Screening

Saleem Ameen [1,*], Ming-Chao Wong [2], Kwang-Chien Yee [1] and Paul Turner [2,*]

1 School of Medicine, College of Health and Medicine, University of Tasmania, Hobart 7000, Australia; kwang.yee@utas.edu.au
2 College of Sciences and Engineering, Information and Communication Technology, University of Tasmania, Hobart 7000, Australia; ming.wong@utas.edu.au
* Correspondence: saleem.ameen@utas.edu.au (S.A.); paul.turner@utas.edu.au (P.T.)

Abstract: Advances in artificial intelligence in healthcare are frequently promoted as 'solutions' to improve the accuracy, safety, and quality of clinical decisions, treatments, and care. Despite some diagnostic success, however, AI systems rely on forms of reductive reasoning and computational determinism that embed problematic assumptions about clinical decision-making and clinical practice. Clinician autonomy, experience, and judgement are reduced to inputs and outputs framed as binary or multi-class classification problems benchmarked against a clinician's capacity to identify or predict disease states. This paper examines this reductive reasoning in AI systems for colorectal cancer (CRC) to highlight their limitations and risks: (1) in AI systems themselves due to inherent biases in (a) retrospective training datasets and (b) embedded assumptions in underlying AI architectures and algorithms; (2) in the problematic and limited evaluations being conducted on AI systems prior to system integration in clinical practice; and (3) in marginalising socio-technical factors in the context-dependent interactions between clinicians, their patients, and the broader health system. The paper argues that to optimise benefits from AI systems and to avoid negative unintended consequences for clinical decision-making and patient care, there is a need for more nuanced and balanced approaches to AI system deployment and evaluation in CRC.

Keywords: artificial intelligence; machine learning; patient outcomes; socio-technical design; algorithmic bias; clinical interaction

1. Introduction

In late 2016, Geoffrey Hinton, arguably one of the most influential researchers in the field of ML and pioneer of neural network architectures and deep learning, evocatively exclaimed that the technology was so profound that "if you work as a radiologist, you are like the cayote already over the edge of the cliff that hasn't yet looked down ... people should stop training radiologists ... it's just completely obvious that within five years deep learning is going to do better than radiologists"; a view that was solidified in a published opinion piece that spoke about how deep learning would fundamentally transform health care as we know it [1,2]. It has been five years since those remarks and clearly AI has not replaced radiologists. To the contrary, radiologists are in higher demand than ever-before [3]. If we trace the long history of healthcare information technologies (HIT), such as the electronic health record (EHR), computerised physician order entry system (CPOE), computer aided decision support system (CAD), e-prescription software, and now AI-enhanced HIT, the narrative has always been the same, that computational systems are introduced with promises of "computational superiority" to the benefit of patient outcomes, by enhancing the safety, quality, personalisation, and efficiency of healthcare services.

However, this hyperbole has been constantly challenged by an extensive body of research in the last three decades that has repeatedly highlighted how HIT results reported in experimental settings are rarely emulated in the real-world of clinical practice. There is also a considerable and growing body of evidence highlighting negative unintended and unanticipated consequences (NUCs) arising at the interface between new HIT tools and socio-organisational systems, leading some to suggest that HIT seems to foster the creation of errors rather than reduce their likelihood [4,5]. These circumstances are no less prevalent in the era of AI, where overly optimistic descriptions of AI systems tend to marginalise possible risks associated with their implementation in real-world practice, particularly when system development is challenged by the nature of contextual and socio-organisational factors in the practice of diagnostic and therapeutic clinical decision-making for the delivery of safe, high quality patient care. This has not prevented technology vendors and AI advocates continuing to promote the view that healthcare is ready for disruption by AI-enhanced HIT and reiterating the standard computational narrative that AI will be the panacea for all problems plaguing the healthcare system. These include but are not limited to problems of misdiagnosis, health costs, time-scarcity, system efficiency, and treatment reproducibility.

Colorectal cancer (CRC) is currently the second leading cause of cancer and cancer-related mortality in the world [6], and therefore there has been significant interest by several IT vendors to promote clinical decision support systems (CDSS) powered by artificial intelligence (AI) and machine learning (ML) to address a subset of discrete challenges in the screening, diagnostic, and therapeutic pathways of clinical practice to improve patient outcomes. These have included preventing missed diagnoses of polyps in CC [7–9], improving reading time efficiency in CE [10], minimising interobserver variability and reproducibility in the histopathological examination of CRC [11,12], or introducing risk-stratification and prognoses prediction for CRC screening or diagnosis more broadly [13–15]. While current evidence suggests these AI tools may help address some of the problems that exist in the application of CRC screening and diagnostic technologies, it has also emerged that these AI enhanced systems themselves have their own limitations that require greater attention, if we are to avoid replacing one set of problems with another set [16]. In particular, these systems are founded on problematic representational, temporal, and cultural biases embedded in end-end data pipelines used to train AI algorithms that become further constrained by the epistemological and ontological limitations inherent to the nature of AI computation that tends to discretely frame problems of the real-world independent of context. Given the tendency for AI system developers to prescribe over-confidence in quantitative metrics produced within experimental settings, this paper explores the potential risks that arise in the absence of adequate socio-technical evaluations of AI system integration across context-dependent clinical interactions that may challenge AI efficacy across socio-cultural and socio-organisational contexts.

Of course, it is acknowledged that technology does have an important role to play in healthcare and that some forms of AI systems do support clinical decision-making and practice. However, this paper highlights how it is very important to recognise that most contemporary AI systems rely on forms of reductive reasoning and computational determinism that embed problematic assumptions about clinical decision-making, which may be problematic depending on the context of clinical practice. It is in the context of these concerns that this paper examines the opportunities and limitations of AI in CRC screening, diagnosis, and treatment. Furthermore, this paper explores whether investment in AI augmentation of CRC diagnostic modalities is misdirected, given that the majority of HIT diagnostic tools that currently support clinicians in the early detection and diagnosis of CRC, such as the Immunochemical Faecal Occult Blood Test (iFOBT) screening test, and diagnostic imaging modalities, such as conventional colonoscopy (CC), CT colonography (CTC), and capsule endoscopy (CE), have done little to change the fact that CRC remains to be the second leading cause of cancer-related death in the world, despite being one of the most preventable diseases [6].

2. Materials and Methods

This paper provides a socio-technical analysis of contemporary research into the use and impact of AI in colorectal cancer (CRC). This analysis is developed through a multi-disciplinary selective review, which identified over 120 papers published post-2018 through medical databases PUBMED, EMBASE, BIOMED, and Cochrane; computer science databases ACM Digital and IEEE Explore; and grey literature through Google Scholar. This approach is adopted in a similar capacity to recently published MDPI research [17,18], in order to offer a balanced critique on the opportunities, limitations, and risks of AI system development and integration in clinical decision-making along CRC screening, diagnostic, and treatment pathways.

The rest of this paper is divided into six main sections. (1) The opportunities presented by AI in health and the problematic assumptions that underpin approaches to AI development, implementation, and evaluation in healthcare are discussed. (2) The limitations and risks of these assumptions are then considered in the context of CRC, through an examination of the multi-faceted dimensions of underlying algorithms in (a) AI and data and (b) AI and models. (3) The social, legal, and ethical implications of these assumptions for AI-mediated clinical decision making are then identified and discussed. (4) Beyond these direct impacts, the paper also considers the broader impact that marginalising socio-technical factors in CRC may have on misdirecting clinical focus in ways that do little to improve patient population outcomes. (5) The paper also briefly looks to the future development of AI systems and the challenges facing regulators and practitioners in responding to the prospect of an era of 'unexplainable' AI. (6) The paper concludes by outlining steps towards building a more nuanced and balanced approach to the deployment of new AI tools in CRC to mitigate the risks to clinicians and patients in CRC diagnosis and treatment pathways. The paper points to the need for greater clarity around policies and procedures for AI clinical system validation encompassing four themes: (a) transparency and auditing of datasets, (b) transparency and reproducibility of algorithmic methodologies and implementations, (c) reproducibility of quantitative metrics through rigorous testing standards across diverse population distributions and under-represented edge cases that are known to challenge AI reliability in clinical practice, and (d) a robust socio-technical framework for AI system evaluation using a systems based approach that is sensitive to (i) the impact of AI system integration on patient outcomes, (ii) the clinical utility of AI system development for health, (iii) the nature of AI integration in the context to existing human computer interaction (HCI) and workflow considerations, and (iv) the nature of clinical interaction with and without AI.

To identify papers, the authors searched key terms relevant to the six sections that included: artificial intelligence, machine learning, deep learning, medicine, health, colorectal cancer, bowel cancer, screening, and participation. Duplicate papers were removed, and subsequent papers were screened according to relevance, application, citation score, and year of publication. Recent research from the last five years was prioritised for the selective review (n = 126 papers). However, historical seminal works were still considered where appropriate. Review papers and opinion pieces were excluded from formal analysis and discussion. However, they were referenced if it provided more context for the reader. Only papers with published results were included in the final analysis. In total, 88 peer-reviewed papers form the main analysis and discussion of this paper.

3. AI in Health: Opportunities and Concerns for Clinical Decision Making

AI in health is a rapidly developing field that has recently demonstrated a remarkable capacity to learn interrelationships within data in a way that offers utility for clinical decision making [19–22]. Most of the recent AI optimism for healthcare has been driven by the phenomenal development and success of deep learning (DL) [21–23]. In this section, we briefly review the different supervised, unsupervised, and reinforcement DL approaches [24,25] that have been used across the screening, diagnostic, therapeutic, and prognostic pathways of clinical decision making. In navigating the application of these methods in medical practice, we introduce some of the problematic assumptions that are embedded in AI system development. Some of the problems are general in nature and implicit to the process of AI system development (e.g., the biases embedded in data used to train AI systems), while others are specific to certain AI algorithmic methodologies that become more visible in the healthcare space of CRC. The purpose of this section is not to undertake an extensive review of AI methodologies, but to highlight that there are inherent methodological considerations that underpin their development that impact on clinical decision making. This indicates that a more nuanced approach to examining AI in CRC is necessary if we are to optimise AI benefits and limit its harms in clinical practice.

The medical literature is ripe with examples that demonstrate the highly efficacious modelling capacity of supervised ML across myriad medical modalities. These have included predicting: (a) benign/malignant cancerous states from pixel data found in photographs of skin lesions [26]; (b) classifications of disease states in chest radiographs (e.g., normal vs. abnormal radiographs, presence of pneumonia, presence of malignant pulmonary nodules) [27–29]; (c) risk stratification and prognosis from whole slide images (WSI) of histopathological tissue specimens that are used to inform therapeutic pathways in areas such as gastroenterology [12,13,30]; (d) arrythmia, atrial fibrillation, or coronary heart disease from wave data in electrocardiograms [31–33]; (e) the likelihood of sepsis based on clinical observation notes and test results found in EHRs [34]; (f) the presence or future onset of neurological diseases, such as brain tumours or Alzheimer's disease, from CT, MRI, or positron emission tomography [35–37]; (g) cardiovascular risk from fundus photography [38]; and (h) colonic polyps in colonoscopy [39], among innumerable other examples [40,41]. Despite the success of supervised ML across myriad medical contexts, researchers have started to identify that there are complex nuances that underpin (a) AI and data, and (b) AI and models, that pose significant challenges to supervised learning systems when modelling the heterogeneity of the real-world, due to its dependency on large volumes of labelled data and narrow task definitions framed by the human observer.

One of these issues includes representational harms introduced through data collection and/or labelling practices [42,43]. For example, in 2019, a landmark study was published in *Science*, where Obermeyer and colleagues [44] revealed how systemic racial biases emerged after auditing a proprietary ML algorithm used routinely on 200 million people in the United States of America each year that was tasked with assigning risk scores on patients that would be eligible for subsided "high-risk care management". While the algorithm was well intentioned, the elusive nature of systemic racial biases meant that the AI was unable to recognise that generational inequalities in healthcare access between two sociodemographic groups resulted in a situation where less money was spent caring for less-healthy Black patients compared to more-healthy White patients. Therefore, at a given risk score, Black patients were considerably more ill than White patients. Interestingly, re-labelling the data with a proxy variable that combined current health status with expenditure was shown to reduce racial bias by 84% and increase the percentage of Black patients receiving additional care from 17.7% to 46.5%.

Beyond systemic biases, another issue that arises is that AI generalisability is dependent on diverse and equitable representation in data distributions, which may not always be achieved by big data. As some genomic studies have shown, marginalised groups may be underrepresented in the data, and their use in practice may lead to confounders and incorrect correlations, as was seen in the prediction of hypertrophic cardiomyopathy in Black versus White patients [45]. Yet, there are public genotype repositories such as the 23AndMe dataset, which is based on 87% European/White representation and only 2% Asian and Black representation respectively [46], and the UK Biobank has a "healthy volunteer" selection bias [47]. Both of these tend to form the basis of training published ML algorithms [48,49]. This could limit the success of the algorithms when used on broader patient cohorts. While there are approaches to mitigate this issue by balancing the data through under/over-sampling techniques and data augmentation [50,51], an accuracy paradox may emerge, since the quality that enabled the AI to perform efficaciously on the dominant class initially (prevalence of large volumes of that class) can be conflated by the prevalence of the newly augmented class. Furthermore, the class that was augmented may have contentious validity, as the nature of synthetic data generation may mean that generated samples do not actually represent the disease state in question [52]. For instance, a chest radiograph that experiences a horizontal flip augmentation can inadvertently result in the depiction of a different medical condition called situs inversus.

More broadly, other issues that have been reported on in the literature include (a) interobserver variability among labellers, which can limit the veracity of the data used to train AI models [53], (b) challenges in delineating the suitable level of abstraction when labelling disease presentations in a way that morphologists agree with [54], and (c) intrinsic biases introduced by the contentious validity of narrow task definitions pre-imposed by the human observer in framing a reductive computational relationship that is maximised between an input X and an output Y independent of broader interrelationships between clinical history, examination, and interaction [55].

Contemporary unsupervised learning and reinforcement learning approaches have attempted to deal with some of these problems in healthcare by approaching computation in a way that is more emblematic of human approaches to knowledge discovery and decision making [56–58]. Unsupervised learning has shown that a data-driven approach independent of human interference can successfully disentangle meaning out of complex data structures, such as learning implicit brain MRI manifolds to enable for better quantitative analysis and observations about the presence and/or development of disease [59], or deriving general-purpose patient representations from electronic health records to predict the onset of future disease states across diverse clinical domains and temporal windows [60]. Similarly, "goal-directed" reinforcement learning has shown much promise in the ICU setting, where optimising decision making for a longitudinal goal that requires extensive personalisation (e.g., patient survival) is highly desired. For example, one study explored how a RL algorithm could use available patient information to define a personalised regime for sedation and weaning off ventilator support in an ICU, by predicting the optimal time to extubation in a way that minimised complications arising from either (a) prolonged dependence on mechanical ventilation on one extreme or (b) premature extubation that requires reintubation on the other extreme [61]. In another study, it was demonstrated that continuous state-space models could learn clinically interpretable treatment policies that could aid ICU physicians in treating septic patients, in a way that improved the likelihood of patient survival [62].

While such studies present an important stride forward in computational clinical decision support that more closely resembles human behaviour, the significance of the results should not be overstated. As Liu et al. [58] highlight in their comprehensive review of RL algorithms developed for critical care settings, while these approaches do mitigate against some of the biases introduced by the human observer in supervised learning approaches, the methods do little to address the fact that data collection itself, may remain biased since (1) the state space used in RL systems are constructed from data constrained by the selection of patient demographics, laboratory tests, and vital signs present in the data; and (2) the task being optimised for is still defined a priori, which means, as in supervised learning, the efficacy of the system is still heavily influenced by the human observer who decides what goal should be optimised for. Most importantly, both unsupervised and reinforcement learning approaches introduce new, more complicated problems around model evaluation in the absence of a labelled benchmark, which has led to researchers such as John Kleinberg to famously declare that unsupervised clustering is so problematic that it's possible to define an "impossibility theorem" for it [63,64].

Given the importance of data and their role in shaping the efficacy of AI predictions, this paper advocates for greater collaboration between the ML, health informatics, and clinical communities to develop a standardised systems-based approach to AI evaluation prior to clinical integration and posits that datasets and algorithms should be thoroughly audited prior to integration into clinical practice. For this to work, transparency from commercial vendor-locked systems and adequate prospective studies must become the norm. Unfortunately, a recent review of 130 FDA-approved AI medical devices found that 126 systems only ever used retrospective studies to report their results, and none of the 54 high-risk devices were evaluated by prospective studies [65]. Unsurprisingly, when one of the commercial algorithms that was being used for the detection of a pneumo-thorax was prospectively evaluated across ethnically diverse population groups, there was a statistically significant difference in performance on the algorithm's ability to accurately predict the pathology in Black versus White patients [65]. Problematically, one meta-analysis also discovered that in 516 publications highlighting the accuracy of medical AI systems, only 6% were externally validated [66]. This may suggest that there is over-optimism on the promise of medical AI and haphazard consequences may arise if sufficient external evaluations of the impact on patient outcomes in varied socio-organisational settings prior to clinical integration do not occur [67].

In the next section, we will deepen our examination of the issues of algorithmic bias in clinical decision making in CRC from a perspective of (a) AI and data, and (b) AI and models. The section integrates a perspective on how socio-technical interactions at the interface of clinical practice in CRC may marginalise the opportunities that AI may provide clinicians, patients, and the healthcare system.

4. AI in CRC: Limitations and Risks of Algorithmic Bias in Clinical Decision Making

Although AI introduces opportunities for clinical decision making, Figure 1 highlights how there are a range of issues that amalgamate to limit model efficacy in the real-world, the most significant of which are related to the interrelationship between: (1) AI and data, through the underlying biases present in data distributions used during model training; and (2) AI and models, through the reductive computational assumptions that emerge out of the translation of medical problems into narrow computational task definitions that are independent of context and that are constrained by limitations in underlying model assumptions. This section examines these issues in the context of CRC screening and diagnosis.

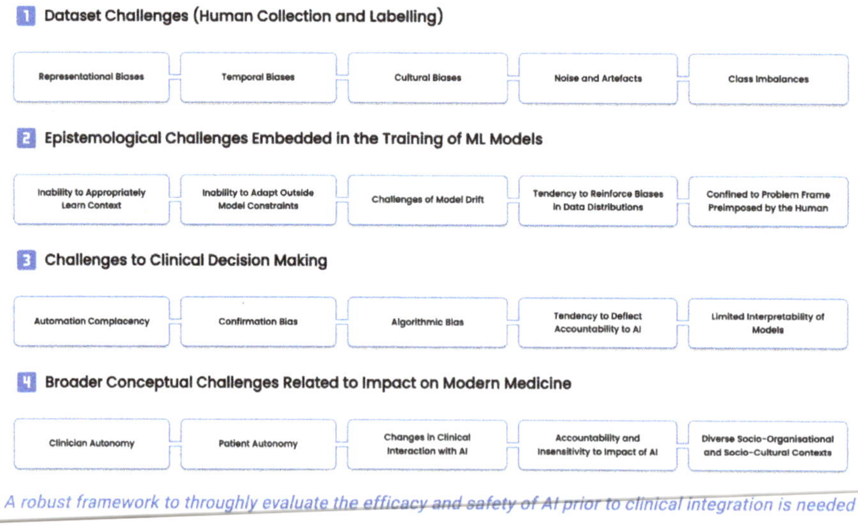
1 Dataset Challenges (Human Collection and Labelling)
Representational Biases
Temporal Biases
Cultural Biases
Noise and Artefacts
Class Imbalances
2 Epistemological Challenges Embedded in the Training of ML Models
Inability to Appropriately Learn Context
Inability to Adapt Outside Model Constraints
Challenges of Model Drift
Tendency to Reinforce Biases in Data Distributions
Confined to Problem Frame Preimposed by the Human
3 Challenges to Clinical Decision Making
Automation Complacency
Confirmation Bias
Algorithmic Bias
Tendency to Deflect Accountability to AI
Limited Interpretability of Models
4 Broader Conceptual Challenges Related to Impact on Modern Medicine
Clinician Autonomy
Patient Autonomy
Changes in Clinical Interaction with AI
Accountability and Insensitivity to Impact of AI
Diverse Socio-Organisational and Socio-Cultural Contexts
A robust framework to throughly evaluate the efficacy and safety of AI prior to clinical integration is needed

Figure 1. This infographic highlights the range of potential challenges associated with AI in clinical decision making and reinforces the need for a robust framework to AI evaluation prior to clinical integration, to maximise confidence in the safety and equity of system use in practice.

4.1. CRC, AI and Data

It is well established that data has the most significant impact on developing efficacious AI models that are robust, performant, fair, safe, and scalable across contexts [68–70]. Access to large-scaled labelled data during model training is so significant that Sun et al. [71] demonstrated that AI model performance increases logarithmically relative to the amount of training data available. However, 'big data' and 'balanced data' are not synonymous. In this section, we explore (1) representational biases and stereotypes that emerge in data relating to race, gender, ethnicity, religion, disability, sexual orientation, and socioeconomic status that alter what AI systems learn, and discuss how they may marginalise patients from backgrounds that tend to be at the highest risk of CRC and have the poorest outcomes [72–78]. Furthermore, we discuss how (2) class imbalances associated with the representation of heterogenous and/or underrepresented disease states in datasets may lead to problematic outcomes for patients with rare diseases, particularly when clinician automation complacency and bias in the presence of AI influence clinical decision making [50,79,80].

4.1.1. Representational Biases in Data and CRC Risk Stratification Algorithms

In CRC screening, it is well known that the patients who participate the least in screening, who have the highest risk of CRC, and who present with the poorest outcomes, tend to be concentrated in groups that have experienced the most social disadvantage, such as people from (a) Indigenous populations, (b) low socio-economic status, (c) diverse cultural backgrounds, or (d) with disability [68–70]. For example, African Americans have the highest incidence of CRC of all ethnic groups in the United States (US), have a mortality rate that is approximately 20% higher than White Americans, and typically have a younger onset of the disease [68]. Yet, such groups tend to either be (a) underrepresented in historical machine learning datasets, or (b) when they are represented, experience algorithmic bias due to systemic inequities embedded in the nature of the data. This poses potential risks to patient care when an algorithmic prediction of patient risk and/or prognosis is clinically implemented to guide clinical decision making around who will benefit from access to treatment interventions.

These representational issues combined with a lack of a standards-based approach to medical AI evaluations poses some interesting challenges in CRC screening, particularly when there is a significant interest in developing ML methods for the screening of early-stage CRC, given that the current two-tiered "Gold Standard" FOBT + colonoscopy approach is challenged by a problem of low patient participation in screening [81]. Wan et al. [82] suggested leveraging ML with whole-genome sequencing of plasma cell-free DNA and demonstrated that is possible to predict the early onset of the disease with a mean area under the curve (AUC) of 0.92 and sensitivity and specificity of 85%. One perspective is that this whole genome approach allows for an unbiased discovery of signals that are not disease specific and can be extended to the monitoring of non-disease states through the detection of biomarker correlations. However, as the authors acknowledge, demographic and institutional biases may impact on the generalisability of the results and the need for prospective trials is emphasised. The issue with prospective trials that are not sensitive to these representational issues, is that they can be designed in a way that unwittingly supports the hypothesis, even when the authors are well intentioned. For example, Chan and colleagues [83] proposed an ensemble ML algorithm to predict recurrence of CRC using historical genomic data from a French population and claimed a sensitivity of 91.18%, which was validated on data from Australia (91.67%) and the United States of America (80%). There are concerns that the AI is therefore optimised for patients with Caucasian ancestry, which could lead to problematic outcomes if these same algorithms are then inappropriately used on patients of different ancestry that they are not optimised for. This is of particular concern when we consider that (a) patients who are often at the highest risk and who demand the most urgent care are often the ones that are least represented in the data, and (b) that clinical decision making, according to some research, can be heavily influenced by the presence of algorithms [15,79,80].

To understand the effects that these algorithms have on clinical decision making, we point to a fascinating study published in *Nature*, where Kostopoulou and colleagues [15] setup an experiment to observe how recommendations for referral to specialised oncology care would change in 157 general practitioners (GP) from the United Kingdom (UK) when presented with 20 vignettes of patients with symptoms that might indicate potential CRC and an unnamed algorithm predicting each of the patient's risk. The researchers observed two things: (1) after receiving the algorithm's estimate, a GP's inclination to refer for specialised care changed 26% of the time, with the greatest impact seen when the GP felt that they underestimated the risk compared to the algorithm; and (2) with continued use, there was a positive GP disposition towards the algorithm, as GPs became better calibrated to the probabilistic way that the algorithm would associate symptoms with risk that they started to inadvertently emulate the same algorithmic approach to deduction and conclusion.

While this study was celebrated as a success with high clinical utility, as GPs seemed to improve their cancer referral decisions to the benefit of the patient, particularly when the AI risk predictor was higher than the clinician; what the study does not thoroughly investigate is the inverse scenario of what happens when patients who are actually high risk are provided with low-risk scores, as witnessed in the previous Obermeyer study [44]. Even though the study does seem to indicate that GPs tend to err on the side of caution and so an incorrect low risk algorithm theoretically should not change a GPs disposition to refer; the effects of these interactions have not been thoroughly investigated. Human factors engineering suggests the opposite may occur, as humans may subconsciously deflect accountability to the machine [84], particularly when the effects of confirmation bias [85,86] and automation complacency [80] set in, where clinicians are believed to lean towards the decision of an automated system and subsequently stop searching for any further confirmatory evidence. This phenomenon has been extensively discussed for two decades in cardiology around the issue of automated electrocardiogram analysis [87,88].

This is concerning, particularly when a close examination of the literature shows examples of representational biases that are both systemic and distributional in nature unwittingly emerge in the absence of a robust methodological framework to address these problems. For example, Nartowt et al. [14] developed an exclusively software-based screening tool for the early identification and prevention of CRC in large populations by training a neural network to classify individuals into low, medium, and high CRC-risk groups using only personal health data found in two public datasets: (1) the National Health Interview Survey (NHIS) dataset and (2) the Prostate, Lung, Colorectal, Ovarian Cancer Screening (PLCO) dataset. To maximise machine performance, the authors converted much of the dataset pertaining to race into a set of binary variables presenting attributes such as "Not Hispanic/Spanish origin", "Black/African American only", "American Indian only", "Other race", "Multiple race", and "Sex factor". However, this reductionism clearly has consequences. Demarcating all other ethnic groups into a single variable of "Other race" is a dangerous assumption, because it implies that there are no differences between all the other rich cultures across the world. Compounding the problem is the fact that systemic disparities that exist across groups due to sociodemographic context are not accounted for, even though it is already known that this can be a significant limitation to predicting accurate outcomes.

4.1.2. Class Imbalance, Heterogeneous Disease States, and Underrepresented Disease

Class imbalances and underrepresentation of rare disease states also presents an interesting challenge for AI in CRC, which is not easily remedied by simply accruing more data. The quality that makes ML so potentially powerful, the ability to learn patterns within data by maximising signals that reinforce distributions in the datasets, is also one that can lead to a situation where an AI optimises for features that are highly predictive of over-represented disease states, at the expense of features that detect or diagnose under-represented rare diseases, even where computational techniques such as data augmentation and regularisation are implemented. For example, in a recent landmark study, Wang and colleagues [11] developed a state-of-the-art deep CNN that capitalised on transfer-learning and demonstrated superior performance to pathologists in the histopathological analysis of CRC tissue specimens, achieving a 0.988 vs. 0.970 AUC. The experimental setup appeared sound and resistant to algorithmic bias: (a) they used a large volume of data (170,099 patches sourced from 14,680 whole slide images, captured from >9631 patients), and (b) the patient cohorts attempted to be clinically representative, by collecting cases from multi-independent sources across China, the USA, and Germany. However, as the authors highlight in their analysis, several histological types were excluded from the study, because they were too rare and had less than a 0.5% incidence. While they acknowledged this limitation and stated that the algorithm would improve over time through the collection of more data, it is important to highlight, again, that balanced data are more important than more data, and the algorithm may remain skewed to the overrepresented class.

This may not be a problem in and of itself, as we acknowledge that rare diseases are difficult for clinicians to diagnose and that the net benefit of these systems may still be incredibly valuable when used as a second observer to ensure common cases are not misdiagnosed and/or missed on account of human error. However, a socio-technical analysis evaluating the system may weigh these benefits against the risk that over-confidence in the AI over time may alter the behaviour of clinical interaction, such that clinicians become less perceptive of signals that an AI is known to be poor at, due to complacency in the presence of the machine. This may mean that more careful consideration to HCI in the development of HIT systems that utilise AI is enacted, or specific clinician retraining around how to approach clinical practice in the presence of AI is mandated.

This may have interesting ramifications in emergent capsule endoscopy technologies, where AI has been heavily promoted to increase small bowel findings while reducing reading time through a mechanism that filters out normal findings and uses image processing techniques to merge similar images together [10]. While this optimisation has largely been lauded as a profound optimisation and improvement to the workflow through the reduced reading time, there are concerns around whether the models will be robust against all possible edge cases, particularly given the highly heterogenous ways that disease can manifest. We do not know the answer to these questions, but it does indicate that, at minimum, we need a rigorous framework around the external validation of AI, specific quantitative testing around edge cases that are expected to be a challenge for AI such as underrepresented classes, and more evaluations of clinician performance with and without the use of AI, to ensure that we optimise the benefits of AI and limit their harm when integrated into clinical practice.

4.2. CRC, AI and Models

In the previous section, the impact of data on AI performance was discussed and it was acknowledged that more sensitive approaches to developing transparent, representative, and equitable datasets could improve the efficacy of AI across diverse patient cohorts and limit potential harms. This section extends on that discussion, to highlight that there are broader contextual factors that impact clinical decision making that poses unique challenges for AI, when consideration is given to the fact that current AI system technology is functionally unable to transcend the epistemological and ontological assumptions embedded in the nature of model design. This tends to leave AI unaware of the nature of clinician, patient, or healthcare interactions and may result in erroneous conclusions by an AI system due to an inability to recognise and appreciate the nuances of (a) temporal context, and/or (b) situational operator context. Consequently, this section re-emphasises the dangers of clinician complacency in the presence of AI system implementation in clinical practice. This section concludes by examining how the inability to adequately explain AI model predictions exacerbates the impact that context has on AI reliability in practice.

4.2.1. Temporal Context

An issue that has been widely discussed in the literature is the problem of model adaptation in the presence of distributional data shift [89], where there is (1) a mismatch between the training data used by an algorithm at one point in time, and unanticipated and/or evolving patient/healthcare contexts that emerge at a later point in time; and (2) an inability of an AI algorithm to accurately adapt to such non-stationary clinical operational environments due to the way that an AI model frames its assumptions of the world [55]. This tends to manifest most when historical EHRs are used to train a ML algorithm and new data are later recorded and captured in the EHR, which was absent in the historical data due to the evolution of clinical practice. This leads to a problem known as model drift [84,90,91]. This is not an easy problem to solve, since historical data cannot suddenly be updated according to new knowledge, and new knowledge is often not voluminous enough to train a new algorithm efficaciously. Even though more contemporary methods allow for continuous learning via a process known as incremental learning [52], it is important to recognise that this process of adaptation is still bound within the initial constraints of the problem definition and an AI algorithm cannot epistemologically adapt outside of the computational model "frame" imposed by the engineer. Importantly, the ML community has not agreed on the best approach to handling class imbalances that emerge during incremental learning, since real-time learning may inadvertently undo any efforts used to balance initial data distributions and may skew the algorithm back too heavily in favour of diseases or population groups that present commonly.

To show how these issues manifest first-hand in a healthcare setting, Davis et al. [92] revealed how decreasing rates of acute kidney injury (AKI) led ML models to drift towards a state of over-prediction of AKI within one year of development and this had the negative unintended consequence of altering clinical decision making in a way that misdirected resource allocation and expenditure. A more extreme example of this problem can be seen in the emergence of the recent COVID-19 pandemic, which witnessed an unprecedented shift in the patient landscape of a typical emergency department (ED), where an exponential increase in ED visits for COVID-19 matched an exponential decline in acute visits for stroke and heart attacks [91]. This presents a potential issue for CRC, given that since the early 1990s, the incidence of colorectal cancer in patients below the age of 50 has nearly doubled, but this population is often not captured by most screening programs [93,94]. While it is true that the absolute number of these patients are currently small and are not necessarily included in screening pathways, it does demonstrate how disease patterns evolve over time, and this has consequences to how AI systems are developed and evaluated. Observations in younger CRC patients who present with more advanced stages of CRC have suggested that there are multifactorial genetic and environmental components that influence the nature of the underlying disease [93]. How does this then influence prognostic model performances, e.g., if the underlying biological mechanisms are discovered to have shifted over time? Therefore, it is important to consider that we need more robust guidelines around how and when algorithms should be re-trained or re-calibrated, to maintain their performance across shifting distributions to ensure that clinical decision making, which is inevitably influenced by algorithmic decisions, remains robust to evolving clinical knowledge and dynamic clinical settings.

The ramifications of temporal context on algorithmic predictability can be quite elusive, particularly when we also consider how AI integration into clinical decision making along therapeutic pathways is quite sensitive to the specific circumstances of the patient's own temporal context, independent of the broader population. For example, it was reported in one study by Jie and colleagues [95], that when IBM's Watson for Oncology (WFO) was used to provide an oncologic treatment recommendation for a colon cancer patient, the WFO did not recommend the usual CapeOX (oxaliplatin + capecitabine) treatment regimen, because WFO assumed it was unsafe for the patient due to a recent biochemical blood test that showed a creatinine clearance rate <30. However, when this was reviewed by the multi-disciplinary team (MDT), the oncologists immediately knew that this was a transient reversible biochemical abnormality due to the treatment, which would organically recover after one week, concluding that it would be irresponsible to stop the CapeOx treatment scheme. On review, the creatinine clearance rate returned to normal as the MDT expected.

4.2.2. Situational and Operator Context

AI algorithms also tend to be unaware of situational context, where environmental factors may have a significant impact on the appropriateness of the predictions, which again reinforces the need for a standardised external validation framework that is sensitive to technical and socio-technical concerns. There have been countless examples in the broader ML literature to show how situationally unaware neural network signal optimisations have led to a model exploiting unreliable artefacts, confounders, or spurious cues in a training dataset to the detriment of its reliability and generalisability in new contexts. The most cited example of this problem in the literature is the classic case where a ML algorithm predicted pneumonia in a chest radiograph due to the type of X-ray machine equipment that was used, rather than any underlying features of pneumonia. By coincidence, the situational context was that patients who were most unwell, and most likely to have pneumonia, were the ones that required point of care imaging by the clinical staff and those radiographs were incidentally stamped with the term "portable" [29]. Given that it is known that an AI may maximise spurious cues to forge incorrect classifications, even at the level of a single pixel perturbation [96], there may be consequences that limit the currently reported success of AI-assisted polyp and/or CRC detection and diagnosis systems used in conventional colonoscopy, when they become more mainstream. In a recent study, Li et al. [97] highlighted the range of situations that contributed to false positive or false negative detections by an AI-assisted polyp detection system, which included: (a) when a polyp had approached the corners of frames when they were about to appear or disappear from the image; (b) when light reflections and shadows were present in the image due to bubbles arising from a patient's sub-optimal bowel preparation; (c) when edges of circular folds could be misconstrued as polyps; or (d) when images were out of focus and blurred.

This introduces an interesting socio-technical question: is the problem here due to the AI, or due to the interaction of the human observer with the AI? One could argue that the AI was performing as intended—it disentangled the factors of variation to demarcate polyps most of the time, as advertised—, but it had some expectations around how the human observer interacted with it. This could include expectations around the endoscopist's pace of movement to limit the likelihood of blur, the patient's minimal bowel preparation, or expectations around the endoscopist's approach to insufflation or irrigation of the bowel. This highlights that clinical decision making may need to be adjusted in the presence of AI and clear guidelines around the expectations and limitations of these systems in-use are needed so that we optimise their benefits and limit their harm.

At times, situational context, patient context, clinician context, temporal context, and representational biases may all interact to affect the relevance of AI decision making. In one WFO feasibility study, Liu's team [98] investigated whether patients with lung cancer who were receiving treatment in China, of Chinese descent, could be provided with treatment recommendations that were consistent with the multidisciplinary team. The authors concluded that the overall consistency was 65.8% and could have been increased to 93.2% had the WFO considered differences between Western and Chinese contexts, such as (1) differences in the presentation of genetic mutations, (2) differences in the sensitivity, tolerance, and metabolism of chemotherapeutic agents due to different physiques that influence treatment regimens between nations (e.g., concurrent vs. sequential chemoradiation), (3) differences in the availability of drugs between markets, and (4) differences between patient preferences, particularly in lieu of treatment prices and medical insurance.

There are different perspectives around why these issues arise and the significance of their impact. Some authors such as Strickland [99] argue that these issues arise due to poor data practices by IBM. However, another perspective could be that the limitation lies in the way that the AI was framed to model the data, and had it been provided with access to the raw data with greater computational capacity, perhaps AI could propose a personalised treatment recommendation (i.e., rather than having a treatment regimen offered according to national guidelines that dismisses concurrent chemoradiation, AI could learn to optimise the dosing of concurrent chemoradiation for the smaller physique). The existence of these competing perspectives validates the position advocated by this paper, that a robust methodology to AI evaluation in healthcare is needed. Furthermore, this example also emphasises that there are clearly dangers when commercial vendors develop algorithms using multi-centre datasets that appear equitable and efficacious on local population distributions but proceed to reductively commercialise that same AI system without any due diligence or oversight to internationally different population distributions.

4.2.3. Interpretability of AI Models

Since AI reliability can be affected by numerous contextual factors that arise in clinical practice, EU regulators have enforced a position through the 2018 European Data Protection Regulation stating that "black box" AI algorithms that have a significant effect on users must be able to explain why a decision was made on-demand, as patients deserve the "right to explanation" [100,101]. As a precedent, this was an important and sensible step towards developing safer AI systems that were operationalised in a way that were more complementary to how clinicians are trained to weigh competing modes of evidence to the contextual circumstances of the patient. The computational community has responded positively to these concerns by enhancing AI system interpretability through integrating (a) gradient-weighted class activation mappings (Grad-CAM) [102–104], (b) replacing singular end-end classification pipelines with sequential segmentation + classification steps [105], (c) extracting highly active neurons to visualise feature detectors [106], (d) gradient feature auditing to estimate the indirect influence a feature has on a prediction [107], and (e) using a process of "deep dreaming" to understand the evolution of a network's layers [108]. However, the diversity of the methods also indicates that "interpretability" exists on a spectrum and knowing what level of interpretation is sufficient to limit the impact of AI bias in clinical practice is unknown.

5. Social, Ethical, and Legal Ramifications of AI Mediated Clinical Decision Making

In the context of the technical and socio-technical critiques discussed above, it is important to delve more deeply into the wider ramifications of the underlying concepts pertaining to computational biases and reductionist assumptions embedded within most contemporary clinical AI systems. Beyond NUCs at the clinical interface, this section highlights that there are potentially broader ethical and moral questions raised by the wide-spread deployment of these systems because of their potential to transform the basis for clinical decisions. We discuss how the socio-technical perspectives provided are not simply 'contextual' concerns but are more deeply grounded in the fundamental limitations and risks embedded within AI systems themselves.

Clinical decision making is not just about treating biological disease, it is about treating a patient with a unique set of psycho-social and cultural factors. It is for this reason that two critical pillars guide the practice of ethical medicine: beneficence (the need for common good and benefit) and nonmaleficence (first, do no harm) [109]. Therefore, clinical care means that even in the absence of evidence, a clinician may choose to "err on the side of caution" and order an investigation, weighing out the risks associated with the potential of a missed diagnosis against the risks of overdiagnosis to the unique circumstances of the patient [84]. AI algorithms are not sensitive to the impact that "absolute" probabilistic decisions around disease, independent of the patient's concerns has on the patient's well-being. While some may argue that this is too strong of a criticism of AI, since AI is not the one making the final decision and is merely "supporting" the physician to make their decision; as we have discussed throughout this paper, clinicians are susceptible to a range of cognitive biases that can influence clinical decision making.

Given the influence algorithms have on clinical decision making, who then is accountable when a clinical error enters clinical practice? Inevitably, the presence of the AI agent will mean that a clinician will always be influenced by its existence, irrespective of whether the human operator chooses to accept or reject the AI. If the AI's deductions are not to be used by the human operator, but are later discovered to have revealed an outcome that could have prevented the loss of human life, is the human operator accountable for choosing to preserve clinical autonomy and ignore the AI? Inversely, if the AI's conclusions are used by the human operator, but are later discovered to have resulted in the loss of human life due to an unexplained statistical error, is the AI or human accountable and can an AI ever understand the concept of accountability? This is further complicated by the fact that the methods used to increase model interpretability are currently constrained to the discrete case of medical imaging and do little to address concerns around more contemporary unsupervised and reinforcement learning approaches that are increasingly being applied to genomics datasets [110–112], the raw text in electronic health records [60], or in some cases across a mixture of data sources sourced longitudinally across different data contexts [113,114]. In these cases, some ethical issues arise from the fact that even if the computational methods were able to explain themselves, there remains the broader problem that there is no guarantee that we may even be able to understand or validate the conclusion that the AI arrives to.

While these issues are beyond the scope of this paper (refer to [67,84,109] for further discussions), we mention them to highlight that, given the fact that we know that (a) there are several potential sources for algorithmic error and bias, (b) algorithms influence clinical decision making, (c) there is an insensitivity to clinical impact by algorithms, and (d) a lack of guidelines around accountability in the presence of an algorithm; it reinforces our position that a more nuanced socio-technical approach to AI system evaluation prior to clinical integration is necessary if we are to avoid a repeated history where negative unintended consequences arise in yet another HIT integration.

6. Further Risks and Limitations from Marginalising Socio-Technical Factors in CRC

In this section, the paper highlights how even if technical and socio-technical concerns are addressed through robust evaluation standards in the interest of patient safety, AI system development and investment should be directed towards problems that have the most measurable impact on patient morbidity and mortality outcomes. Much of the AI optimism in CRC screening has been driven by the fact that it presents a potential solution to the problem that in a routine screening colonoscopy, between 17–28% of colorectal polyps (adenomas) are missed, which is concerning given that for every 1% increase in a clinician's adenoma detection rate (ADR), there is a 3% decrease in the risk of interval cancer [115–117]. Several of the vendor-backed AI augmented diagnostic systems have proposed to address this issue by providing clinicians with a real-time AI polyp detection system, and the evidence provided by recent RCTs is promising. It suggests that the ADR increases by up to 50% with the inclusion of an AI detection system, with the most pronounced effect on trainee gastroenterologists [7–9]. Similarly, in AI-enhanced capsule endoscopy (CE), experimental evidence suggests that AI augmentation consistently outperforms a conventional CE reader in terms of both accuracy and time, showing a 99.88% vs. 74.57% sensitivity in the per-patient detection of abnormalities and, significantly, a 5.9 vs. 96.6-min recording on per-patient reading time between the AI vs. human respectively [10].

While such results are exciting and show some promise in improving patient outcomes, it is also important to recognise that one of the biggest influences on CRC-related mortality is not fundamentally due to the nature of the current technology, but rather due to the prevalence of low rates of participation in CRC screening [118]. Various studies from Australia, which implemented one of the first national approaches to bowel cancer screening, have suggested that at the current participation rate of ~40%, a 15–36% reduction in CRC-related mortality can be expected, and if participation rates in the screening population were to increase to 70%, a 59% reduction in CRC-related mortality would be observed [119–124]. The problem is that several high-income nations have failed to reach their desired target of 65–80% screening coverage, even in the presence of wide-scale public health campaigns to raise awareness about its importance [81,125]. Unfortunately, it seems that these rates are not likely to increase, given that the rate of FOBT-based screening coverage has plateaued in Australia over the last five years [126]. Participation in follow-up colonoscopy, where many of the AI-enhanced methods are poised to transform outcomes are equally discouraging. Studies from Europe, the United States, Canada, and Australia show that even in the presence of a positive FOBT, only between 50–70% of patients proceed for a diagnostic examination via colonoscopy [126–129]. Participation among the most marginalised groups that have historically experienced social disadvantage, such as those from Indigenous populations, low socio-economic status, cultural and ethnic diversity, or disability, tends to be the lowest in either stage of the screening process [69,130,131].

Consequently, it is possible that the extensive focus of AI adoption and integration into the CRC diagnostic pathway may not have the drastic impact it has promised on patient outcomes. In the following sections, we highlight how the barriers to participation in CRC screening is permeated by human factors, and that if we are sensitive to these factors, we can capitalise on AI methods in a way that can lead to a more significant impact to patient outcomes by developing technology that increases the uptake of screening coverage in high-risk population groups.

6.1. Interaction between Patient & Healthcare System

Several international qualitative studies [132–138] have concluded that there are numerous psycho-social and cultural factors that interact and accumulate to impact on a patient's willingness to participate in CRC screening. Barriers include low awareness and a misunderstanding of the medical guidelines around the need for CRC screening and/or believing that screening was only required in the presence of symptoms, which is exacerbated by a lower perception of risk associated with bowel cancer compared with other more high-profile cancers [139]. There has also tended to be limited promotion in community languages among culturally and linguistically diverse populations, which contributes to challenges around the understanding of the purpose of testing and/or how to apply the test kit instructions even if patients choose to proceed [69]. Even where promotion has occurred, screening programme administrators have tended to have limited awareness of how factors, such as culture or gender, influence the way individuals interpret and receive information [132,133]. Additional factors have included the logistics relating to a lack of time to get screened or lack of transportation. For those in urban areas, lack of time could be related to extensive work commitments and a perception of inefficiency by the healthcare system, while for those in rural and remote areas, lack of time may relate to distance and access to healthcare services [134]. Furthermore, fear, anxiety, stigma, shame, uneasiness, or embarrassment in engaging with a procedure that involves stool collection (e.g., the FOBT), or an invasive visualisation of the bowels (e.g., the colonoscopy), both of which may lead to a positive diagnosis of cancer, have been suggested to exacerbate an unwillingness to get screened regardless of sociodemographic context [132].

6.2. Interaction between Patient & Clinician

Given the problematic issues around sensitivity and rates of false positives arising from FOBT tests [140,141], patients and clinicians have also been found to convince themselves (in the absence of evidence) that a positive FOBT reading is a false positive attributed to an alternative source of bleeding (e.g., haemorrhoids, menstruation, and straining due to constipation), dietary factors (consumption of beets or orange juice), or medications (e.g., the use of blood thinners). In more extreme cases, some patients more speculatively reported that they believed the toilet was contaminated with someone else's blood, even if the toilet had been cleaned prior [142]. Interestingly, despite the established guidelines around the importance of FOBT-based screening, one qualitative study involving interviews of general practitioner (GP) perceptions of CRC screening in Australia found that many GPs reinforced negative attitudes towards the FOBT, leading patients to either reject undertaking the FOBT or reject the result of the FOBT in the presence of a positive result. For example, GPs were found to use low risk of bowel cancer arguments to negate the significance of screening, and where a patient returned a positive FOBT, provided explanations that implied that the positive FOBT was more likely the result of a benign source of bleeding [143].

6.3. *Interaction between Clinician & Healthcare System*

System based factors have also been implicated in having a significant role in the management of patients that require CRC screening. Primary care physicians play an important role in the advocacy, facilitation, support, education, and counselling of patients [144]. However, since screening is typically managed outside of the practice setting by a broader national bowel cancer screening infrastructure, there are inconsistencies in the way that results are recorded in patient health records and the availability of that information in the primary care setting. This introduces complexities in the way that GPs flag patients who are overdue for screening, particularly given that FOBT-based screening should occur biennially to achieve its purported benefits. Some studies have suggested that even when the information is made available in the EHR and made accessible in the primary care setting, poor HIT practices have led to workarounds and the under-utilisation of these systems by practitioners [145]. These issues are only compounded in busy primary care settings, where there exists a limited capacity and/or unwillingness to discuss the importance of screening with patients when other more immediate acute and chronic conditions need to be managed in a short consultation session [143].

7. The Future of AI and Potential Implications for Clinical Decision Making

In recent years, extensive research and investment has gone into developing (1) novel AI methods that are more emblematic of human reasoning, (2) cloud computing infrastructure to support the storage and retrieval of large volumes of structured and unstructured data through data lakes, and (3) the acceleration of computational processing power in both the domains of super computing and quantum computing. For AI researchers, the belief is that the union of these three fields will result in the holy grail of AI research, artificial general intelligence (AGI). Whether the advancements will correspond to achieving this esoteric goal of human hubris is yet to be seen. However, it does indicate that AI systems are here to stay and both regulators and medical practitioners are likely going to need to grapple with ethical issues surrounding patient autonomy in the presence of contemporary unexplainable AI systems, where some end-of-life patients may argue that they prefer to experiment with an algorithmically inspired personalised therapy that we do not understand, and which may have no evidence.

There is some evidence in the literature to suggest that AI is capable of remarkable feats that can paradoxically be incapable of explanation, problematic for interpretation, yet remain useful to clinical application. The first was an unsupervised learning algorithm known as Deep Patient that was trained on data aggregated from approximately 700,000 patients to broadly predict the health state of an individual by assessing their probability to develop various diseases. The algorithm was evaluated on 76,214 patients comprising 78 diseases across diverse clinical contexts and temporal distributions [60]. Interestingly, the model managed to predict the onset of psychiatric disorders that are notoriously difficult to detect and diagnose by physicians, such as schizophrenia, with remarkable precision, significantly outperforming prior efforts. However, as the lead researcher concedes in an interview, "we can build these models … but we don't know how they work" [146]. Similarly, in the field of computational biology, researchers from Google achieved a phenomenal leap forward in the 50-year-old "protein-folding challenge", using an algorithm, AlphaFold, to determine the structure of a protein based solely on its amino acid sequence, achieving an accuracy of 92.4 on the Global Distance Test (GDT) [112]. This has significant ramifications for developing new therapeutics, given that it is the closest attempt to solving Levintha's paradox, which describes the peculiar situation where there are 10^{300} possible configurations of a protein from a typical sequence of amino acids, yet nature folds proteins spontaneously to a consistently exact configuration. The success of such approaches has already found its way into CRC, where deep reinforcement learning has been applied to understand the association between human MicroRNA and colorectal cancer disease progression [147].

It is important to remember that the way AI perceives, interprets, and "senses" reality across millions of data points is epistemologically different to the way humans do, and therefore there may always remain a divide between our understanding of AI and the AI's understanding of the world. Is there a quantitative threshold with which we can "trust" the AI in favour of human judgement in the absence of understanding if the AI is consistently correct across longitudinal observation? This is an open question we currently have no answer to. From the perspective of the EU regulators, a system that cannot explain itself and one that we do not understand has no place in clinical practice. This view is certainly one that seems sensible for the time-being, as it would appear as though the systems that act with profundity are currently the exception, not the rule. However, as more evidence evolves in the near future, it may be the case that persisting with this position may itself be an ethical danger, as preventing individuals from access to personalised algorithmically inspired medical interventions that may be life altering, even in the absence of understanding, will invite new questions around patient autonomy, as some patients may simply prefer to take the risk.

8. A Way Forward to Enhancing Clinical Decision Making in CRC: A More Nuanced Approach to AI Systems Development, Implementation, and Evaluation

This paper has presented a socio-technical analysis of contemporary research into the use and impact of AI enhanced HIT in healthcare broadly and in colorectal cancer, specifically to offer a balanced critique on the opportunities, limitations, and risks of AI system development and integration in clinical decision-making. Through this approach, the paper has highlighted socio-technical perspectives on the important contextual nuances that arise from problematic assumptions embedded in the development, implementation, and evaluation of AI systems when applied along the screening, diagnostic, and treatment pathways of CRC.

In Section 3, a series of problematic assumptions underpinning approaches to AI development and implementation in health were identified. These included the general data problems associated with systemic representational biases that manifest elusively through data and the way that unbalanced data distributions tend to marginalise underrepresented groups even in the presence of "big data". An examination of specific issues that permeate supervised learning (intractability of labelling, veracity of labels, and the computational reductionism intrinsic to narrow task definitions), unsupervised learning (the "impossibility" of evaluation and interpretation), and reinforcement learning (selection biases in the framing of environmental data and goals) was then provided. Having examined these issues and in recognition of the fact that minimal external validation of AI in health has existed in both academic research and commercial FDA-approved systems, this paper advocates that, moving forward, it is critical that datasets that are used for ML learning training are independently audited in a transparent way. While the authors do acknowledge that data are perceived as the currency of ML and many vendors have locked commercial agreements in place that are also protected by legislation around patient privacy, it is important to remember that the aircraft industry is supported by an extensive amount of vendor-backed software and hardware components that have managed to cooperate with one another in the interests of safety while maintaining competitiveness. Some researchers, therefore, have advocated that independent auditing analogous to the Aviation Safety Reporting System should exist in healthcare [148].

In Section 4, these issues in the context of AI in CRC were examined and additional nuances were identified in the nature of AI through an evaluation of problematic data and model assumptions. In data, it was highlighted that there was significant interest in using ML for the purpose of risk stratification and prognostic prediction, particularly given that participation in the existing paradigm of CRC screening was low. However, it was uncovered that several studies reinforced racial biases and used distributions that underrepresented the most marginalised patients, who tend to have the poorest CRC outcomes. It was also observed that class imbalances in modelling the heterogeneity of disease presentation remained a problem, similar to problems that have been identified in the broader AI in health literature. In models, the frame problem of AI was revisited and it was observed that the epistemological and ontological assumptions embedded in ML algorithms were often not resistant to the impact that context-dependent clinical interactions between the patient, clinician, and health system had on clinical decision making. These interactions included the way that knowledge and operational practices evolved over time to create a problem of temporally-influenced model drift; the way that transient effects in the patient circumstances could obfuscate model conclusions in oncologic treatment; the way that spurious cues in data due to situational context could lead to erroneous signal optimisation; the way that operator interactions with AI systems influenced prediction outputs in colonoscopy; the way that a model built for one local populace but commercialised in an international market could not synthesise differences in national guidelines to treatment; and the broader issue where many approaches were not explainable or interpretable.

In examining these issues, the theme that pervaded the multifaceted discussion was that human behavioural studies had identified that clinical decision making had a tendency to be influenced by confirmation bias, algorithmic bias, and automation complacency. Therefore, there was a risk that even small system errors could have major ramifications to patient safety. In recognising these issues, it was identified that the emphasis of the ML literature was on quantitative outcomes, but very few works existed that explored the qualitative socio-technical impact that this would have on patient outcomes. When the issue was discussed, it tended to only ever be conjectured as a potential problem, while studies focused on reporting quantitative outcomes to justify their integration into clinical practice were often not reproduced. This paper therefore suggests that, moving forward, ML studies in health and in CRC have strict standards around: (a) the reproducibility of algorithms prior to publication, (b) reproducibility of quantitative metrics across different socio-organisational settings, (c) a definition for what "interpretability" should look like, given the myriad methodologies that claim to achieve machine interpretability in various ways, and (d) a systems-based approach to the qualitative evaluation that carefully examines: (i) the impact of AI system integration on patient outcomes, (ii) the clinical utility of an AI system, (iii) the nature of AI integration in context to existing HCI and workflow considerations across varied socio-organisational and cultural settings, and (iv) the nature of clinical interaction with and without AI. Further research into a unified quantitative and qualitative methodological framework for AI-enhanced HIT evaluation is urgently required. Indeed, this is something that the broader ML community has identified, motivating an upcoming dedicated conference (ICLR2022 ML Evaluation Standards) to deal with this exact issue [149].

In Section 5, the discussion on AI and clinical decision making was broadened to introduce the fact that there were additional social, ethical, and legal ramifications around the integration of AI systems into clinical practice. It was highlighted that there were problems around the fact that AI itself is insensitive to impact, particularly when probabilistic approaches to clinical decision making that discretise diseases upend decades of medical dogma that has identified health as an interplay that is influenced by complex psycho-social and cultural interactions. Issues pertaining to clinical accountability were also discussed. It was highlighted that the philosophical and ethical debates remain ongoing, particularly around issues of culpability in the presence of machine and/or human error. Given that this research suggests that AI errors are inevitable and will have undue influence on the human observer, moving forward, the authors advocate that careful consideration of the socio-technical interactions of system use, particularly around the nature of human–computer interaction is examined. The ML model is only one component, whereas how and when the prediction is relayed to the clinician is entirely dependent on the nature of HCI. Therefore, careful examination of how AI is rendered in-use is as critical as the model development, and well-crafted product design solutions inspired by participatory design principles can limit some of the complications that may arise from automation complacency.

In Section 6, the paper reasserted the view that AI efficacy and investment need to be moderated against their impact on patient outcomes. It was identified that the last three decades of technological advancement have done little to perturb the rate of CRC mortality, and that in the presence of increased incidence, it is critical that the one factor that is known to have the most measurable effect on mortality, namely increasing rates of screening participation, should be the context that future AI technology should attempt to address. Complex human factors emerged in the interactions between (a) the patient and healthcare system (misunderstanding, miscommunication, accessibility, cultural sensitivity and broader psycho-social dimensions), (b) the patient and clinician (trust and perception of inefficacy of FOBT), and (c) the clinician and healthcare system (poor interoperability between national and community infrastructure, and poor HIT practices with the EHR). In recognising these issues, the authors emphasise that sensitivity to socio-technical factors in the design and implementation of new technologies is critical. One solution that has not yet been considered in the literature is whether capsule-based technology can be creatively repurposed, reimagined, and repositioned as a tool for the screening of precancerous lesions from home, which may address patient anxieties around (a) the anxiety of a cancer diagnosis, (b) the inconclusiveness of a FOBT result, (c) concerns around the invasiveness of a colonoscopic investigation, and (d) accessibility to healthcare centres both in terms of distance and time.

In Section 7, the paper concluded with a brief look into the future to suggest that the union of big data, high performance computation, and contemporary approaches to unsupervised and reinforcement learning means that regulators may be required to grapple with complex issues around patient autonomy in the era of unexplainable AI. Early evidence suggests that more modern approaches may unlock immense power to the benefit of the patient through personalised medicine. However, this is complicated by the fact that these methods are not interpretable, and even if they were, may never be understood. Where this leaves clinical decision making and clinical autonomy in the presence of patients who may prefer algorithmic clinical decision making needs to be discussed.

9. Conclusions

Through a socio-technical analysis of the contemporary literature on AI in CRC, it is evident that a more nuanced approach to AI development and implementation is required. While there is no doubt that AI itself is a transformative technology that has the capacity to positively impact clinical practice to the benefit of the patient, AI optimism needs to be balanced against a thorough understanding of the limitations that also permeate the underlying nature of the technology. This paper highlighted how there are concerns around: (a) biases in end-end data pipelines and technical issues associated with algorithmic model assumptions in the design and development of AI systems; (b) socio-technical issues relating to confirmation bias, automation complacency, interpretability, and the clinician workflow that arises from the interaction with AI systems; (c) ethical and legal implications around accountability and autonomy for both the clinician and the patient; and (d) the potential for misdirected AI investment in the specific context of CRC, where there may be less of an impact on patient mortality and morbidity outcomes, given that the larger issue that proliferates CRC screening is the problem of patient participation that AI currently does little to address. Through the amalgamation of these issues, the authors conclude that the way forward is to develop a more robust mixed methods framework around the auditing and evaluation of AI systems prior to system integration in clinical practice. Such a framework should be guided by principles of data transparency, the reproducibility of

ML models, and more balanced evaluation metrics that weigh quantitative ML metrics against important qualitative clinical considerations, such as (i) the impact of AI system integration on patient outcomes, (ii) the clinical utility of the system, (iii) HCI and clinical workflow considerations across varied socio-cultural and socio-organisational contexts, and (iv) the nature of clinical interaction. In this way, there can be increased confidence that the future of AI in CRC is safe, effective, equitable, and beneficial to clinicians, patients, and the broader health system.

Author Contributions: Conceptualization, S.A., P.T., K.-C.Y. and M.-C.W.; methodology, S.A. and P.T.; formal analysis, S.A. and P.T.; investigation, S.A. and P.T.; resources, S.A., P.T., K.-C.Y. and M.-C.W.; data curation, S.A. and P.T.; writing—original draft preparation, S.A. and P.T.; writing—review and editing, S.A., P.T., K.-C.Y. and M.-C.W.; supervision, P.T., K.-C.Y. and M.-C.W.; project administration, S.A., P.T., K.-C.Y. and M.-C.W. All authors have read and agreed to the published version of the manuscript.

Funding: This research received no external funding.

Institutional Review Board Statement: Not applicable.

Informed Consent Statement: Not applicable.

Data Availability Statement: Not applicable.

Acknowledgments: This research was supported by an Australian Government Research Training Program Scholarship.

Conflicts of Interest: The authors declare no conflict of interest.

References

1. Hinton, G. Deep Learning—A Technology with the Potential to Transform Health Care. *JAMA* **2018**, *320*, 1101. [CrossRef] [PubMed]
2. Geoff Hinton: On Radiology. 2016. Available online: https://www.youtube.com/watch?v=2HMPRXstSvQ (accessed on 22 January 2022).
3. International Radiology Societies Tackle Radiologist Shortage. Available online: https://www.rsna.org/news/2020/february/international-radiology-societies-and-shortage (accessed on 22 January 2022).
4. Harrison, M.I.; Koppel, R.; Bar-Lev, S. Unintended Consequences of Information Technologies in Health Care—an Interactive Sociotechnical Analysis. *J. Am. Med. Inform. Assoc. JAMIA* **2007**, *14*, 542–549. [CrossRef] [PubMed]
5. Ash, J.S.; Berg, M.; Coiera, E. Some Unintended Consequences of Information Technology in Health Care: The Nature of Patient Care Information System-Related Errors. *J. Am. Med. Inform. Assoc.* **2004**, *11*, 104–112. [CrossRef] [PubMed]
6. Sung, H.; Ferlay, J.; Siegel, R.L.; Laversanne, M.; Soerjomataram, I.; Jemal, A.; Bray, F. Global Cancer Statistics 2020: GLOBOCAN Estimates of Incidence and Mortality Worldwide for 36 Cancers in 185 Countries. *CA A Cancer J. Clin.* **2021**, *71*, 209–249. [CrossRef] [PubMed]
7. Yoshida, N.; Inoue, K.; Tomita, Y.; Kobayashi, R.; Hashimoto, H.; Sugino, S.; Hirose, R.; Dohi, O.; Yasuda, H.; Morinaga, Y.; et al. An Analysis about the Function of a New Artificial Intelligence, CAD EYE with the Lesion Recognition and Diagnosis for Colorectal Polyps in Clinical Practice. *Int. J. Colorectal Dis.* **2021**, *36*, 2237–2245. [CrossRef] [PubMed]
8. Barua, I.; Vinsard, D.G.; Jodal, H.C.; Løberg, M.; Kalager, M.; Holme, Ø.; Misawa, M.; Bretthauer, M.; Mori, Y. Artificial Intelligence for Polyp Detection during Colonoscopy: A Systematic Review and Meta-Analysis. *Endoscopy* **2020**, *53*, 277–284. [CrossRef]
9. Hassan, C.; Spadaccini, M.; Iannone, A.; Maselli, R.; Jovani, M.; Chandrasekar, V.T.; Antonelli, G.; Yu, H.; Areia, M.; Dinis-Ribeiro, M.; et al. Performance of Artificial Intelligence in Colonoscopy for Adenoma and Polyp Detection: A Systematic Review and Meta-Analysis. *Gastrointest. Endosc.* **2021**, *93*, 77–85. [CrossRef]
10. Ding, Z.; Shi, H.; Zhang, H.; Meng, L.; Fan, M.; Han, C.; Zhang, K.; Ming, F.; Xie, X.; Liu, H.; et al. Gastroenterologist-Level Identification of Small-Bowel Diseases and Normal Variants by Capsule Endoscopy Using a Deep-Learning Model. *Gastroenterology* **2019**, *157*, 1044–1054. [CrossRef]
11. Wang, K.S.; Yu, G.; Xu, C.; Meng, X.H.; Zhou, J.; Zheng, C.; Deng, Z.; Shang, L.; Liu, R.; Su, S.; et al. Accurate Diagnosis of Colorectal Cancer Based on Histopathology Images Using Artificial Intelligence. *BMC Med.* **2021**, *19*, 76. [CrossRef]
12. Skrede, O.-J.; Raedt, S.D.; Kleppe, A.; Hveem, T.S.; Liestøl, K.; Maddison, J.; Askautrud, H.A.; Pradhan, M.; Nesheim, J.A.; Albregtsen, F.; et al. Deep Learning for Prediction of Colorectal Cancer Outcome: A Discovery and Validation Study. *Lancet* **2020**, *395*, 350–360. [CrossRef]
13. Bychkov, D.; Linder, N.; Turkki, R.; Nordling, S.; Kovanen, P.E.; Verrill, C.; Walliander, M.; Lundin, M.; Haglund, C.; Lundin, J. Deep Learning Based Tissue Analysis Predicts Outcome in Colorectal Cancer. *Sci. Rep.* **2018**, *8*, 3395. [CrossRef] [PubMed]

14. Nartowt, B.J.; Hart, G.R.; Muhammad, W.; Liang, Y.; Stark, G.F.; Deng, J. Robust Machine Learning for Colorectal Cancer Risk Prediction and Stratification. *Front. Big Data* **2020**, *3*, 6. [CrossRef] [PubMed]
15. Kostopoulou, O.; Arora, K.; Pálfi, B. Using Cancer Risk Algorithms to Improve Risk Estimates and Referral Decisions. *Commun. Med.* **2022**, *2*, 2. [CrossRef]
16. Mori, Y.; Bretthauer, M.; Kalager, M. Hopes and Hypes for Artificial Intelligence in Colorectal Cancer Screening. *Gastroenterology* **2021**, *161*, 774–777. [CrossRef] [PubMed]
17. Abdul Halim, A.A.; Andrew, A.M.; Mohd Yasin, M.N.; Abd Rahman, M.A.; Jusoh, M.; Veeraperumal, V.; Rahim, H.A.; Illahi, U.; Abdul Karim, M.K.; Scavino, E. Existing and Emerging Breast Cancer Detection Technologies and Its Challenges: A Review. *Appl. Sci.* **2021**, *11*, 10753. [CrossRef]
18. Avanzo, M.; Trianni, A.; Botta, F.; Talamonti, C.; Stasi, M.; Iori, M. Artificial Intelligence and the Medical Physicist: Welcome to the Machine. *Appl. Sci.* **2021**, *11*, 1691. [CrossRef]
19. Panch, T.; Szolovits, P.; Atun, R. Artificial Intelligence, Machine Learning and Health Systems. *J. Glob. Health* **2018**, *8*, 020303. [CrossRef]
20. Beam, A.L.; Kohane, I.S. Big Data and Machine Learning in Health Care. *JAMA* **2018**, *319*, 1317. [CrossRef]
21. Goodfellow, I.; Bengio, Y.; Courville, A. *Deep Learning*; The Mit Press: Cambridge, MA, USA, 2016.
22. Litjens, G.; Kooi, T.; Bejnordi, B.E.; Setio, A.A.A.; Ciompi, F.; Ghafoorian, M.; van der Laak, J.A.W.M.; van Ginneken, B.; Sánchez, C.I. A Survey on Deep Learning in Medical Image Analysis. *Med. Image Anal.* **2017**, *42*, 60–88. [CrossRef]
23. Selvikvåg Lundervold, A.; Lundervold, A. An Overview of Deep Learning in Medical Imaging Focusing on MRI. *Z. Für Med. Phys.* **2018**, *29*, 102–127. [CrossRef]
24. Sarker, I.H. Machine Learning: Algorithms, Real-World Applications and Research Directions. *SN Comput. Sci.* **2021**, *2*, 160. [CrossRef] [PubMed]
25. LeCun, Y.; Bengio, Y.; Hinton, G. Deep Learning. *Nature* **2015**, *521*, 436–444. [CrossRef] [PubMed]
26. Esteva, A.; Kuprel, B.; Novoa, R.A.; Ko, J.; Swetter, S.M.; Blau, H.M.; Thrun, S. Dermatologist-Level Classification of Skin Cancer with Deep Neural Networks. *Nature* **2017**, *542*, 115–118. [CrossRef] [PubMed]
27. Nam, J.G.; Park, S.; Hwang, E.J.; Lee, J.H.; Jin, K.-N.; Lim, K.Y.; Vu, T.H.; Sohn, J.H.; Hwang, S.; Goo, J.M.; et al. Development and Validation of Deep Learning–Based Automatic Detection Algorithm for Malignant Pulmonary Nodules on Chest Radiographs. *Radiology* **2019**, *290*, 218–228. [CrossRef] [PubMed]
28. Nabulsi, Z.; Sellergren, A.; Jamshy, S.; Lau, C.; Santos, E.; Kiraly, A.P.; Ye, W.; Yang, J.; Pilgrim, R.; Kazemzadeh, S.; et al. Deep Learning for Distinguishing Normal versus Abnormal Chest Radiographs and Generalization to Two Unseen Diseases Tuberculosis and COVID-19. *Sci. Rep.* **2021**, *11*, 15523. [CrossRef]
29. Zech, J.R.; Badgeley, M.A.; Liu, M.; Costa, A.B.; Titano, J.J.; Oermann, E.K. Variable Generalization Performance of a Deep Learning Model to Detect Pneumonia in Chest Radiographs: A Cross-Sectional Study. *PLoS Med.* **2018**, *15*, e1002683. [CrossRef]
30. Yoshida, H.; Shimazu, T.; Kiyuna, T.; Marugame, A.; Yamashita, Y.; Cosatto, E.; Taniguchi, H.; Sekine, S.; Ochiai, A. Automated Histological Classification of Whole-Slide Images of Gastric Biopsy Specimens. *Gastric Cancer Off. J. Int. Gastric Cancer Assoc. Jpn. Gastric Cancer Assoc.* **2018**, *21*, 249–257. [CrossRef]
31. Hannun, A.Y.; Rajpurkar, P.; Haghpanahi, M.; Tison, G.H.; Bourn, C.; Turakhia, M.P.; Ng, A.Y. Cardiologist-Level Arrhythmia Detection and Classification in Ambulatory Electrocardiograms Using a Deep Neural Network. *Nat. Med.* **2019**, *25*, 65–69. [CrossRef]
32. Attia, Z.I.; Noseworthy, P.A.; Lopez-Jimenez, F.; Asirvatham, S.J.; Deshmukh, A.J.; Gersh, B.J.; Carter, R.E.; Yao, X.; Rabinstein, A.A.; Erickson, B.J.; et al. An Artificial Intelligence-Enabled ECG Algorithm for the Identification of Patients with Atrial Fibrillation during Sinus Rhythm: A Retrospective Analysis of Outcome Prediction. *Lancet* **2019**, *394*, 861–867. [CrossRef]
33. Al-Zaiti, S.; Besomi, L.; Bouzid, Z.; Faramand, Z.; Frisch, S.; Martin-Gill, C.; Gregg, R.; Saba, S.; Callaway, C.; Sejdić, E. Machine Learning-Based Prediction of Acute Coronary Syndrome Using Only the Pre-Hospital 12-Lead Electrocardiogram. *Nat. Commun.* **2020**, *11*, 3966. [CrossRef]
34. Desautels, T.; Calvert, J.; Hoffman, J.; Jay, M.; Kerem, Y.; Shieh, L.; Shimabukuro, D.; Chettipally, U.; Feldman, M.D.; Barton, C.; et al. Prediction of Sepsis in the Intensive Care Unit with Minimal Electronic Health Record Data: A Machine Learning Approach. *JMIR Med. Inform.* **2016**, *4*, e28. [CrossRef] [PubMed]
35. Kamnitsas, K.; Ferrante, E.; Parisot, S.; Ledig, C.; Nori, A.V.; Criminisi, A.; Rueckert, D.; Glocker, B. DeepMedic for Brain Tumor Segmentation. In *Brainlesion: Glioma, Multiple Sclerosis, Stroke and Traumatic Brain Injuries, Proceedings of the Third International Workshop, BrainLes 2017, Quebec City, QC, Canada, 14 September 2017*; Springer: Cham, Switzerland, 2016; pp. 138–149. [CrossRef]
36. Ding, Y.; Sohn, J.H.; Kawczynski, M.G.; Trivedi, H.; Harnish, R.; Jenkins, N.W.; Lituiev, D.; Copeland, T.P.; Aboian, M.S.; Mari Aparici, C.; et al. A Deep Learning Model to Predict a Diagnosis of Alzheimer Disease by Using 18F-FDG PET of the Brain. *Radiology* **2019**, *290*, 456–464. [CrossRef] [PubMed]
37. Chilamkurthy, S.; Ghosh, R.; Tanamala, S.; Biviji, M.; Campeau, N.G.; Venugopal, V.K.; Mahajan, V.; Rao, P.; Warier, P. Deep Learning Algorithms for Detection of Critical Findings in Head CT Scans: A Retrospective Study. *Lancet* **2018**, *392*, 2388–2396. [CrossRef]
38. Poplin, R.; Varadarajan, A.V.; Blumer, K.; Liu, Y.; McConnell, M.V.; Corrado, G.S.; Peng, L.; Webster, D.R. Prediction of Cardiovascular Risk Factors from Retinal Fundus Photographs via Deep Learning. *Nat. Biomed. Eng.* **2018**, *2*, 158–164. [CrossRef] [PubMed]

39. Lee, J.Y.; Jeong, J.; Song, E.M.; Ha, C.; Lee, H.J.; Koo, J.E.; Yang, D.-H.; Kim, N.; Byeon, J.-S. Real-Time Detection of Colon Polyps during Colonoscopy Using Deep Learning: Systematic Validation with Four Independent Datasets. *Sci. Rep.* **2020**, *10*, 8379. [CrossRef] [PubMed]
40. Miotto, R.; Wang, F.; Wang, S.; Jiang, X.; Dudley, J.T. Deep Learning for Healthcare: Review, Opportunities and Challenges. *Brief. Bioinform.* **2018**, *19*, 1236–1246. [CrossRef]
41. Aggarwal, R.; Sounderajah, V.; Martin, G.; Ting, D.S.W.; Karthikesalingam, A.; King, D.; Ashrafian, H.; Darzi, A. Diagnostic Accuracy of Deep Learning in Medical Imaging: A Systematic Review and Meta-Analysis. *NPJ Digit. Med.* **2021**, *4*, 65. [CrossRef]
42. Paullada, A.; Raji, I.D.; Bender, E.M.; Denton, E.; Hanna, A. Data and Its (Dis)Contents: A Survey of Dataset Development and Use in Machine Learning Research. *Patterns* **2021**, *2*, 100336. [CrossRef]
43. Sambasivan, N.; Kapania, S.; Highfill, H.; Akrong, D.; Paritosh, P.; Aroyo, L. Everyone Wants to Do the Model Work, Not the Data Work: Data Cascades in High-Stakes AI. In Proceedings of the 2021 CHI Conference on Human Factors in Computing Systems, Yokohama, Japan, 8–13 May 2021. [CrossRef]
44. Obermeyer, Z.; Powers, B.; Vogeli, C.; Mullainathan, S. Dissecting Racial Bias in an Algorithm Used to Manage the Health of Populations. *Science* **2019**, *366*, 447–453. [CrossRef]
45. Manrai, A.K.; Funke, B.H.; Rehm, H.L.; Olesen, M.S.; Maron, B.A.; Szolovits, P.; Margulies, D.M.; Loscalzo, J.; Kohane, I.S. Genetic Misdiagnoses and the Potential for Health Disparities. *New Engl. J. Med.* **2016**, *375*, 655–665. [CrossRef]
46. Shaw, R.J.; Corpas, M. A Collection of 2280 Public Domain (CC0) Curated Human Genotypes. *bioRxiv* **2017**. [CrossRef]
47. Fry, A.; Littlejohns, T.J.; Sudlow, C.; Doherty, N.; Adamska, L.; Sprosen, T.; Collins, R.; Allen, N.E. Comparison of Sociodemographic and Health-Related Characteristics of UK Biobank Participants with Those of the General Population. *Am. J. Epidemiol.* **2017**, *186*, 1026–1034. [CrossRef] [PubMed]
48. Zhou, Y.; Zhao, L.; Zhou, N.; Zhao, Y.; Marino, S.; Wang, T.; Sun, H.; Toga, A.W.; Dinov, I.D. Predictive Big Data Analytics Using the UK Biobank Data. *Sci. Rep.* **2019**, *9*, 6012. [CrossRef] [PubMed]
49. Abbasi, J. 23andMe, Big Data, and the Genetics of Depression. *JAMA* **2017**, *317*, 14. [CrossRef]
50. Kaur, H.; Pannu, H.S.; Malhi, A.K. A Systematic Review on Imbalanced Data Challenges in Machine Learning. *ACM Comput. Surv.* **2019**, *52*, 1–36. [CrossRef]
51. Nalepa, J.; Marcinkiewicz, M.; Kawulok, M. Data Augmentation for Brain-Tumor Segmentation: A Review. *Front. Comput. Neurosci.* **2019**, *13*, 83. [CrossRef]
52. Luo, Y.; Yin, L.; Bai, W.; Mao, K. An Appraisal of Incremental Learning Methods. *Entropy* **2020**, *22*, 1190. [CrossRef]
53. Ahmad, Z.; Rahim, S.; Zubair, M.; Abdul-Ghafar, J. Artificial Intelligence (AI) in Medicine, Current Applications and Future Role with Special Emphasis on Its Potential and Promise in Pathology: Present and Future Impact, Obstacles Including Costs and Acceptance among Pathologists, Practical and Philosophical Considerations. A Comprehensive Review. *Diagn. Pathol.* **2021**, *16*, 24. [CrossRef]
54. Liu, Y.; Geipel, M.M.; Tietz, C.; Buettner, F. TIMELY: Improving Labelling Consistency in Medical Imaging for Cell Type Classification. *arXiv* **2020**, arXiv:2007.05307.
55. Yu, K.-H.; Kohane, I.S. Framing the Challenges of Artificial Intelligence in Medicine. *BMJ Qual. Saf.* **2018**, *28*, 238–241. [CrossRef]
56. Dike, H.U.; Zhou, Y.; Deveerasetty, K.K.; Wu, Q. Unsupervised Learning Based on Artificial Neural Network: A Review. In Proceedings of the 2018 IEEE International Conference on Cyborg and Bionic Systems (CBS), Shenzhen, China, 25–27 October 2018. [CrossRef]
57. Montague, P.R. Reinforcement Learning: An Introduction, by Sutton, RS and Barto, AG. *Trends Cogn. Sci.* **1999**, *3*, 360. [CrossRef]
58. Liu, S.; See, K.C.; Ngiam, K.Y.; Celi, L.A.; Sun, X.; Feng, M. Reinforcement Learning for Clinical Decision Support in Critical Care: Comprehensive Review. *J. Med. Internet Res.* **2020**, *22*, e18477. [CrossRef] [PubMed]
59. Plassard, A.J.; Davis, L.T.; Newton, A.T.; Resnick, S.M.; Landman, B.A.; Bermudez, C. Learning Implicit Brain MRI Manifolds with Deep Learning. In Proceedings of the Medical Imaging 2018: Image Processing, Houston, TX, USA, 10–15 February 2018. [CrossRef]
60. Miotto, R.; Li, L.; Kidd, B.A.; Dudley, J.T. Deep Patient: An Unsupervised Representation to Predict the Future of Patients from the Electronic Health Records. *Sci. Rep.* **2016**, *6*, 26094. [CrossRef]
61. Prasad, N.; Cheng, L.-F.; Chivers, C.; Draugelis, M.; Engelhardt, B.E. A Reinforcement Learning Approach to Weaning of Mechanical Ventilation in Intensive Care Units. *arXiv* **2017**, arXiv:1704.06300.
62. Raghu, A.; Komorowski, M.; Ahmed, I.; Celi, L.; Szolovits, P.; Ghassemi, M. Deep Reinforcement Learning for Sepsis Treatment. *arXiv* **2017**, arXiv:1711.09602.
63. Palacio-Niño, J.-O.; Berzal, F. Evaluation Metrics for Unsupervised Learning Algorithms. *arXiv* **2019**, arXiv:1905.05667.
64. Kleinberg, J. An Impossibility Theorem for Clustering. In Proceedings of the 15th International Conference on Neural Information Processing Systems, Cambridge, MA, USA, 1 January 2002; MIT Press: Cambridge, MA, USA, 2002.
65. Wu, E.; Wu, K.; Daneshjou, R.; Ouyang, D.; Ho, D.E.; Zou, J. How Medical AI Devices are Evaluated: Limitations and Recommendations from an Analysis of FDA Approvals. *Nat. Med.* **2021**, *27*, 582–584. [CrossRef]
66. Kim, D.W.; Jang, H.Y.; Kim, K.W.; Shin, Y.; Park, S.H. Design Characteristics of Studies Reporting the Performance of Artificial Intelligence Algorithms for Diagnostic Analysis of Medical Images: Results from Recently Published Papers. *Korean J. Radiol.* **2019**, *20*, 405. [CrossRef]

67. Kelly, C.J.; Karthikesalingam, A.; Suleyman, M.; Corrado, G.; King, D. Key Challenges for Delivering Clinical Impact with Artificial Intelligence. *BMC Med.* **2019**, *17*, 195. [CrossRef]
68. Macrae, F.A. Colorectal Cancer: Epidemiology, Risk Factors, and Protective Factors. UpToDate. 2022. Available online: https://www.uptodate.com/contents/colorectal-cancer-epidemiology-risk-factors-and-protective-factors (accessed on 24 January 2022).
69. Lotfi-Jam, K.; O'Reilly, C.; Feng, C.; Wakefield, M.; Durkin, S.; Broun, K. Increasing Bowel Cancer Screening Participation: Integrating Population-Wide, Primary Care and More Targeted Approaches. *Public Health Res. Pract.* **2019**, *29*, 2921916. [CrossRef]
70. Brenner, H.; Chen, C. The Colorectal Cancer Epidemic: Challenges and Opportunities for Primary, Secondary and Tertiary Prevention. *Br. J. Cancer* **2018**, *119*, 785–792. [CrossRef] [PubMed]
71. Sun, C.; Shrivastava, A.; Singh, S.; Gupta, A. Revisiting Unreasonable Effectiveness of Data in Deep Learning Era. In Proceedings of the 2017 IEEE International Conference on Computer Vision (ICCV), Venice, Italy, 22–29 October 2017. [CrossRef]
72. Raji, I.D.; Fried, G. About Face: A Survey of Facial Recognition Evaluation. *arXiv* **2021**, arXiv:2102.00813.
73. Zhao, J.; Wang, T.; Yatskar, M.; Ordonez, V.; Chang, K.-W. Gender Bias in Coreference Resolution: Evaluation and Debiasing Methods. In Proceedings of the 2018 Conference of the North American Chapter of the Association for Computational Linguistics: Human Language Technologies, Volume 2 (Short Papers), New Orleans, LA, USA, 1–6 June 2018. [CrossRef]
74. Garg, N.; Schiebinger, L.; Jurafsky, D.; Zou, J. Word Embeddings Quantify 100 Years of Gender and Ethnic Stereotypes. *Proc. Natl. Acad. Sci. USA* **2018**, *115*, E3635–E3644. [CrossRef] [PubMed]
75. van Miltenburg, E. Stereotyping and Bias in the Flickr30K Dataset. *arXiv* **2016**, arXiv:1605.06083.
76. Hutchinson, B.; Prabhakaran, V.; Denton, E.; Webster, K.; Zhong, Y.; Denuyl, S. Social Biases in NLP Models as Barriers for Persons with Disabilities. *arXiv* **2020**, arXiv:2005.00813.
77. De, M. *Closing the Gap in a Generation: Health Equity through Action on the Social Determinants of Health*; WHO Press: Geneva, Switzerland, 2008.
78. Showell, C.; Turner, P. The PLU Problem: Are We Designing Personal Ehealth for People like Us? *Stud. Health Technol. Inform.* **2013**, *183*, 276–280.
79. Zerilli, J.; Knott, A.; Maclaurin, J.; Gavaghan, C. Algorithmic Decision-Making and the Control Problem. *Minds Mach.* **2019**, *29*, 555–578. [CrossRef]
80. Parasuraman, R.; Manzey, D.H. Complacency and Bias in Human Use of Automation: An Attentional Integration. *Hum. Factors J. Hum. Factors Ergon. Soc.* **2010**, *52*, 381–410. [CrossRef]
81. Navarro, M.; Nicolas, A.; Ferrandez, A.; Lanas, A. Colorectal Cancer Population Screening Programs Worldwide in 2016: An Update. *World J. Gastroenterol.* **2017**, *23*, 3632. [CrossRef]
82. Wan, N.; Weinberg, D.; Liu, T.-Y.; Niehaus, K.; Ariazi, E.A.; Delubac, D.; Kannan, A.; White, B.; Bailey, M.; Bertin, M.; et al. Machine Learning Enables Detection of Early-Stage Colorectal Cancer by Whole-Genome Sequencing of Plasma Cell-Free DNA. *BMC Cancer* **2019**, *19*, 832. [CrossRef]
83. Chan, H.-C.; Chattopadhyay, A.; Chuang, E.Y.; Lu, T.-P. Development of a Gene-Based Prediction Model for Recurrence of Colorectal Cancer Using an Ensemble Learning Algorithm. *Front. Oncol.* **2021**, *11*, 631056. [CrossRef] [PubMed]
84. Challen, R.; Denny, J.; Pitt, M.; Gompels, L.; Edwards, T.; Tsaneva-Atanasova, K. Artificial Intelligence, Bias and Clinical Safety. *BMJ Qual. Saf.* **2019**, *28*, 231–237. [CrossRef] [PubMed]
85. Elston, D.M. Confirmation Bias in Medical Decision-Making. *J. Am. Acad. Dermatol.* **2020**, *82*, 572. [CrossRef] [PubMed]
86. Dawson, N.V.; Arkes, H.R. Systematic Errors in Medical Decision Making. *J. Gen. Intern. Med.* **1987**, *2*, 183–187. [CrossRef]
87. Bond, R.R.; Novotny, T.; Andrsova, I.; Koc, L.; Sisakova, M.; Finlay, D.; Guldenring, D.; McLaughlin, J.; Peace, A.; McGilligan, V.; et al. Automation Bias in Medicine: The Influence of Automated Diagnoses on Interpreter Accuracy and Uncertainty When Reading Electrocardiograms. *J. Electrocardiol.* **2018**, *51*, S6–S11. [CrossRef]
88. Tsai, T.L.; Fridsma, D.B.; Gatti, G. Computer Decision Support as a Source of Interpretation Error: The Case of Electrocardiograms. *J. Am. Med. Inform. Assoc.* **2003**, *10*, 478–483. [CrossRef]
89. Nestor, B.; McDermott, M.B.A.; Chauhan, G.; Naumann, T.; Hughes, M.C.; Goldenberg, A.; Ghassemi, M. Rethinking Clinical Prediction: Why Machine Learning Must Consider Year of Care and Feature Aggregation. *arXiv* **2018**, arXiv:1811.12583.
90. Davis, S.E.; Greevy, R.A.; Fonnesbeck, C.; Lasko, T.A.; Walsh, C.G.; Matheny, M.E. A Nonparametric Updating Method to Correct Clinical Prediction Model Drift. *J. Am. Med. Inform. Assoc.* **2019**, *26*, 1448–1457. [CrossRef]
91. Duckworth, C.; Chmiel, F.P.; Burns, D.K.; Zlatev, Z.D.; White, N.M.; Daniels, T.W.V.; Kiuber, M.; Boniface, M.J. Using Explainable Machine Learning to Characterise Data Drift and Detect Emergent Health Risks for Emergency Department Admissions during COVID-19. *Sci. Rep.* **2021**, *11*, 23017. [CrossRef]
92. Davis, S.E.; Lasko, T.A.; Chen, G.; Siew, E.D.; Matheny, M.E. Calibration Drift in Regression and Machine Learning Models for Acute Kidney Injury. *J. Am. Med. Inform. Assoc.* **2017**, *24*, 1052–1061. [CrossRef]
93. Done, J.Z.; Fang, S.H. Young-Onset Colorectal Cancer: A Review. *World J. Gastrointest. Oncol.* **2021**, *13*, 856–866. [CrossRef] [PubMed]
94. Saad El Din, K.; Loree, J.M.; Sayre, E.C.; Gill, S.; Brown, C.J.; Dau, H.; De Vera, M.A. Trends in the Epidemiology of Young-Onset Colorectal Cancer: A Worldwide Systematic Review. *BMC Cancer* **2020**, *20*, 288. [CrossRef] [PubMed]
95. Jie, Z.; Zhiying, Z.; Li, L. A Meta-Analysis of Watson for Oncology in Clinical Application. *Sci. Rep.* **2021**, *11*, 5792. [CrossRef] [PubMed]

96. Su, J.; Vargas, D.V.; Sakurai, K. One Pixel Attack for Fooling Deep Neural Networks. *IEEE Trans. Evol. Comput.* **2019**, *23*, 828–841. [CrossRef]
97. Li, J.W.; Chia, T.; Fock, K.M.; Chong, K.D.W.; Wong, Y.J.; Ang, T.L. Artificial Intelligence and Polyp Detection in Colonoscopy: Use of a Single Neural Network to Achieve Rapid Polyp Localization for Clinical Use. *J. Gastroenterol. Hepatol.* **2021**, *36*, 3298–3307. [CrossRef]
98. Liu, C.; Liu, X.; Wu, F.; Xie, M.; Feng, Y.; Hu, C. Using Artificial Intelligence (Watson for Oncology) for Treatment Recommendations amongst Chinese Patients with Lung Cancer: Feasibility Study. *J. Med. Internet Res.* **2018**, *20*, e11087. [CrossRef]
99. Strickland, E. IBM Watson, Heal Thyself: How IBM Overpromised and Underdelivered on AI Health Care. *IEEE Spectr.* **2019**, *56*, 24–31. [CrossRef]
100. Holzinger, A.; Biemann, C.; Pattichis, C.S.; Kell, D.B. What Do We Need to Build Explainable AI Systems for the Medical Domain? *arXiv* **2017**, arXiv:1712.09923.
101. Goodman, B.; Flaxman, S. European Union Regulations on Algorithmic Decision-Making and a Right to Explanation. *AI Mag.* **2017**, *38*, 50–57. [CrossRef]
102. Selvaraju, R.R.; Cogswell, M.; Das, A.; Vedantam, R.; Parikh, D.; Batra, D. Grad-CAM: Visual Explanations from Deep Networks via Gradient-Based Localization. *Int. J. Comput. Vis.* **2020**, *128*, 336–359. [CrossRef]
103. Rajpurkar, P.; Irvin, J.; Ball, R.L.; Zhu, K.; Yang, B.; Mehta, H.; Duan, T.; Ding, D.; Bagul, A.; Langlotz, C.P.; et al. Deep Learning for Chest Radiograph Diagnosis: A Retrospective Comparison of the CheXNeXt Algorithm to Practicing Radiologists. *PLoS Med.* **2018**, *15*, e1002686. [CrossRef] [PubMed]
104. Panwar, H.; Gupta, P.K.; Siddiqui, M.K.; Morales-Menendez, R.; Bhardwaj, P.; Singh, V. A Deep Learning and Grad-CAM Based Color Visualization Approach for Fast Detection of COVID-19 Cases Using Chest X-Ray and CT-Scan Images. *Chaos Solitons Fractals* **2020**, *140*, 110190. [CrossRef] [PubMed]
105. De Fauw, J.; Ledsam, J.R.; Romera-Paredes, B.; Nikolov, S.; Tomasev, N.; Blackwell, S.; Askham, H.; Glorot, X.; O'Donoghue, B.; Visentin, D.; et al. Clinically Applicable Deep Learning for Diagnosis and Referral in Retinal Disease. *Nat. Med.* **2018**, *24*, 1342–1350. [CrossRef] [PubMed]
106. Yosinski, J.; Clune, J.; Nguyen, A.; Fuchs, T.; Lipson, H. Understanding Neural Networks through Deep Visualization. *arXiv* **2015**, arXiv:1506.06579.
107. Adler, P.; Falk, C.; Friedler, S.A.; Rybeck, G.; Scheidegger, C.; Smith, B.; Venkatasubramanian, S. Auditing Black-Box Models for Indirect Influence. *arXiv* **2016**, arXiv:1602.07043.
108. Spratt, E.L. Dream Formulations and Deep Neural Networks: Humanistic Themes in the Iconology of the Machine-Learned Image. *arXiv* **2018**, arXiv:1802.01274.
109. Currie, G.; Hawk, K.E. Ethical and Legal Challenges of Artificial Intelligence in Nuclear Medicine. *Semin. Nucl. Med.* **2020**, *51*, 120–125. [CrossRef]
110. Ma, J.; Sheridan, R.P.; Liaw, A.; Dahl, G.E.; Svetnik, V. Deep Neural Nets as a Method for Quantitative Structure–Activity Relationships. *J. Chem. Inf. Modeling* **2015**, *55*, 263–274. [CrossRef]
111. Alipanahi, B.; Delong, A.; Weirauch, M.T.; Frey, B.J. Predicting the Sequence Specificities of DNA- and RNA-Binding Proteins by Deep Learning. *Nat. Biotechnol.* **2015**, *33*, 831–838. [CrossRef]
112. Jumper, J.; Evans, R.; Pritzel, A.; Green, T.; Figurnov, M.; Ronneberger, O.; Tunyasuvunakool, K.; Bates, R.; Žídek, A.; Potapenko, A.; et al. Highly Accurate Protein Structure Prediction with AlphaFold. *Nature* **2021**, *596*, 583–589. [CrossRef]
113. Goh, K.H.; Wang, L.; Yeow, A.Y.K.; Poh, H.; Li, K.; Yeow, J.J.L.; Tan, G.Y.H. Artificial Intelligence in Sepsis Early Prediction and Diagnosis Using Unstructured Data in Healthcare. *Nat. Commun.* **2021**, *12*, 711. [CrossRef]
114. Yala, A.; Mikhael, P.G.; Strand, F.; Lin, G.; Satuluru, S.; Kim, T.; Banerjee, I.; Gichoya, J.; Trivedi, H.; Lehman, C.D.; et al. Multi-Institutional Validation of a Mammography-Based Breast Cancer Risk Model. *J. Clin. Oncol.* **2021**, JCO2101337. [CrossRef]
115. Yu, C.; Helwig, E.J. The Role of AI Technology in Prediction, Diagnosis and Treatment of Colorectal Cancer. *Artif. Intell. Rev.* **2021**, *55*, 323–343. [CrossRef]
116. Kim, N.H.; Jung, Y.S.; Jeong, W.S.; Yang, H.-J.; Park, S.-K.; Choi, K.; Park, D.I. Miss Rate of Colorectal Neoplastic Polyps and Risk Factors for Missed Polyps in Consecutive Colonoscopies. *Intest. Res.* **2017**, *15*, 411–418. [CrossRef]
117. Corley, D.A.; Jensen, C.D.; Marks, A.R.; Zhao, W.K.; Lee, J.K.; Doubeni, C.A.; Zauber, A.G.; de Boer, J.; Fireman, B.H.; Schottinger, J.E.; et al. Adenoma Detection Rate and Risk of Colorectal Cancer and Death. *New Engl. J. Med.* **2014**, *370*, 1298–1306. [CrossRef]
118. Gini, A.; Jansen, E.E.L.; Zielonke, N.; Meester, R.G.S.; Senore, C.; Anttila, A.; Segnan, N.; Mlakar, D.N.; de Koning, H.J.; Lansdorp-Vogelaar, I.; et al. Impact of Colorectal Cancer Screening on Cancer-Specific Mortality in Europe: A Systematic Review. *Eur. J. Cancer* **2020**, *127*, 224–235. [CrossRef]
119. Lew, J.-B.; St John, D.J.B.; Xu, X.-M.; Greuter, M.J.E.; Caruana, M.; Cenin, D.R.; He, E.; Saville, M.; Grogan, P.; Coupé, V.M.H.; et al. Long-Term Evaluation of Benefits, Harms, and Cost-Effectiveness of the National Bowel Cancer Screening Program in Australia: A Modelling Study. *Lancet Public Health* **2017**, *2*, e331–e340. [CrossRef]
120. Li, M.; Olver, I.; Keefe, D.; Holden, C.; Worthley, D.; Price, T.; Karapetis, C.; Miller, C.; Powell, K.; Buranyi-Trevarton, D.; et al. Pre-Diagnostic Colonoscopies Reduce Cancer Mortality—Results from Linked Population-Based Data in South Australia. *BMC Cancer* **2019**, *19*, 856. [CrossRef]

121. Pignone, M.P.; Flitcroft, K.L.; Howard, K.; Trevena, L.J.; Salkeld, G.P.; St John, D.J.B. Costs and Cost-Effectiveness of Full Implementation of a Biennial Faecal Occult Blood Test Screening Program for Bowel Cancer in Australia. *Med. J. Aust.* **2011**, *194*, 180–185. [CrossRef]
122. Cole, S.R.; Tucker, G.R.; Osborne, J.M.; Byrne, S.E.; Bampton, P.A.; Fraser, R.J.L.; Young, G.P. Shift to Earlier Stage at Diagnosis as a Consequence of the National Bowel Cancer Screening Program. *Med. J. Aust.* **2013**, *198*, 327–330. [CrossRef]
123. Ananda, S.S.; McLaughlin, S.J.; Chen, F.; Hayes, I.P.; Hunter, A.A.; Skinner, I.J.; Steel, M.C.A.; Jones, I.T.; Hastie, I.A.; Rieger, N.A.; et al. Initial Impact of Australia's National Bowel Cancer Screening Program. *Med. J. Aust.* **2009**, *191*, 378–381. [CrossRef]
124. Howe, M. The National Bowel Cancer Screening Program: Time to Achieve Its Potential to Save Lives | PHRP. Available online: https://www.phrp.com.au/issues/july-2019-volume-29-issue-2/the-national-bowel-cancer-screening-program-time-to-achieve-its-potential-to-save-lives/ (accessed on 4 January 2022).
125. European Guidelines for Quality Assurance in Colorectal Cancer Screening and Diagnosis: Overview and Introduction to the Full Supplement Publication. *Endoscopy* **2012**, *45*, 51–59. [CrossRef]
126. National Bowel Cancer Screening Program Monitoring Report 2021. Summary. Available online: https://www.aihw.gov.au/reports/cancer-screening/nbcsp-monitoring-report-2021/summary (accessed on 12 January 2022).
127. Rao, S.K.; Schilling, T.F.; Sequist, T.D. Challenges in the Management of Positive Fecal Occult Blood Tests. *J. Gen. Intern. Med.* **2009**, *24*, 356–360. [CrossRef]
128. Levin, B.; Lieberman, D.A.; McFarland, B.; Smith, R.A.; Brooks, D.; Andrews, K.S.; Dash, C.; Giardiello, F.M.; Glick, S.; Levin, T.R.; et al. Screening and Surveillance for the Early Detection of Colorectal Cancer and Adenomatous Polyps, 2008: A Joint Guideline from the American Cancer Society, the US Multi-Society Task Force on Colorectal Cancer, and the American College of Radiology. *CA Cancer J. Clin.* **2018**, *58*, 130–160. [CrossRef]
129. Green, B.B.; Baldwin, L.-M.; West, I.I.; Schwartz, M.; Coronado, G.D. Low Rates of Colonoscopy Follow-up after a Positive Fecal Immunochemical Test in a Medicaid Health Plan Delivered Mailed Colorectal Cancer Screening Program. *J. Prim. Care Community Health* **2020**, *11*, 215013272095852. [CrossRef]
130. Shahidi, N.; Cheung, W.Y. Colorectal Cancer Screening: Opportunities to Improve Uptake, Outcomes, and Disparities. *World J. Gastrointest. Endosc.* **2016**, *8*, 733. [CrossRef]
131. Hurtado, J.L.; Bacigalupe, A.; Calvo, M.; Esnaola, S.; Mendizabal, N.; Portillo, I.; Idigoras, I.; Millán, E.; Arana-Arri, E. Social Inequalities in a Population Based Colorectal Cancer Screening Programme in the Basque Country. *BMC Public Health* **2015**, *15*, 1021. [CrossRef]
132. Plumb, A.A.; Ghanouni, A.; Rainbow, S.; Djedovic, N.; Marshall, S.; Stein, J.; Taylor, S.A.; Halligan, S.; Lyratzopoulos, G.; von Wagner, C. Patient Factors Associated with Non-Attendance at Colonoscopy after a Positive Screening Faecal Occult Blood Test. *J. Med. Screen.* **2016**, *24*, 12–19. [CrossRef]
133. Earl, V.; Beasley, D.; Ye, C.; Halpin, S.N.; Gauthreaux, N.; Escoffery, C.; Chawla, S. Barriers and Facilitators to Colorectal Cancer Screening in African-American Men. *Dig. Dis. Sci.* **2021**, *67*, 463–472. [CrossRef]
134. Muthukrishnan, M.; Arnold, L.D.; James, A.S. Patients' Self-Reported Barriers to Colon Cancer Screening in Federally Qualified Health Center Settings. *Prev. Med. Rep.* **2019**, *15*, 100896. [CrossRef]
135. Turner, B.; Myers, R.E.; Hyslop, T.; Hauck, W.W.; Weinberg, D.; Brigham, T.; Grana, J.; Rothermel, T.; Schlackman, N. Physician and Patient Factors Associated with Ordering a Colon Evaluation after a Positive Fecal Occult Blood Test. *J. Gen. Intern. Med.* **2003**, *18*, 357–363. [CrossRef]
136. Jones, R.M.; Woolf, S.H.; Cunningham, T.D.; Johnson, R.E.; Krist, A.H.; Rothemich, S.F.; Vernon, S.W. The Relative Importance of Patient-Reported Barriers to Colorectal Cancer Screening. *Am. J. Prev. Med.* **2010**, *38*, 499–507. [CrossRef]
137. Wangmar, J.; Wengström, Y.; Jervaeus, A.; Hultcrantz, R.; Fritzell, K. Decision-Making about Participation in Colorectal Cancer Screening in Sweden: Autonomous, Value-Dependent but Uninformed? *Patient Educ. Couns.* **2020**, *104*, 919–926. [CrossRef]
138. Nielsen, J.B.; Berg-Beckhoff, G.; Leppin, A. To Do or Not to Do—A Survey Study on Factors Associated with Participating in the Danish Screening Program for Colorectal Cancer. *BMC Health Serv. Res.* **2021**, *21*, 43. [CrossRef]
139. Clinical Practice Guidelines for the Prevention, Early Detection and Management of Colorectal Cancer—Cancer Guidelines Wiki. Available online: https://wiki.cancer.org.au/australia/Guidelines:Colorectal_cancer (accessed on 12 January 2022).
140. Hubbard, R.A.; Johnson, E.; Hsia, R.; Rutter, C.M. The Cumulative Risk of False-Positive Fecal Occult Blood Test after 10 Years of Colorectal Cancer Screening. *Cancer Epidemiol. Biomark. Prev. A Publ. Am. Assoc. Cancer Res. Cosponsored Am. Soc. Prev. Oncol.* **2013**, *22*, 1612–1619. [CrossRef]
141. Meklin, J.; Syrjänen, K.; Eskelinen, M. Fecal Occult Blood Tests in Colorectal Cancer Screening: Systematic Review and Meta-Analysis of Traditional and New-Generation Fecal Immunochemical Tests. *Anticancer Res.* **2020**, *40*, 3591–3604. [CrossRef]
142. Llovet, D.; Serenity, M.; Conn, L.G.; Bravo, C.A.; McCurdy, B.R.; Dubé, C.; Baxter, N.N.; Paszat, L.; Rabeneck, L.; Peters, A.; et al. Reasons for Lack of Follow-up Colonoscopy among Persons with a Positive Fecal Occult Blood Test Result: A Qualitative Study. *Am. J. Gastroenterol.* **2018**, *113*, 1872–1880. [CrossRef]
143. Dawson, G.; Crane, M.; Lyons, C.; Burnham, A.; Bowman, T.; Perez, D.; Travaglia, J. General Practitioners' Perceptions of Population Based Bowel Screening and Their Influence on Practice: A Qualitative Study. *BMC Fam. Pract.* **2017**, *18*, 36. [CrossRef]
144. Hanks, H.; Veitch, C.; Harris, M. Colorectal Cancer Management—The Role of the GP. *Aust. Fam. Physician* **2008**, *37*, 259–261.
145. Baus, A.; Wright, L.E.; Kennedy-Rea, S.; Conn, M.E.; Eason, S.; Boatman, D.; Pollard, C.; Calkins, A.; Gadde, D. Leveraging Electronic Health Records Data for Enhanced Colorectal Cancer Screening Efforts. *J. Appalach. Health* **2020**, *2*, 53–63.

146. Knight, W. The Dark Secret at the Heart of AI. Available online: https://www.technologyreview.com/2017/04/11/5113/the-dark-secret-at-the-heart-of-ai/ (accessed on 16 January 2022).
147. Cui, L.; Lu, Y.; Sun, J.; Fu, Q.; Xu, X.; Wu, H.; Chen, J. RFLMDA: A Novel Reinforcement Learning-Based Computational Model for Human MicroRNA-Disease Association Prediction. *Biomolecules* **2021**, *11*, 1835. [CrossRef]
148. Middleton, B.; Bloomrosen, M.; Dente, M.A.; Hashmat, B.; Koppel, R.; Overhage, J.M.; Payne, T.H.; Rosenbloom, S.T.; Weaver, C.; Zhang, J. Enhancing Patient Safety and Quality of Care by Improving the Usability of Electronic Health Record Systems: Recommendations from AMIA. *J. Am. Med. Inform. Assoc.* **2013**, *20*, e2–e8. [CrossRef]
149. ML Evaluation Standards. Available online: https://ml-eval.github.io (accessed on 31 January 2022).

applied sciences

MDPI

Article

Exploring Early Prediction of Chronic Kidney Disease Using Machine Learning Algorithms for Small and Imbalanced Datasets

Andressa C. M. da Silveira [1,†], Álvaro Sobrinho [2,3,*,†], Leandro Dias da Silva [3,†], Evandro de Barros Costa [4,†], Maria Eliete Pinheiro [4,†] and Angelo Perkusich [5,†]

1 Electrical Engineering Department, Federal University of Campina Grande, Campina Grande 58428-830, Brazil; andressa.queiroz@ee.ufcg.edu.br
2 Computer Science, Federal University of the Agreste of Pernambuco, Garanhuns 55292-270, Brazil
3 Computing Institute, Federal University of Alagoas, Maceió 57072-900, Brazil; leandrodias@ic.ufal.br
4 Faculty of Medicine, Federal University of Alagoas, Maceió 57072-900, Brazil; evandro@ic.ufal.br (E.d.B.C.); elietepinheiro@uol.com.br (M.E.P.)
5 Virtus Research, Development and Innovation Center, Federal University of Campina Grande, Campina Grande 58428-830, Brazil; perkusic@virtus.ufcg.edu.br
* Correspondence: alvaro.alvares@ufape.edu.br
† These authors contributed equally to this work.

Abstract: Chronic kidney disease (CKD) is a worldwide public health problem, usually diagnosed in the late stages of the disease. To alleviate such issue, investment in early prediction is necessary. The purpose of this study is to assist the early prediction of CKD, addressing problems related to imbalanced and limited-size datasets. We used data from medical records of Brazilians with or without a diagnosis of CKD, containing the following attributes: hypertension, diabetes mellitus, creatinine, urea, albuminuria, age, gender, and glomerular filtration rate. We present an oversampling approach based on manual and automated augmentation. We experimented with the synthetic minority oversampling technique (SMOTE), Borderline-SMOTE, and Borderline-SMOTE SVM. We implemented models based on the algorithms: decision tree (DT), random forest, and multi-class AdaBoosted DTs. We also applied the overall local accuracy and local class accuracy methods for dynamic classifier selection; and the k-nearest oracles-union, k-nearest oracles-eliminate, and META-DES for dynamic ensemble selection. We analyzed the models' performances using the hold-out validation, multiple stratified cross-validation (CV), and nested CV. The DT model presented the highest accuracy score (98.99%) using the manual augmentation and SMOTE. Our approach can assist in designing systems for the early prediction of CKD using imbalanced and limited-size datasets.

Keywords: primary care; machine learning; limited size datasets; public health; imbalanced datasets

1. Introduction

The high prevalence and mortality rates of persons with chronic diseases, such as chronic kidney disease (CKD) [1], are real-world public health problems. The world health organization (WHO) estimated that chronic diseases would cause 60 percent of the deaths reported in 2005, 80 percent in low-income and lower-middle-income countries, increasing to 66.7 percent in 2020 [2]. According to the WHO health statistics 2019 [3], people who live in low-income and lower-middle-income countries have a higher probability of dying prematurely from known chronic diseases such as diabetes mellitus (DM). Estimates reveal that in 2045, about 628.6 million people will have DM, with 79% of them living in low-income and lower-middle-income countries [4].

For CKD's specific case, the early prediction and monitoring of this disease and its risk factors reduce the CKD progression and prevent adverse events, such as sudden development of diabetic nephropathy. Thus, this study considers CKD early prediction and monitoring focusing on a dataset from people who live in Brazil, a continental-size developing country. Developing countries stand for low- and middle-income regions, while developed countries are high-income regions, such as the USA [5]. Developing countries suffer from increased mortality rates caused by chronic diseases, e.g., CKD, arterial hypertension (AH), and DM [6]. AH and DM are two of the most common CKD risk factors. People with type 1 or type 2 DM are at high risk of developing diabetic nephropathy [7], while severe AH cases may increase kidney damage. For example, in 2019, about 10 percent of the adult Brazilian population was aware of having kidney damage, while about 70 percent remained undiagnosed [8].

The CKD is characterized by permanent damage, reducing the kidneys' excretory function, measured using glomerular filtration [9]. However, the diagnosis usually occurs during more advanced stages because it is asymptomatic, postponing the application of countermeasures, decreasing people's quality of life, and possibly leading to lethal kidney damage. For example, in 2010, about 500–650 people per million of the Brazilian population faced dialysis and kidney transplantation [10]. This number has grown, warning governments about the relevance of the CKD early prediction. In 2016, according to the Brazilian chronic dialysis survey, the number of patients under dialysis was 122,825.00, increasing this number by 31,000.00 in the last five years [11]. In 2017, the prevalence and incidence rates of patients under dialysis were 610 and 194 per million [12]. The incidence continued to be high in 2018 (133,464.00) [13]. Estimates also indicate that, in 2030, about 4 million patients will be under dialysis worldwide [14].

The high prevalence and incidence of dialysis and kidney transplantation increase public health costs. Therefore, CKD has an expressive impact on the health economics perspective [15]. For instance, the Brazilian Ministry of Health reported that transplantation and its procedures spent about 720 million reais in 2008 and 1.3 billion in 2015 [16]. According to the Brazilian Ministry of Health, in 2020, the Brazilian government spent more than 1.4 billion reais for hemodialysis procedures. The costs and the high rates of persons waiting for transplantation suggest the increased public spending on kidney diseases. Preventing CKD has a relevant role in reducing mortality rates and public health costs [17]. The CKD early prediction is even more challenging for people who live in remote and hard-to-reach settings because of either lack of or precarious primary care. CKD early prediction is relevant to improve CKD screening and reduce public health costs.

In this study, we address four problems. The first problem is size limitation, in which training models using small datasets can result in skewed performance estimates [18]. The second problem is the imbalance problem [19], in which models may underperform in minority classes, producing misleading results [20]. The third problem is the choice of the algorithm to address imbalanced and limited-size datasets. The fourth problem is the early prediction of CKD using risk levels (low risk, moderate risk, high risk, and very high risk) and a reduced number of biomarkers. CKD datasets with risk level evaluation are very scarce and of limited size. The majority of available datasets are composed of binary classes. The analyses based on risk levels enable patients to have more detailed explanations about the evaluation results. In the medical area, the availability of imbalanced and limited-size datasets is common. Although the usage of limited-size datasets may be questioned, it is already evidenced that such datasets can be relevant for the medical area [21].

Our study relies on data from medical records of Brazilians to provide classification models to assist in the early prediction of CKD in developing countries. We performed comparisons between machine learning (ML) models, considering ensemble and non-ensemble approaches. This work complements the results presented in our previous study [5], where a comparative analysis was performed with the following ML techniques: decision tree (DT), random forest (RF), naive Bayes, support vector machine (SVM), multilayer perceptron, and k-nearest neighbor (KNN). In such a previous study, DT and RF presented the highest performances. However, in our previous experiments, we did not apply automated oversampling techniques.

Notwithstanding, in the current study, we used the same Brazilian CKD dataset to enable the implementation and validation of the models: DT, RF, and multi-class AdaBoosted DTs. We conduct further experiments to improve the state-of-the-art by presenting an approach based on oversampling techniques. We applied the overall local accuracy (OLA) and local class accuracy (LCA) methods for dynamic classifier selection (DCS). We used the k-nearest oracles-union (KNORA-U), k-nearest oracles- eliminate (KNORA-E), and META-DES methods for dynamic ensemble selection (DES). We used such methods due to their usual high performance with imbalanced and limited size datasets [22]. The definitions of frequently used acronyms are presented in Table 1.

Table 1. Summary of main acronyms.

Acronyms	Definition
CKD	Chronic Kidney Disease
WHO	World Health Organization
DM	Diabetes Mellitus
AH	Arterial Hypertension
ML	Machine Learning
DT	Decision Tree
RF	Random Forest
SVM	Support Vector Machine
KNN	K-Nearest Neighbor
OLA	Overall Local Accuracy
LCA	Local Class Accuracy
DCS	Dynamic Classifier Selection
KNORA-U	K-Nearest Oracles-Union
KNORA-E	K-Nearest Oracles-Eliminate
DES	Dynamic Ensemble Selection
SMOTE	Synthetic Minority Oversampling Technique
ROC	Receiver Operating Characteristic
PRC	Precision-Recall Curve
MCC	Matthew's Correlation Coefficient
FMI	Fowlkes-Mallows
GFR	Glomerular Filtration Rate
ANN	Artificial Neural Network
OCT	Optical Coherence Tomography
PR	Precision
ACC	Accuracy score
PHR	Personal Health Records
DSS	Decision Support System
CDA	Clinical Document Architecture
GUI	Graphical User Interface
CV	Cross-Validation

For the implemented ensemble models, we prioritized the attributes of the dataset by applying the multi-class feature selection framework proposed by Pineda-Bautista et al. [23], including class binarization and balancing with the synthetic minority oversampling technique (SMOTE), evaluated with the receiver operating characteristic (ROC) curve and precision-recall curve (PRC) areas.

To address problems related to imbalanced and limited-size datasets, it is relevant to carry out data oversampling by rebalancing the classes before training the ML models [24,25]. We conducted experiments by oversampling the data from the medical records of Brazilian patients and comparing methods for resampling the data. We also used dynamic selection methods for further addressing such problems.

Besides, to deploy our approach, we developed a decision support system (DSS) to embed the ML model with the highest performance. In this article, the development of a DSS was relevant to discuss a clinical practice context, showing how our approach can be reused in a real-world scenario.

This work provides insights for developers of medical systems to assist in the early prediction of CKD to reduce the impacts of the late diagnosis, mainly in low-income and hard-to-reach locations, when using imbalanced and limited-size datasets. The main contributions of this work are: (1) the presentation of an approach for data oversampling (i.e., a combination of manual augmentation with automated augmentation); (2) the comparison of data oversampling techniques; (3) the comparison of validation methods; and (4) the comparison of ML models to assist the CKD early prediction in developing countries using imbalanced and limited size datasets. Therefore, one of the main technical novelties of this article relates to the presentation and evaluation of our oversampling approach that combines manual augmentation and automated augmentation.

2. Preliminaries

The research methodology of this study consists of data preprocessing, model implementation, validation methods, data augmentation, and multi-class classification metrics (Figure 1). Firstly, we preprocessed the Brazilian CKD dataset (i.e., binarization of attributes) and translated it to English.

We implemented ensemble (Figure 1a) and non-ensemble (Figure 1b) models using the algorithms DT, RF, and multi-class AdaBoosted DTs. We also selected the DCS (OLA and LCA) and DES (KNORA-U, KNORA-E, and META-DES) methods. We used the default configuration with a pool of classifiers of 10 decision trees. We chose this configuration because decision tree-based algorithms usually present high performance in imbalanced datasets. We implemented the ensemble models based on the framework proposed by Pineda-Bautista et al. [23].

We applied three ensemble and non-ensemble models validation methods: hold-out validation, multiple stratified CV, and nested CV. We used these methods to investigate whether they satisfactorily control overfitting caused due to the limited size of our dataset [26]. We applied the multiple stratified CV and nested CV with 10 folds and five repetitions. For the hold-out method, we split our dataset into 70% for training and 30% for testing. Thus, we conducted data augmentation only for the training set to ensure that the test set contained only real data. Our approach combines the data oversampling using: (1) manual augmentation, validated by an experienced nephrologist, and (2) automated augmentation (experimenting with the SMOTE, Borderline-SMOTE, and Borderline-SMOTE SVM).

Hence, we applied the following multi-class classification metrics: precision, accuracy score, recall, weighted F-score (F1), macro F1, Matthew's correlation coefficient (MCC), Fowlkes-Mallows (FMI), ROC, and PRC. We used the python scikit-learn library [27] to implement the models and to apply the validation methods and metrics. For dynamic selection techniques, we used the DESlib library [22].

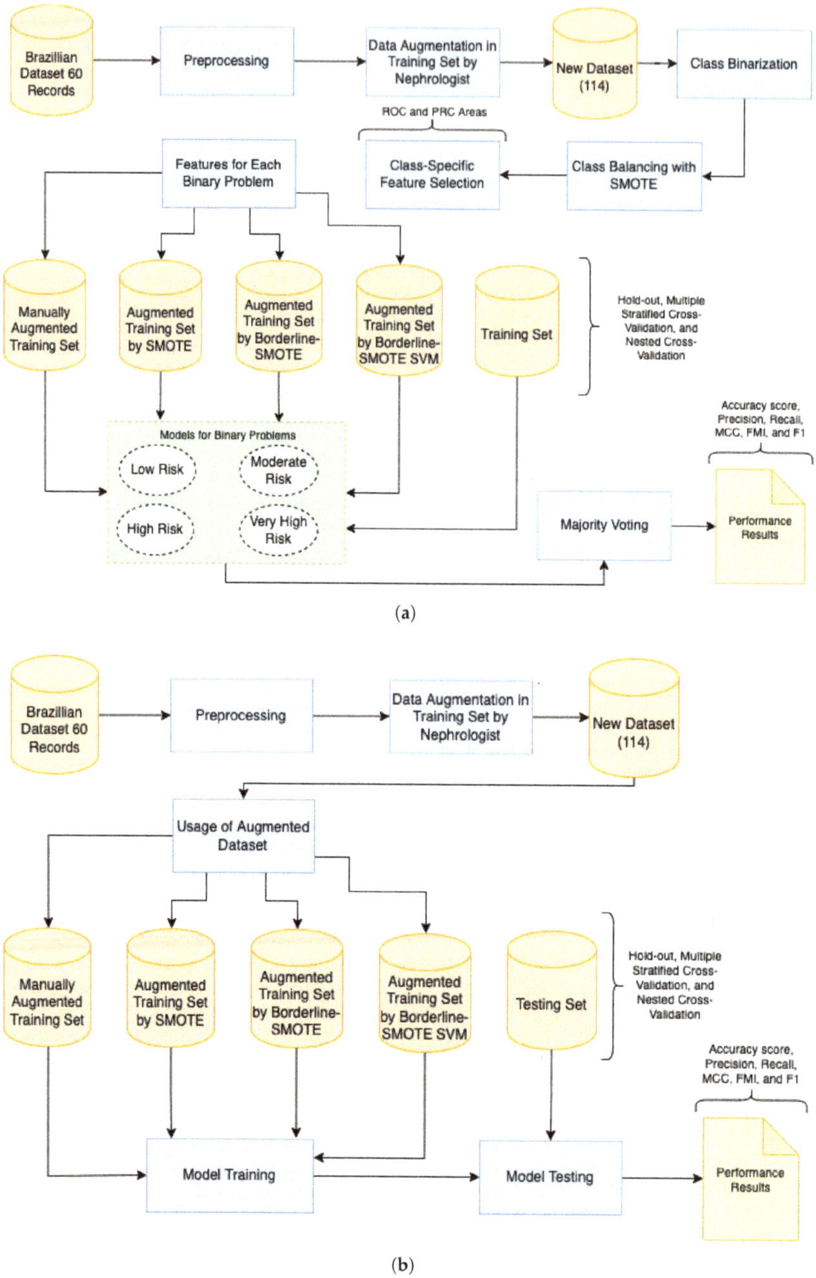

Figure 1. (**a**) Research steps based on the framework proposed by Pineda-Bautista et al. [23]: data preprocessing, model implementation, validation methods, data augmentation, and multi-class classification metrics. (**b**) Research steps based on simple approach: data preprocessing, model implementation, validation methods, data augmentation, and multi-class classification metrics.

2.1. Data Collection and Preprocessing

In a previous study [28], we collected medical data (60 real-world medical records) from physical medical records of adult subjects (age $\geq$ 18) under the treatment of University Hospital Prof. Alberto Antunes of the UFAL, Brazil. The data collection from medical records maintained in a non-electronic format at the hospital was approved by the Brazilian ethics committee of UFAL and conducted between 2015 and 2016. The dataset comprises 16 subjects with no kidney damage, 14 subjects diagnosed only with CKD, and 30 subjects diagnosed with CKD, AH, and/or DM. In general, the sample included subjects with ages between 18 and 79 years; approximately 94.5% of the subjects were diagnosed with AH, and 58.82% were diagnosed with DM (Table 2). With over 30 years of experience in CKD treatment and diagnosis in Brazil, a nephrologist labeled the risk classifications based on the KDIGO guideline [29]. The dataset with 60 medical records from the real world was classified into four risk classes: low risk (30 records), moderate risk (11 records), high risk (16 records), and very high risk (3 records).

We primarily selected dataset features based on medical guidelines. Specifically, the KDIGO guideline [29], the national institute for health and care excellence guideline [30], and the KDOQI guideline [31]. Besides, we interviewed a set of Brazilian nephrologists to confirm the relevance of the features in Brazil's context. The final set of CKD features focusing on Brazilian communities included AH, DM, creatinine, urea, albuminuria, age, gender, and glomerular filtration rate (GFR). The dataset did not contain duplicated and missing values. We only translated the dataset to English and converted the gender of subjects from string to a binary representation to enable the DT algorithm's usage.

Table 2. Demographic, laboratory tests, and commodities of patients from the 60 real-world medical records.

Features	Patients
Gender (%)	F(41) M (19)
Age	Between 18 and 79 years
Creatinine, *n* (%)	60 (100%)
Urea, *n* (%)	60 (100%)
Albuminuria, *n* (%)	60 (100%)
Albuminuria, *n* (%)	60 (100%)
GFR, *n* (%)	60 (100%)
DM	Yes (15) No (45)
AH	Yes (29) No (31)

2.2. Manual Augmentation

In our previous study [5], only for the training set, we manually augmented the dataset to decrease the impacts of using a small number of instances, including more than 54 records, by duplicating real-world medical records and carefully modifying the features, i.e., increasing each CKD biomarker by 0.5. We selected the constant 0.5 with no other purpose than to differentiate the instances and maintain the new one with the correct label. The perturbation of the data did not result in unacceptable ranges of values and incorrect labeling. An experienced nephrologist verified the augmented data's validity by analyzing each record regarding the correct risk classification (i.e., low, moderate, high, or very high risk). As stated above, the experienced nephrologist also evaluated the 60 real-world medical records. The preprocessed original dataset (60 records) and augmented dataset (54 records) are freely available in our public repository [32]. As an experienced nephrologist evaluated the new 54 records, all training and testing are conducted using more than 100 records (an acceptable number of instances for a small dataset). In this article, we propose the usage of such a manual step, along with automated augmentation (e.g., SMOTE), to address extremely small and imbalanced datasets.

2.3. Automated Augmentation

In the current study, based on the Python imbalanced-learn library [33], we conducted the automated data augmentation using the SMOTE, Borderline-SMOTE, and Borderline-SMOTE SVM. The SMOTE is one of the most used oversampling techniques and consists of oversampling the minority class by generating synthetic data through feature space. The method draws a line between the k-neighbors closest to the minority class and creates a synthetic sample at one point along that line [34]. Borderline-SMOTE is a widely used variation of SMOTE and consists of selecting samples from the minority class wrongly classified using the KNN classifier [35]. Finally, Borderline-SMOTE SVM uses the SVM classifier to identify erroneously classified samples in the decision limit [36]. In our implementation, due to a limited amount of data from the minority class, we use k = 3 to create a new synthetic sample.

2.4. Multi-Class Feature Selection

As stated, we conducted manual data augmentation to improve the original dataset. Besides, we binarized the translated, preprocessed, and manually augmented dataset to enable the multi-class feature selection for implementing ensemble models. The multi-class feature selection included an additional data augmentation using SMOTE to balance each binary problem (low risk, moderate risk, high risk, and very high risk). We solve each binary problem with feature selection based on the framework proposed by Pineda-Bautista et al. [23]. The framework considers multi-class feature selection using class binarization and balancing. Thus, we applied the one-against-all class strategy and the SMOTE. Our main objective with the multi-class feature selection is to verify the importance of features and improve the ML ensemble models' implementation. We used the ROC and PRC areas to conduct evaluations during the multi-class feature selection. Although ROC and PRC areas are typically used in binary classification, it is possible to extend them to evaluate multi-class classification problems using the one-against-all class strategy, as is the case of our multi-class feature selection. This enabled the definition of an ensemble model to solve our original multi-class problem by voting, trained based on the feature selection results for each binary problem.

2.5. Hold-Out Validation

We applied the hold-out method by splitting the original dataset into 70% for training and 30% for testing. For the manual augmentation, a dataset with 54 records, used in our previous study [5], was added to the training set composed of the original data, resulting in 96 records: low risk (51 records), moderate risk (18 records), high risk (24 records), and very high risk (3 records). We used the dataset generated by the manual augmentation for the automated augmentation and applied the SMOTE, Borderline-SMOTE, and Borderline-SMOTE SVM. The resampling using the SMOTE and Borderline-SMOTE resulted in 204 records, in which each class contained 51 records. The usage of Borderline-SMOTE SVM resulted in 181 records: low risk (51 records), moderate risk (51 records), high risk (51 records), and very high risk (28 records). The test sets, for all approaches, contained 18 records: low risk (7 records), moderate risk (1 record), high risk (8 records), and very high risk (2 records). The test set only contains non-augmented data. Thus, we only conducted data augmentation for the training set to ensure that the test set contained real data. We conducted comparisons using the following datasets: Only Manual Augmentation, Manual Augmentation + Augmentation with SMOTE, Manual Augmentation + Augmentation with Borderline-SMOTE, and Manual Augmentation + Augmentation with Borderline-SMOTE SVM.

2.6. Multiple Stratified Cross-Validation and Nested Cross-Validation

For the multiple stratified CV and nested CV methods, we split the original dataset into 10-folds, resulting in 54 records for training and 6 for testing. For the manual augmentation, we included 54 records in each of the 10-folds, in which each fold contained 108 data for training and 6 for testing. Training folds from 1 to 6 contained: low risk (55 records), moderate risk (18 records), high risk (30 records), and very high risk (5 records). The 7th-fold contained: low risk (55 records), moderate risk (17 records), high risk (31 records), and very high risk (5 records). From the 8th to 10th folds: low risk (55 records), moderate risk (18 records), high risk (31 records), and very high risk (4 records). We used the dataset generated by the manual augmentation for the automated augmentation and applied the SMOTE, Borderline-SMOTE, and Borderline-SMOTE SVM. The resampling using SMOTE and Borderline-SMOTE resulted in 220 records, in which all folds contained 55 records for each class. The Borderline-SMOTE SVM resulted in training folds, from 1st to 7th, with 196 records: low risk (55 records), moderate risk (55 records), high risk (55 records), and very high risk (31 records). Besides, from the 8th to 10th folds, it resulted in 195 records: low risk (55 records), moderate risk (55 records), high risk (55 records), and very high risk (30 records).

Besides investigating whether such methods satisfactorily control overfitting for our dataset (by comparison), in this article, the evaluation results are relevant to increase confidence in the ML model embedded in our developed DSS (Section 5—clinical context scenario). Therefore, they enabled us to evaluate the quality of our approach.

2.7. Algorithms

We experimented with supervised learning and the DT, RF, and multi-class AdaBoosted DTs classification models. We also apply methods for DCS (OLA and LCA) and methods for DES (KNORA-U, KNORA-E, and META-DES).

A DT uses the divide-and-conquer technique to solve classification and regression problems. It is an acyclic graph where each node is a division node or leaf node. The rules are based on information gain, which uses the concept of entropy to measure the randomness of a discrete random variable A (with domain $a_1, a_2, \ldots, a_n$) [37]. Entropy is used to calculate the difficulty of predicting the target attribute, where the entropy of A can be calculated by:

$$A = -\sum_{i=1}^{n} p_i log_2(p_i) \quad (1)$$

where, p_i is the probability of observing each value $a_1, a_2, \ldots, a_n$. In the literature, DT has performed well with imbalanced datasets. Different algorithms generate the DT, such as ID3, C4.5, C5.0, and CART. The Scikit-learn library uses the CART algorithm.

The RF algorithm is used to combine DTs, generating several random trees. The algorithm assists modelers in preventing overfitting, being more robust when compared to a DT. It uses the Gini impurity criterion to conduct the feature selection, in which the following equation [38] guides the split of a node:

$$i(w) = \sum_{l=1}^{L} p_w^l (1 - p_w^l) \quad (2)$$

where p_j is the relative frequency of class j [33].

The multi-class AdaBoosted DTs algorithm creates a set of classifiers that contribute to the classification of test samples through weighted voting. With each new iteration, the weight of the training samples is changed considering the error of the set of classifiers previously implemented [37]. A multi-class AdaBoosted DTs performs the combination of predictions from all DTs in the set for multi-class problems.

Finally, a dynamic selection technique measures the performance level of each classifier in a classifier pool. If a classifier pool is not defined, a BaggingClassifier generates a pool containing 10 DTs. For the DCS method, the classifier that has achieved the highest performance level when classifying the samples in the test set is selected [22]. For the DES method, a set of classifiers that provide a minimum performance level is selected.

2.8. Classification Metrics

We computed the performance of the classification models using the python scikit-learn library [39] and the following metrics: precision, accuracy score, recall, balanced F score, MCC, ROC, and PRC. Precision represents the classifier's ability of not label a sample incorrectly and is given by the equation:

$$Precision = \frac{TP}{TP + FP} \tag{3}$$

where, TP represents the true positives and FP represents the false positives. The accuracy score calculates the total performance of the model using the equation:

$$A(y, \hat{y}) = \frac{1}{n} \sum_{i=0}^{n-1} 1(\hat{y}_i = y_i) \tag{4}$$

where, $\hat{y}_i$ represents the value that the model classified the sample, y_i represents the real value of the sample, n is the total number of samples, and $I(x)$ is the indicator function [27].

The recall corresponds to the hit rate in the positive class and is given by

$$Recall = \frac{TP}{TP + FN} \tag{5}$$

where, FN represents the false negatives. The balanced F-score or F measure is a weighted average between precision and recall:

$$F1 = 2 * \frac{Precision * Recall}{Precision + Recall} \tag{6}$$

The *MCC* is used to assess the quality of ratings and is highly recommended for imbalanced data [40], given by the following equation:

$$MCC = \frac{TP * TN - FP * FN}{\sqrt{(TP + FP)(TP + FN)(TN + FP)(TN + FN)}} \tag{7}$$

where, TN represents the true negative. Besides, the *FMI* is used to measure the similarity between two clusters, the measure varies between 0 and 1, where a high value indicates a good similarity [41]. *FMI* is defined as the geometric mean between precision and recall, given by the equation:

$$FMI = \sqrt{\frac{TP}{TP + FP} * \frac{TP}{TP + FN}} \tag{8}$$

The ROC calculates the probability estimates that a sample belongs to a specific class [42]. For multi-class problems, ROC uses two approaches: one-vs-one and one-vs-rest. Finally, the PRC is a widely used metric for imbalanced datasets that provides a clear visualization of the performance of a classifier [43].

3. Related Works

3.1. Early Prediction and DSS

ML models' usage to assist in decision making has received the attention of researchers in the last years. For instance, Hsu [28] describes a framework based on a ranking and feature selection algorithm to assist physicians' decision-making on cardiovascular diseases' most relevant risk factors. The author also applies machine learning techniques to enable identifying the risk factors.

Walczak and Velanovich [29] developed an artificial neural network (ANN) system to assist physicians and patients in selecting pancreatic cancer treatment. The system determines the 7-month survival or mortality of patients based on a specific treatment decision. Topuz et al. [31] propose a decision support methodology guided by a Bayesian belief network algorithm to predict kidney transplantation's graft survival. The authors use a database with more than 31,000 U.S. patients and argue that the methodology can be reused in other datasets.

Wang et al. [30] evaluate a murine model, induced by intravenous Adriamycin injection, using optical coherence tomography (OCT) to assess the CKD progression by images of rat kidneys. The authors highlight that OCT images contain relevant data about kidney histopathology. Jahantigh, Malmir, and Avilaq [32] propose a fuzzy expert system to assist the medical diagnosis, focusing initially on kidney diseases. The system is guided by the experience of physicians to indicate disease profiles. Neves et al. [34] present a DSS to identify acute kidney injury and CKD using knowledge representation and reasoning procedures based on logic programming and ANN. Polat et al. [33] used the support vector machine technique and the two-feature selection methods wrapper and filter to conduct the CKD identification early. The authors justify the computer-aided diagnosis based on high mortality rates of CKD. Finally, Arulanthu and Perumal [35] presented a DSS for CKD prediction (CKD or non-CKD) using a logistic regression model.

However, these CKD studies have some limitations. For example, relevant topics are the ML technique used to identify the disease and the costs of required examinations (predictors). Most of the studies use many predictors and apply complex analysis, increasing costs and making physician double-checking results problematic. Indeed, this type of functionality is relevant because other clinical conditions influence CKD, and the diagnosis is usually improved when physicians collaborate to conclude.

3.2. Oversampling Methods

As mentioned earlier, the growing use of ML in the medical field brings challenges such as limited and imbalanced data. Despite this, the use of such datasets can be quite relevant for the medical field [21] and studies have been carried out to deal with such limitations. Some methods use ML algorithms, probability, or weights to define the samples to be resampled, while some methods perform the combination of oversampling and undersampling [44]. Some of these works will be reported below.

One of the best-known techniques for dealing with this type of problem is SMOTE [34]. The purpose of SMOTE is to generate new synthetic minority class data, thus selecting a sample of the minority class randomly and its k nearest neighbors of the same class are calculated (by default 5) as a line is drawn around the selected samples and new synthetic data is generated.

Chawla et al. [34] performed a combination of subsampling and supersampling techniques. The subsampling technique was proposed in conjunction with supersampling to increase the sensitivity of a classifier to the minority class. Thus, in the proposed method, samples from the majority class were taken randomly and samples from the minority class were synthetically generated until it has a specific proportion of the majority class. In another work, Chawla et al. [45] performed a combination of the SMOTE algorithm with the boosting procedure, changing the update weights and compensating for skewed distributions of misclassified instances to generate synthetic data, thus creating the SMOTE-Boost algorithm.

Unlike other methods that resample all examples from the minority class or that randomly select a subset, Han et al. [35] in their study, selects only the minority class samples that are Borderline and most likely to be misclassified, thus developing a variation of the SMOTE oversampling method called Borderline-SMOTE. While Nguyen and Kamei [36] used the SVM classifier to find the boundary region, combined with extrapolation and interpolation techniques for oversampling the minority boundary instances.

Das et al. [46] addressed two types of oversampling, namely, RACOG and wRACOG, where it used joint probability distribution of data attributes and Gibbs sampling to choose and generate the samples of minority classes synthetically. Wang [44] used the SMOTE oversampling method only to support minority class vectors that were found by training the cost-sensitive SVM classifier.

In contrast, we address very limited datasets by combining manual augmentation and automated augmentation. To verify the best combination, we experiment with manual augmentation along with automated augmentation using SMOTE, Borderline-SMOTE, and Borderline-SMOTE SVM.

3.3. Validation Methods

Some studies conduct comparisons of validation methods for ML models. For example, Varma and Simon [26] compared the multiple stratified CV and nested CV methods. The authors conclude that CV presents significantly biased estimates, in contrast with nested CV, that provides an almost unbiased estimate of the true error.

Moreover, Vabalas et al. [18] investigated whether bias, identified in some studies in the literature when reporting classification accuracy, could be caused by the use of specific validation methods. The authors also conclude that multiple stratified CV produces strongly biased performance estimates with small sample sizes. However, they also state that nested CV and hold-out present unbiased estimates. In another study, Varoquaux [47] also highlights the possibility of obtaining underestimated performance evaluation using CV.

Krstajic et al. [48] address best practices to improve reliability and confidence during the evaluation of ML models. The authors describe a repeated grid-search V-fold cross-validation approach and define a repeated nested cross-validation algorithm. They highlight the relevance of repeating cross-validation during model evaluation.

3.4. Comparison of ML Algorithms

Furthermore, some studies focus on the comparison of ML models to predict CKD. For example, Ilyas et al. [49] compared ML models for early prediction of CKD. They used the UCI machine learning repository, which consists of two classes (i.e., CKD affected and NOTCKD, indicating people with no CKD). However, the authors subdivide the CKD class into stages: Stage 1, Stage 2, Stage 3A, Stage 3B, Stage 4, and Stage 5. The prediction focuses on such stages.

Qin et al. [50] also used the UCI machine learning repository to assist the early detection of CKD as a binary problem. The authors apply KNN imputation to fill in the missing values of the dataset. They implemented ML models using logistic regression, RF, SVM, KNN, naive Bayes, and feed-forward neural network.

Chittora et al. [51] implemented ML models using ANN, C5.0, Chi-square Automatic interaction detector, logistic regression, linear SVM with penalty L1 and L2, and random tree. As a binary problem, the authors apply feature selection and oversampling techniques based on the UCI machine learning repository.

Chaurasia et al. [52] compared ensemble and non-ensemble models for the prediction of CKD as a binary problem. They evaluated the models using performance metrics such as accuracy rate, recall rate, F1 score, and support value. The ensemble models outperformed non-ensemble models.

4. Experiments

4.1. Statistical Significance

We conducted a correlation analysis to verify the relationship between the variables. Firstly, we analyze the correlation matrix generated through Person's coefficients, where the measures vary between 1 and -1. On the one hand, a value closer to 1 indicates a strong correlation between two variables. On the other hand, a value close to -1 indicates an inverse correlation. The values are represented by means of colors. Thus, the lighter the color, the greater the correlation between the variables.

Figure 2 shows a sample of the correlation matrix coefficients using our CKD datasets. Figure 2a presents the correlation matrix from the dataset with the 60 real-world records and 54 manually augmented data. Samples of correlation matrix coefficients from the datasets related to the application of the hold-out method are also presented, with data further resampled with SMOTE (Figure 2b), borderline-SMOTE (Figure 2c), and borderline-SMOTE SVM (Figure 2d). Figure 2e presents the correlation matrix associated with the CV method with data further resampled with SMOTE. In general, the highest correlation coefficients relate to creatinine, urea, albuminuria, and age.

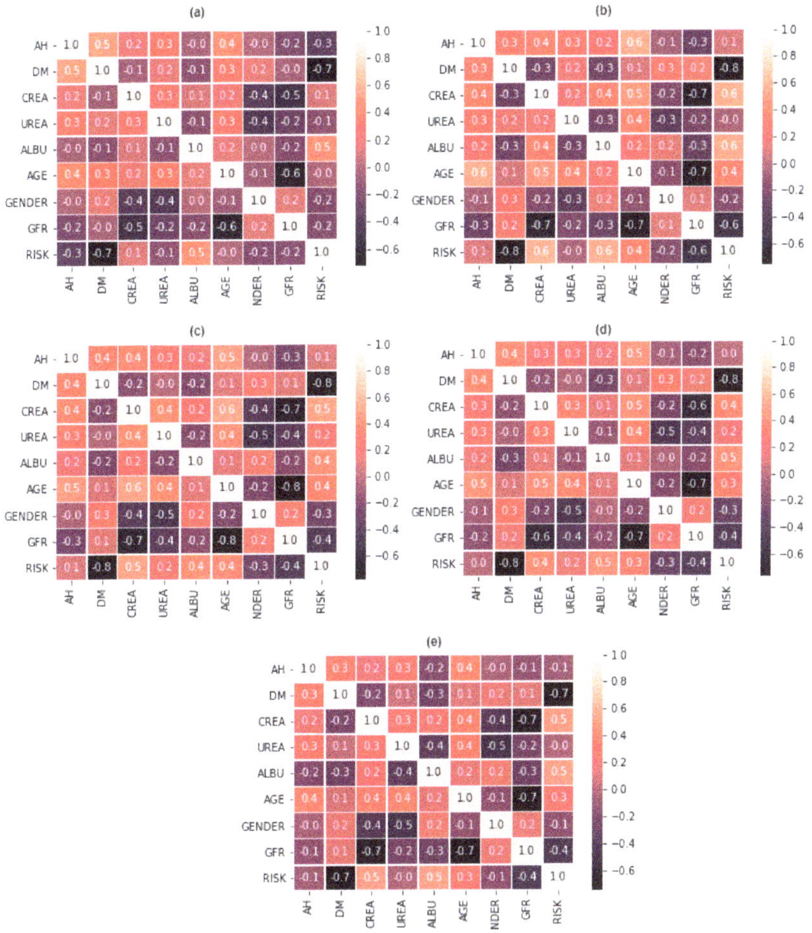

Figure 2. Sample of correlation matrix coefficients. (**a**) Dataset with the 60 real-world records and 54 manually augmented data. (**b**) Dataset with the application of the hold-out method and data further resampled with SMOTE. (**c**) Dataset with the application of the hold-out method and data further resampled with borderline-SMOTE. (**d**) Dataset with the application of the hold-out method and data further resampled with borderline-SMOTE SVM. (**e**) Dataset with CV method with data further resampled with SMOTE

Moreover, we used linear regression to conduct a hypothesis test to verify statistical significance. We calculated the p-value to quantify statistical significance and analyze whether our hypothesis had any correlation between the features and the target. We consider a p-value < 0.05, as a strong relationship between the feature and the target. We also calculated the F-statistic to analyze the significance of the model implemented using the datasets (must be greater than 1). We used the R-Squared statistic to complement the analysis of the relationship between two variables, between 0 and 1 (indicates a strong correlation).

A sample of p-value, F-statistic, and R-Squared results is presented in Table S1 of Supplementary Materials. We identified a strong correlation between variables. For example, when using the dataset that relates to the application of the CV method, with data resampled using the manual approach and SMOTE, the null hypothesis was refuted for AH, DM, creatinine, albuminuria, and age. Besides, the F-statistic resulted in 126.90 and the R-Squared in 0.828, indicating a strong relationship between the variables and the target.

4.2. Implementation and Evaluation

We implemented the classification models using the DT, RF, and multi-class AdaBoosted DTs algorithms. Besides, we used dynamic selection methods: OLA, LCA, KNORA-E, KNORA-U, and META-DES. As mentioned before, we used the validation methods hold-out, multiple stratified CV, and nested CV, comparing resampling approaches: only manual augmentation, SMOTE, Borderline-SMOTE, and Borderline-SMOTE SVM. For the hold-out method, without the usage of the framework proposed by Pineda-Bautista et al. [23], dynamic selection (OLA, KNORA-E, and META-DES) and the DT model presented the highest performances using the mean values of precision (PR), accuracy score (ACC), recall, FMI, MCC, and F1 (e.g., with an equal ACC of 94.44% using the Borderline-SMOTE SVM). For the other resampling techniques, such models presented lower performances, with an ACC between 83.33% and 88.88%. We present such results in Table S2 of the Supplementary Materials. Due to the imbalance and limited size of the test set used for the hold-out method, we also applied the multiple stratified CV and nested CV as validation methods. Such methods evaluate the generalization of a model to a new dataset, using the whole data for training and testing.

Then, we applied the gridSearchCV tool with 5 repetitions for the multiple stratified CV and nested CV methods. We used such a tool to automate the combination of the best parameters and obtain the best performance from each algorithm. We used multiple stratified CV and nested CV with 10-folds and five repetitions. The multiple stratified CV method obtained a very similar result when compared to the nested CV, in some cases, with a difference of up to 6%. There is a difference because the multiple stratified CV uses the entire dataset to perform the best fit, producing optimistic performance estimates [53]. However, the nested CV splits the data into training, validation, and testing, using the gridSearchCV tool to set the best parameters only for the training data to produce unbiased performance estimates.

The DT, RF, and multi-class AdaBoosted DTs models presented stable results, obtaining high performance for all resampling methods. For multiple stratified CV and nested CV, the models achieved an ACC that ranged between 92.33% and 98.99%. The DT model presented the best performance, with an ACC of 98.99%, using SMOTE (see Tables S3 and S4 of our Supplementary Materials).

Furthermore, to improve the experiments, we implemented ensemble models based on the framework proposed by Pineda-Bautista et al. [23]. We split the original dataset into 70% for training and 30% for testing to select features from multiple classes. We improved the data using 38 records from the augmented dataset available in our public repository [32]. Afterward, we conducted the binarization of the training and test sets using the one-against-all classes strategy. We conducted the binarization for each class of our multi-class problem to obtain four different binary problems (low risk, moderate risk, high risk, and very high risk). We applied the SMOTE to handle imbalanced data for each binary problem; however, the usage of SMOTE did not improve the results. Finally, we used the CfsSubsetEval attribute evaluator and the BestFist research method to select the features of our binary problems. The feature selection results, for each binary problem, resulted in a maximum of five features for each class (Table 3).

Table 3. Results of feature selection for each binary problem generated using the low risk, moderate risk, high risk, and very high risk classes.

Importance	Low	Moderate	High	Very High
1	AH	DM	AH	Crea
2	DM	Albu	DM	Age
3	Albu	-	Albu	GFR
4	Age	-	Age	-
5	GFR	-	Gender	-

The resulting ensemble model is composed of four submodels (one per class). Each submodel is trained based on the augmented dataset and the feature selection results for a specific class. Thus, each submodel may assign different classes to a new instance. To conduct the final classifications, we used the majority vote strategy.

We also applied the hold-out, multiple stratified CV, and nested CV validation methods for the ensemble models, comparing the resampling approaches: manual augmentation, SMOTE, Borderline-SMOTE, and Borderline-SMOTE SVM. In the hold-out validation method (Table 4), models implemented based on dynamic selection (KNORA-E and KNORA-U) and the DT algorithm presented the highest performances. KNORA-E and KNORA-U achieved the highest accuracy score for the Borderline-SMOTE SVM and Borderline-SMOTE resampling techniques, respectively. The DT model showed stability for all resampling techniques, with an accuracy score of 94.44%.

Table 4. Results for the hold-out method for the ensemble models implemented based on the framework proposed by Pineda-Bautista et al. [23].

	ACC	PR	Recall	Weighted F1	Macro F1	MCC	FMI
Manual Augmentation Only							
Decision Tree	94.44	0.95	0.94	0.93	0.90	0.91	0.92
Random Forest	94.44	0.95	0.94	0.93	0.90	0.91	0.92
AdaBoosted DT	88.88	0.91	0.88	0.88	0.86	0.83	0.78
OLA	88.88	0.91	0.88	0.89	0.77	0.83	0.89
LCA	88.88	0.81	0.88	0.84	0.65	0.83	0.90
KNORA-U	88.88	0.81	0.88	0.84	0.65	0.83	0.90
KNORA-E	83.33	0.77	0.83	0.79	0.61	0.75	0.77
META-DES	83.33	0.80	0.83	0.80	0.59	0.75	0.82
Manual Augmentation + Augmentation with SMOTE							
Decision Tree	94.44	0.95	0.94	0.93	0.90	0.91	0.92
Random Forest	94.44	0.95	0.94	0.93	0.90	0.91	0.92
AdaBoosted DT	94.44	0.95	0.94	0.93	0.90	0.91	0.91
OLA	88.88	0.89	0.88	0.88	0.84	0.83	0.84
LCA	88.88	0.91	0.88	0.89	0.77	0.83	0.89
KNORA-U	94.44	0.96	0.94	0.94	0.93	0.91	0.90
KNORA-E	94.44	0.97	0.94	0.95	0.90	0.92	0.91
META-DES	94.44	0.96	0.94	0.94	0.93	0.91	0.90
Manual Augmentation + Augmentation with Borderline-SMOTE							
Decision Tree	94.44	0.95	0.94	0.93	0.90	0.91	0.92
Random Forest	88.88	0.91	0.88	0.88	0.86	0.83	0.78
AdaBoosted DT	88.88	0.89	0.88	0.88	0.86	0.82	0.80

Table 4. *Cont.*

	ACC	PR	Recall	Weighted F1	Macro F1	MCC	FMI
OLA	88.88	0.89	0.88	0.88	0.84	0.83	0.84
LCA	88.88	0.91	0.88	0.88	0.86	0.83	0.78
KNORA-U	100.00	1.00	1.00	1.00	1.00	1.00	1.00
KNORA-E	94.44	0.95	0.94	0.93	0.90	0.91	0.91
META-DES	88.88	0.91	0.88	0.88	0.80	0.83	0.84
Manual Augmentation + Augmentation with Borderline-SMOTE SVM							
Decision Tree	94.44	0.95	0.94	0.93	0.90	0.91	0.92
Random Forest	94.44	0.96	0.94	0.94	0.93	0.91	0.90
AdaBoosted DT	88.88	0.91	0.88	0.88	0.86	0.83	0.78
OLA	88.88	0.89	0.88	0.88	0.84	0.83	0.84
LCA	88.88	0.92	0.88	0.88	0.79	0.83	0.84
KNORA-U	88.88	88.88	88.88	88.88	0.84	0.82	0.84
KNORA-E	100.00	1.00	1.00	1.00	1.00	1.00	1.00
META-DES	94.44	0.96	0.94	0.94	0.93	0.91	0.90

Finally, we applied the multiple stratified CV and nested CV validation methods, in which the DT and multi-class AdaBoosted DTs models demonstrated stability (the highest performances for all resampling methods). The multiple stratified CV method achieved an accuracy score between 95.00% and 97.66% (Table 5), while the nested CV method achieved an accuracy score between 94.98% and 96.66% (Table 6).

Table 5. Results for the multiple stratified CV method for the ensemble models implemented based on the framework proposed by Pineda-Bautista et al. [23].

	ACC	PR	Recall	Weighted F1	Macro F1	MCC	FMI
Manual Augmentation Only							
Decision Tree	95.66	0.92	0.95	0.93	0.90	0.93	0.94
Random Forest	91.00	0.84	0.91	0.87	0.80	0.86	0.87
AdaBoosted DT	95.00	0.93	0.95	0.93	0.91	0.93	0.91
OLA	90.33	0.84	0.90	0.86	0.79	0.86	0.88
LCA	87.33	0.80	0.87	0.82	0.74	0.81	0.83
KNORA-U	89.33	0.83	0.89	0.68	0.78	0.84	0.85
KNORA-E	91.33	0.85	0.91	0.87	0.81	0.87	0.88
META-DES	91.66	0.86	0.91	0.88	0.81	0.88	0.89
Manual Augmentation + Augmentation with SMOTE							
Decision Tree	94.44	0.95	0.94	0.93	0.93	0.91	0.92
Random Forest	94.44	0.95	0.94	0.93	0.84	0.91	0.92
AdaBoosted DT	97.66	0.97	0.97	0.97	0.97	0.96	0.94
OLA	92.66	0.90	0.92	0.90	0.85	0.89	0.89
LCA	91.33	0.89	0.91	0.89	0.93	0.87	0.87
KNORA-U	94.99	0.94	0.95	0.94	0.89	0.93	0.94
KNORA-E	93.66	0.91	0.93	0.92	0.86	0.90	0.91
META-DES	93.33	0.92	0.93	0.92	0.87	0.90	0.89
Manual Augmentation + Augmentation with Borderline-SMOTE							
Decision Tree	96.00	0.94	0.96	0.94	0.92	0.94	0.93
Random Forest	93.33	0.90	0.93	0.91	0.87	0.90	0.89
AdaBoosted DT	95.00	0.93	0.95	0.93	0.91	0.93	0.91
OLA	92.33	0.91	0.92	0.91	0.85	0.89	0.88
LCA	91.33	0.89	0.91	0.89	0.84	0.88	0.85
KNORA-U	94.33	0.93	0.94	0.93	0.88	0.92	0.93

Table 5. *Cont.*

	ACC	PR	Recall	Weighted F1	Macro F1	MCC	FMI
KNORA-E	94.00	0.92	0.94	0.92	0.88	0.91	0.91
META-DES	94.33	0.93	0.94	0.93	0.87	0.92	0.93
Manual Augmentation + Augmentation with Borderline-SMOTE SVM							
Decision Tree	96.66	0.94	0.96	0.95	0.92	0.95	0.95
Random Forest	91.66	0.87	0.91	0.88	0.85	0.88	0.84
AdaBoosted DT	95.33	0.93	0.95	0.93	0.91	0.93	0.92
OLA	88.88	0.89	0.88	0.88	0.85	0.83	0.84
LCA	90.66	0.85	0.90	0.87	0.80	0.86	0.87
KNORA-U	94.00	0.91	0.94	0.92	0.87	0.91	0.92
KNORA-E	93.33	0.92	0.93	0.92	0.86	0.90	0.91
META-DES	93.00	0.92	0.93	0.91	0.86	0.90	0.91

Table 6. Results for the nested CV method for the ensemble models implemented based on the framework proposed by Pineda-Bautista et al. [23].

	ACC	PR	Recall	Weighted F1	Macro F1	MCC	FMI
Manual Augmentation Only							
Decision Tree	95.66	0.94	0.95	0.93	0.90	0.93	0.94
Random Forest	91.66	0.85	0.91	0.88	0.81	0.87	0.88
AdaBoosted DT	95.00	0.93	0.95	0.93	0.91	0.93	0.91
OLA	89.00	0.82	0.89	0.85	0.77	0.84	0.87
LCA	83.99	0.75	0.84	0.78	0.69	0.76	0.78
KNORA-U	88.00	0.81	0.88	0.83	0.76	0.82	0.84
KNORA-E	91.66	0.87	0.91	0.89	0.82	0.87	0.88
META-DES	90.00	0.83	0.90	0.86	0.78	0.85	0.87
Manual Augmentation + Augmentation with SMOTE							
Decision Tree	94.98	0.92	0.94	0.93	0.90	0.92	0.91
Random Forest	90.00	0.85	0.90	0.86	0.80	0.85	0.84
AdaBoosted DT	96.66	0.94	0.96	0.95	0.93	0.95	0.95
OLA	92.66	0.92	0.92	0.91	0.85	0.89	0.90
LCA	91.33	0.89	0.91	0.89	0.85	0.87	0.85
KNORA-U	92.66	0.92	0.92	0.91	0.86	0.86	0.89
KNORA-E	90.00	0.88	0.90	0.88	0.80	0.89	0.85
META-DES	92.66	0.90	0.92	0.91	0.85	0.89	0.90
Manual Augmentation + Augmentation with Borderline-SMOTE							
Decision Tree	96.00	0.93	0.94	0.94	0.92	0.94	0.93
Random Forest	92.66	0.89	0.92	0.90	0.85	0.89	0.88
AdaBoosted DT	96.66	0.95	0.96	0.95	0.93	0.95	0.94
OLA	90.00	0.88	0.90	0.88	0.82	0.85	0.83
LCA	90.66	0.88	0.90	0.89	0.83	0.87	0.85
KNORA-U	92.33	0.91	0.92	0.91	0.85	0.89	0.89
KNORA-E	92.66	0.91	0.92	0.91	0.85	0.89	0.90
META-DES	92.66	0.90	0.92	0.90	0.84	0.89	0.90
Manual Augmentation + Augmentation with Borderline-SMOTE SVM							
Decision Tree	91.33	0.89	0.92	0.88	0.82	0.87	0.86
Random Forest	90.66	0.85	0.90	0.87	0.82	0.86	0.84
AdaBoosted DT	92.66	0.90	0.92	0.90	0.86	0.89	0.87
OLA	90.33	0.86	0.90	0.87	0.81	0.86	0.85
LCA	88.66	0.84	0.88	0.85	0.79	0.84	0.82

Table 6. *Cont.*

	ACC	PR	Recall	Weighted F1	Macro F1	MCC	FMI
KNORA-U	92.66	0.91	0.92	0.91	0.86	0.89	0.89
KNORA-E	91.33	0.89	0.91	0.89	0.82	0.87	0.88
META-DES	93.00	0.92	0.93	0.91	0.86	0.90	0.91

As stated above, our comparisons also considered the results without using the framework proposed by Pineda-Bautista et al. [23] (see Tables S2–S4 of our Supplementary Materials). To summarize our findings, we present the decision tree results (from Tables S2–S4 of our Supplementary Materials) in Table 7.

Table 7. Decision tree results for the hold-out, multiple stratified CV, and nested CV methods without using the framework proposed by Pineda-Bautista et al. [23].

	ACC	PR	Recall	Weighted F1	Macro F1	MCC	FMI
Manual Augmentation Only							
Hold-out	83.33	0.77	0.83	0.79	0.61	0.74	0.77
Multiple stratified CV	92.33	0.92	0.92	0.91	0.88	0.90	0.86
Nested CV	92.33	0.92	0.92	0.91	0.90	0.90	0.82
Manual Augmentation + Augmentation with SMOTE							
Hold-out	83.33	0.86	0.83	0.84	0.80	0.74	0.78
Multiple stratified CV	98.99	0.99	0.99	0.98	0.98	0.98	0.98
Nested CV	98.99	1.00	0.99	0.99	0.98	0.98	0.99
Manual Augmentation + Augmentation with Borderline-SMOTE							
Hold-out	88.88	0.88	0.88	0.88	0.84	0.82	0.84
Multiple stratified CV	98.00	0.98	0.98	0.97	0.96	0.97	0.98
Nested CV	95.00	0.95	0.95	0.95	0.94	0.93	0.88
Manual Augmentation + Augmentation with Borderline-SMOTE SVM							
Hold-out	94.44	0.95	0.94	0.93	0.90	0.91	0.91
Multiple stratified CV	95.00	0.93	0.95	0.93	0.91	0.93	0.91
Nested CV	96.00	0.94	0.96	0.95	0.91	0.94	0.95

Besides, we calculated the ROC and PRC curves using a one-against-all classes strategy. We identified the trade-offs between sensitivity (true positive rate) and specificity (true negative rate) to show the model's diagnostic abilities using the ROC area. For example, for the ROC curve performance of the DT model, which relates to the usage of SMOTE and the nested CV methods, high discriminatory power was achieved for all folds. One can also identify that the curves are closer to the upper left corner of each graphic (Figures 3 and 4). In addition, the PRC area shows the relationship between accuracy and recall and is relevant to analyze imbalanced datasets (see Figures S1–S3 of our Supplemental Materials). The precision-recall curve shows the trade-off between precision and recall for different thresholds. For the performance of the DT model, which is related to the use of SMOTE and nested CV methods, high discriminatory power was achieved for all folds, increasing confidence in the results presented with ROC curves. The source codes of the experiments are available in our repository [54].

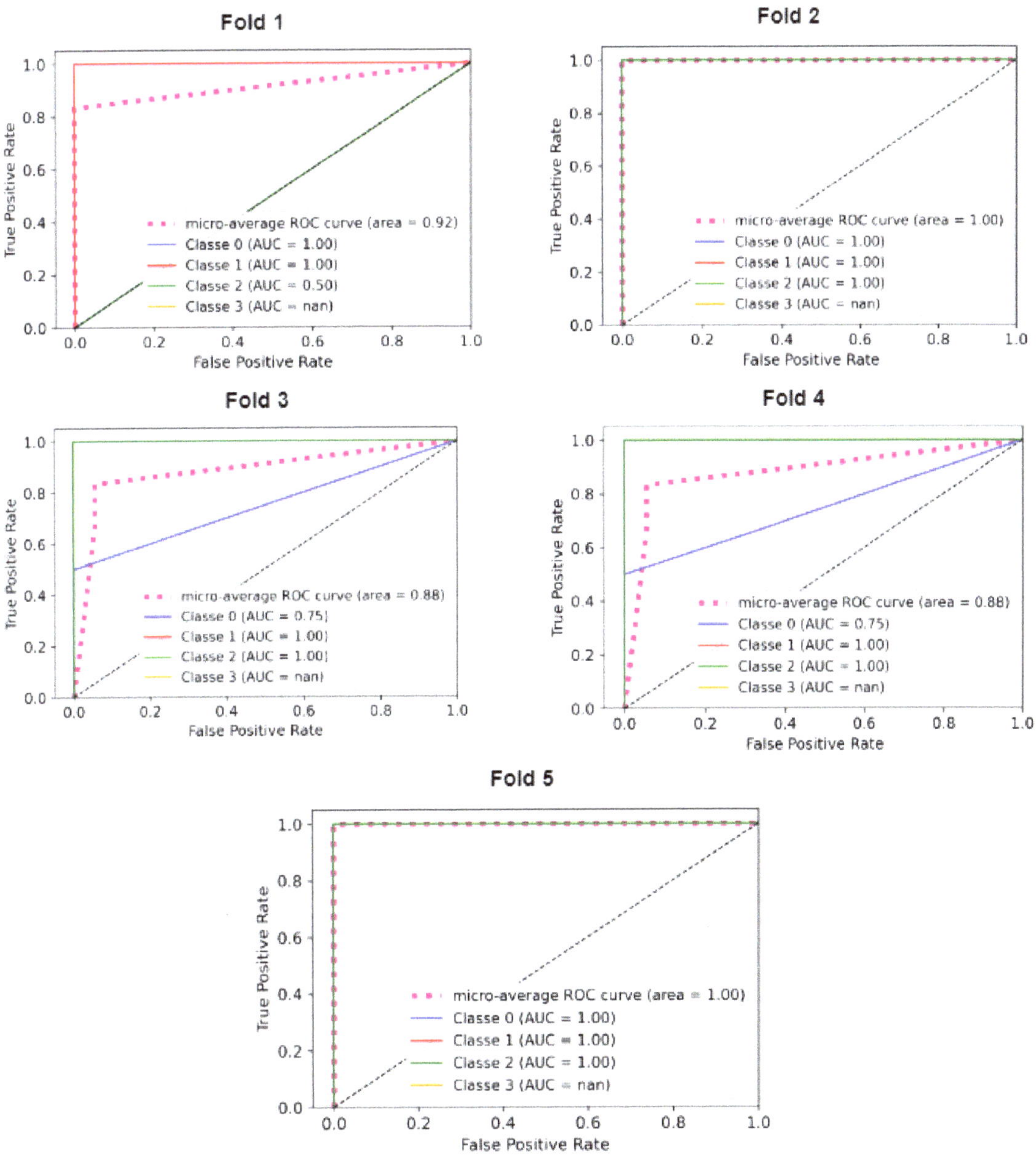

Figure 3. ROC curves of the DT model using SMOTE and the nested CV method for the five first folds. Each graphic represents one of the ten folds.

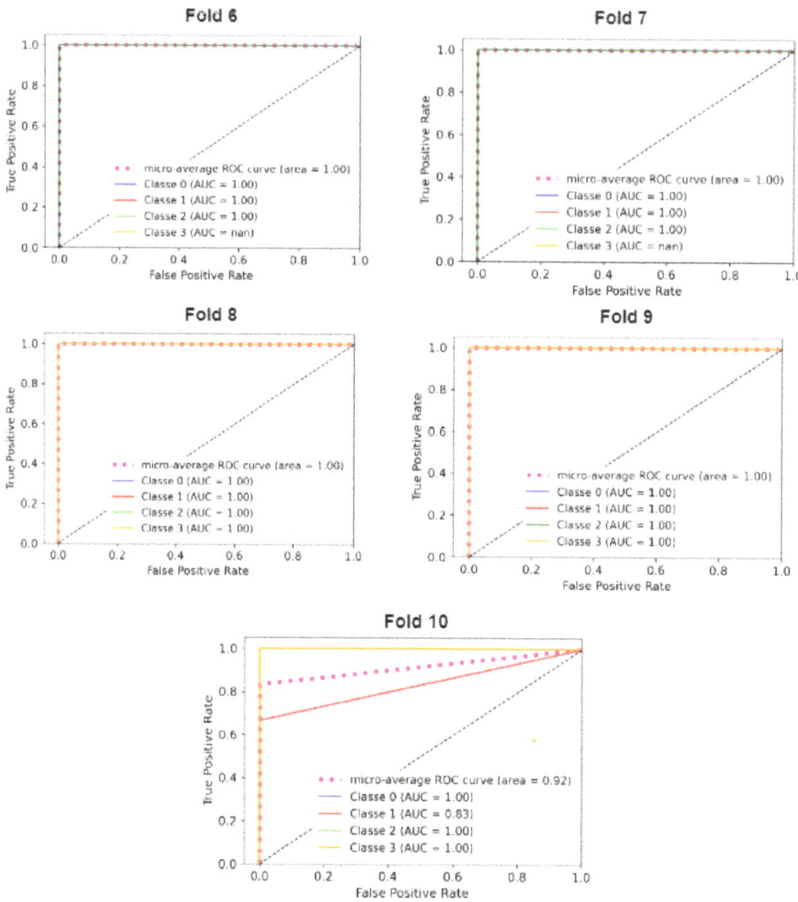

Figure 4. ROC curves of the DT model using SMOTE and the nested CV method for the sixth, seventh, eighth, ninth, and tenth folds. Each graphic represents one of the ten folds.

5. Clinical Practice Context

Using eHealth and mHealth systems to aid in the treatment and identification of chronic diseases can be one way to reduce high mortality rates through monitoring chronic diseases such as CKD. This situation refers to using information and technologies intelligently and effectively to guide those whom public health systems will eventually assist. Early computer-aided identification of CKD can help people living in the countryside and environments with difficult access to primary care. In addition, mobile health apps (i.e., mHealth), which generate personal health records (PHR), can be used to reduce issues (i.e., store a patient's complete medical history with diagnosis, administered medications, plans for treatment, vaccination dates, allergies) related to primary health care in remote locations.

Therefore, the presented classification models can be used to develop eHealth and mHealth systems that assist patients, clinicians, and the government in monitoring CKD and its risk factors. Using the Brazilian CKD dataset, we recommend applying the DT model with data resampled with the SMOTE technique to develop a DSS. The DT model achieved high performance, and it is considered a white box analysis approach with a straightforward interpretation of results. Interpreting the results helps doctors understand how the model achieved a specific risk rating, increasing these professionals' confidence in the results.

The ML model can be the basis for developing a DSS to identify and monitor CKD in Brazilian communities, where the interaction between three actors is proposed: doctor, patient, and public health system (Figure 5). The system used by patients is presented as a web-based system divided into front-end and back-end, which contains PHR and CKD risk assessment functionality. The risk assessment is performed after inputting the results of exams, where the classification of risk of CKD is based on the DT model. After the user's clinical evaluation, the system can send a clinical document, structured from the HL7 clinical document architecture (CDA) to the doctor responsible for monitoring the patient. The HL7 CDA document is an XML file that contains the risk analysis data, a risk analysis DT, and the PHR.

The medical system receives the CDA document to confirm the risk assessment by analyzing the classification, the DT, and the PHR data. In an uncertain diagnosis, the doctor can send the CDA document to other doctors for a second opinion. The patient and medical subsystems use web services provided by the Server subsystem to update the PHR of patients as part of the medical records available at a healthcare facility. We provide a more detailed explanation of this type of system for CKD and related technologies in our previous publication [28].

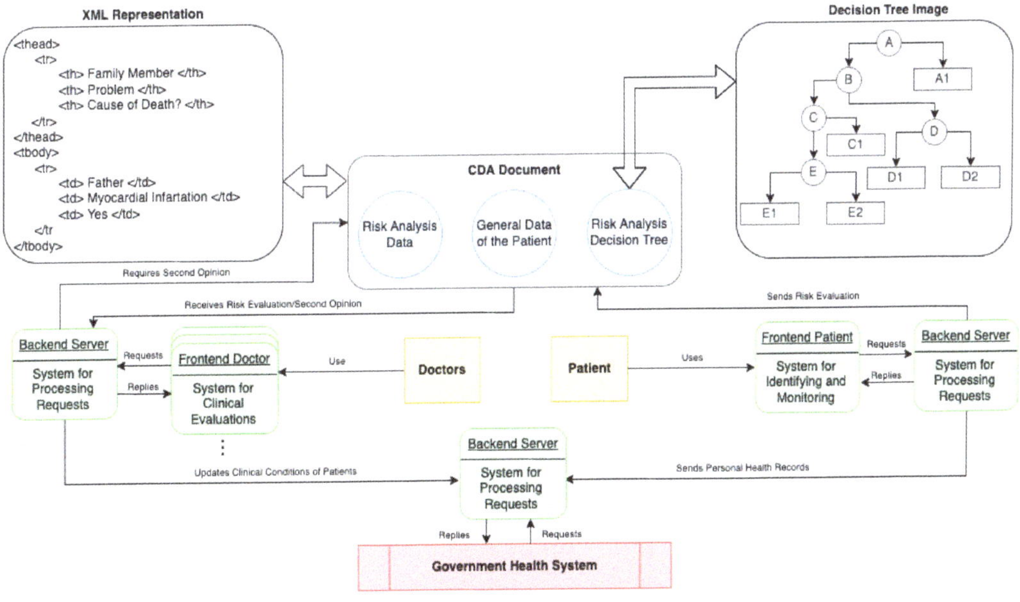

Figure 5. DSS methodology schema of identification and monitoring of CKD in developing countries.

Therefore, we implemented a web-based application considering the system used by patients, as an improvement of the results presented in [28]. The back-end of such subsystem was implemented using the Java programming language and web services. The subsystem comprises the following main features: access control, management of ingested drugs, management of allergies, management of examinations, monitoring of hypertension and DM, execution of risk analysis, generation and sharing CDA documents, and analysis of the emergency. In contrast, the front-end of the subsystem is implemented using HTML 5, Bootstrap, JavaScript, and Vue.js. For the graphical user interface (GUI) for recording a new CKD test result (the main inputs for the risk assessment model), the user can also upload an XML file containing the test results to present a large number of manual inputs. Once the patient provides the current test results, the main GUI of the subsystem is updated, showing the test results available for the risk assessment.

Figure 6 illustrates the main GUI of the patient sub-system, describing the creatinine, urea, albuminuria, and GFR (i.e., the main attributes used by the risk assessment model). This study reduces the number of required test results to conduct the CKD risk analysis from 5 to 4 compared to the previously published research [16]. This is critical for low-income populations using the sub-system because a very large number of biomarkers increases costs, that usually cannot be afforded by such people. Indeed, a reduced number of biomarkers can include more users for this type of DSS that would be possibly excluded due to their limited financial resources. The sub-system provides a new CKD risk analysis when the patient inputs all CKD attributes.

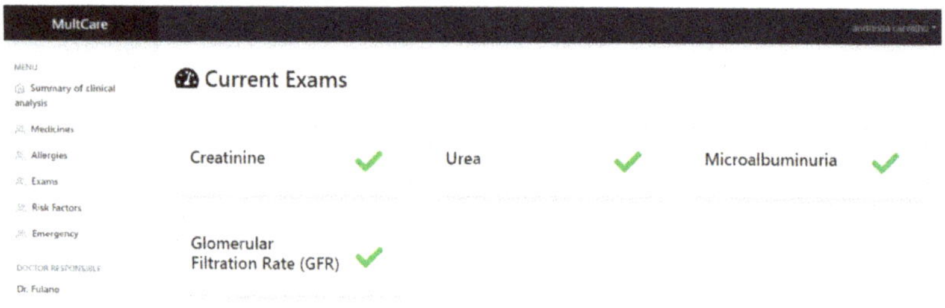

Figure 6. Screenshot of the main GUI for the patient sub-system.

During the CKD risk analysis (conducted when all tests are available), and based on the presence/absence of DM, presence/absence of hypertension, age, and gender, the J48 decision tree algorithm classifies the patient's situation considering four classes: low risk, moderate risk, high risk, and very high risk. In case of moderate risk, high risk, or very high risk, the sub-system packages the classification results as a CDA document, along with the decision tree graphic and general data of the patient. The sub-system alerts the physician responsible for the patient and sends the complete CDA document (i.e., the main output of the DSS) for further clinical analysis. In the case of low risk, the sub-system only records the risk analysis results to keep track of the patient's clinical situation. It does not send the physician alert, automating the risk analysis and sharing. This illustrates an example of scenario that shows how the definition of risk levels can provide more details on the patients' clinical conditions.

Results presented in this article justify the usage of the DT algorithm and attributes (i.e., presence/absence of DM, presence/absence of AH, creatinine, urea, albuminuria, age, gender, and GFR) to conduct risk analyses in developing countries. The physician responsible for the healthcare of a specific patient can, remotely, access the CDA document by a medical sub-system, re-evaluate or confirm the risk analysis (i.e., preliminary diagnosis) provided by the patient sub-system, and share the data with other physicians to get second opinions. If the physician confirms the preliminary diagnosis, the patient can continue using the patient sub-system to prevent the CKD progression, including the monitoring of risk factors (DM and AH), CKD stage, and risk level.

We also implemented the medical and server sub-systems using web technologies based on Figure 5. However, the description of such sub-systems is not in the scope of this article.

6. Discussion

When dealing with imbalanced and limited-size datasets, the evaluation of resampling and validation methods is essential to verify the stability of ML models. Our results indicated the non-ensemble DT model with data resampled with manual augmentation + SMOTE, with the best performance, obtaining a mean accuracy score of 98.99% for multiple stratified CV (see Table S2 of our Supplementary Materials) and nested CV (see Table S3 of our Supplementary Materials). The DT is followed by the multi-class AdaBoosted DTs model with a mean accuracy score of 97.99% for multiple stratified CV (see Table S2 of our Supplementary Materials) and 98% for nested CV (see Table S3 of our Supplementary Materials).

During CKD monitoring, based on the non-ensemble DT model with data resampled with manual augmentation + SMOTE, assuming the previous DM evaluation, the user only needs to perform two blood tests: creatinine and urea periodically. Albuminuria is measured using a urine test, while GFR can be calculated using the Cockcroft-Gault equation. The reduced number of exams is relevant for developing countries like Brazil due to the high poverty levels.

From the misclassified instances identified when testing the non-ensemble DT model, with data resampled with manual augmentation + SMOTE, the model disagreed with the experienced nephrologist, declaring very high risk rather than high risk (only one individual). However, the model did not lead to any critical underestimation of individuals' at-risk status (e.g., low risk rather than moderate risk). This situation would be a critical issue because the patient is usually referred to a nephrologist at moderate or high risk. Misleading classifications are less harmful to the patient as they still result in the patient being referred for evaluation, even if the risk is overestimated.

Along with using a reduced number of features and the absence of critical underestimations, another advantage of the DT model is the direct interpretation of results. A more straightforward interpretation of the CKD risk analysis by nephrologists and primary care doctors who need to perform additional tests to confirm a patient's clinical status is critical to reusing the model in real-world situations. The tree generated by the DT model encompasses each CKD biomarker considered and the related classification. A doctor follows the decisions to interpret the logic of classification. Of the 8 CKD features, only 5 were used by the non-ensemble DT model with data resampled with manual augmentation + SMOTE, to classify the risk (i.e., creatinine, gender, HA, urea, and albuminuria), requiring one blood test and one urine test when DM has already been evaluated, at the cost of one misclassified instance.

However, one of the main limitations of this study is the usage of the gridSearchCV tool to find the best parameters for each algorithm. We faced processing limitations, mainly for the ensemble models, because the parameter search was conducted for each ML model. The usage of gridSearchCV with 5 folds for the DT model is one example of such a situation. We handled 960 candidates, resulting in 4800 adjustments. However, when using the META-DES model, we handle 8640 candidates, resulting in 43,200 adjustments for the ensemble model, presenting a higher processing cost to adjust the parameters.

Besides, the reduced amount of manually augmented instances may also be considered a limitation. For example, the number of instances for the very high risk class in the test set is too reduced, which can have a negative impact on the performance evaluation for such class. The nested CV assisted us in reducing this limitation. We did not provide more augmented data because it is a time-consuming task for the nephrologist. However, given that one of the main purposes of this study is to address limited size datasets, the manual augmentation provided by the nephrologist was enough to conduct the experiments.

7. Conclusions and Future Work

The approach presented in this article can help design DSS to identify CKD in Brazilian communities. Such a system is relevant because low-income populations in Brazil generally suffer from the lack/precariousness of primary care. We develop and evaluate ensemble and non-ensemble models using different data resampling techniques for our CKD datasets. The result of the DT model with data resampled with the SMOTE technique improves the results of previous works. The remote identification of chronic diseases through DSS is even more relevant, considering the epidemics that prevent face-to-face care. For example, in Brazil, the COVID-19 epidemic negatively impacted the health assistance of low-income populations with chronic diseases, increasing mortality rates.

As future work, we envision applying formal modeling languages, such as coloured Petri nets, aiming to improve the accuracy of decision rules extracted from ML models. The formal modeling of decision rules is relevant, for example, to solve conflicting rules.

Supplementary Materials: The following supporting information can be downloaded at: https://bit.ly/3iwcwpK, Table S1: Sample of results from the analysis of statistical significance, Table S2: Results for the hold-out method without using the framework proposed by Pineda-Bautista et al. [23], Table S3: Results for the multiple stratified CV method without using the framework proposed by Pineda-Bautista et al. [23], Table S4: Results for the nested CV method without using the framework proposed by Pineda-Bautista et al. [23], Figure S1: PRC curves for the DT model using SMOTE and the nested CV method for the four first folds, Figure S2: PRC curves for the DT model using SMOTE and the nested CV method for the fifth, sixth, seventh, and eighth folds, Figure S3: PRC curves for the DT model using SMOTE and the nested CV method for the ninth and tenth folds.

Author Contributions: All authors contributed equally to this work. All authors have read and agreed to the published version of the manuscript.

Funding: The APC was funded by Federal University of Campina Grande and Virtus Research, Development and Innovation Center.

Institutional Review Board Statement: Not applicable.

Informed Consent Statement: Not applicable.

Data Availability Statement: Not applicable.

Acknowledgments: The authors would like to thank the Conselho Nacional de Desenvolvimento Científico e Tecnológico (CNPq); Virtus Research, Development and Innovation Center; and Programa de Pós-Graduação em Engenharia Elétrica, Federal University of Campina Grande for supporting this research. This study was financed in part by the Coordenação de Aperfeiçoamento de Pessoal de Nível Superior—Brazil: Project 88881.507204/2020-01.

Conflicts of Interest: The authors declare no conflict of interest.

References

1. Bikbov, B.; Purcell, C.A.; Levey, A.S.; Smith, M.; Abdoli, A.; Abebe, M.; Adebayo, O.M.; Afarideh, M.; Agarwal, S.K.; Agudelo-Botero, M.; et al. Global, regional, and national burden of chronic kidney disease, 1990–2017: A systematic analysis for the global burden of disease study 2017. *Lancet* **2020**, *395*, 709–733. [CrossRef]
2. Abegunde, D.; Stanciole, A. *Preventing Chronic Diseases: A Vital Investment: Who Global Report*; World Health Organization: Geneva, Switzerland, 2006.
3. World Health Organization. *World Health Statistics Overview 2019: Monitoring Health for the SDGS, Sustainable Development Goals*; World Health Organization: Geneva, Switzerland, 2019.
4. Sociedade Brasileira de Diabetes. *Guidelines of the Brazilian Society of Diabetes 2019–2020*; Sociedade Brasileira de Diabetes: São Paulo, Brazil, 2019.
5. Sobrinho, A.; Queiroz, A.C.M.D.S.; Silva, L.D.D.; Costa, E.D.B.; Pinheiro, M.E.; Perkusich, A. Computer-aided diagnosis of chronic kidney disease in developing countries: A comparative analysis of machine learning techniques. *IEEE Access* **2020**, *8*, 25407–25419. [CrossRef]
6. Levey, A.; Inker, L.; Coresh, J. Chronic kidney disease in older people. *J. Am. Med. Assoc.* **2015**, *314*, 557–558. [CrossRef] [PubMed]
7. Kinaan, M.; Yau, H.; Martinez, S.Q.; Kar, P. Concepts in diabetic nephropathy: From pathophysiology to treatment. *J. Ren. Hepatic Disord.* **2017**, *1*, 10–24. [CrossRef]

8. Sesso, R.C.C.; Lopes, A.A.; Thomé, F.S.; Lugon, J.R.; Burdmann, E.A. Brazilian dialysis census 2009. *Braz. J. Nephrol.* **2010**, *32*, 380–384. [CrossRef]
9. Webster, A.C.; Nagler, E.V.; Morton, R.L.; Masson, P. Chronic kidney disease. *Lancet* **2017**, *389*, 1238–1252. [CrossRef]
10. Sesso, R.C.; Lopes, A.A.; Thomé, F.S.; Lugon, J.R.; dos Santos, D.R. 2010 report of the brazilian dialysis census. *Braz. J. Nephrol.* **2011**, *33*, 442–447. [CrossRef]
11. Sesso, R.C.; Lopes, A.A.; Thomé, F.S.; Lugon, J.R.; Martins, C.T. Brazilian chronic dialysis survey 2016. *Braz. J. Nephrol.* **2017**, *39*, 380–384. [CrossRef]
12. Thomé, F.S.; Sesso, R.C.; Lopes, A.A.; Lugon, J.R.; Martins, C.T. Brazilian chronic dialysis survey 2017. *Braz. J. Nephrol.* **2019**, *41*, 208–214. [CrossRef]
13. Neves, P.D.M.M.; Sesso, R.C.C.; Thomé, F.S.; Lugon, J.R.; Nascimento, M.M. Brazilian dialysis census: Analysis of data from the 2009–2018 decade. *Braz. J. Nephrol.* **2020**, *42*, 191–200. [CrossRef]
14. Chan, C.T.; Blankestijn, P.J.; Dember, L.M.; Gallieni, M.; Harris, D.C.; Lok, C.E.; Mehrotra, R.; Stevens, P.E.; Wang, A.Y.M.; Cheung, M.; et al. Dialysis initiation, modality choice, access, and prescription: Conclusions from a Kidney Disease: Improving Global Outcomes (KDIGO) Controversies Conference. *Kidney Int.* **2019**, *96*, 37–47. [CrossRef] [PubMed]
15. Elshahat, S.; Cockwell, P.; Maxwell, A.P.; Griffin, M.; O'Brien, T.; O'Neill, C. The impact of chronic kidney disease on developed countries from a health economics perspective: A systematic scoping review. *PLoS ONE* **2020**, *15*, e0230512. [CrossRef] [PubMed]
16. Brazilian Ministry of Health. Available online: https://bit.ly/3uNAS3Y (accessed on 1 April 2020).
17. Cha'on, U.; Wongtrangan, K.; Thinkhamrop, B.; Tatiyanupanwong, S.; Limwattananon, C.; Pongskul, C.; Panaput, T.; Chalermwat, C.; Lert-Itthiporn, W.; Sharma, A.; et al. Ckdnet, a quality improvement project for prevention and reduction of chronic kidney disease in the northeast Thailand. *BMC Public Health* **2020**, *20*, 1–11. [CrossRef] [PubMed]
18. Vabalas, A.; Gowen, E.; Poliakoff, E.; Casson, A.J. Machine learning algorithm validation with a limited sample size. *PLoS ONE* **2019**, *14*, e0224365. [CrossRef] [PubMed]
19. Sun, Y.; Wong, A.K.C.; Kamel, M.S. Classification of imbalanced data: A review. *Int. J. Pattern Recognit. Artif. Intell.* **2009**, *23*, 687–719. [CrossRef]
20. Jeni, L.A.; Cohn, J.F.; De La Torre, F. Facing imbalanced data–recommendations for the use of performance metrics. In Proceedings of the 2013 Humaine Association Conference on Affective Computing and Intelligent Interaction, Geneva, Switzerland, 2–5 September 2013; pp. 245–251.
21. Choi, M.Y.; Christopher, M. Making a big impact with small datasets using machine-learning approaches. *Lancet Rheumatol.* **2020**, *2*, e451–e452. [CrossRef]
22. Cruz, R.M.O.; Hafemann, L.G.; Sabourin, R.; Cavalcanti, G.D.C. DESlib: A Dynamic ensemble selection library in Python. *J. Mach. Learn. Res.* **2020**, *21*, 1–5.
23. Pineda-Bautista, B.B.; Carrasco-Ochoa, J.; Martınez-Trinida, J.F. General framework for class-specific feature selection. *Expert Syst. Appl.* **2011**, *38*, 10018–10024. [CrossRef]
24. Hulse, J.V.; Khoshgoftaar, T.M.; Napolitano, A. Experimental perspectives on learning from imbalanced data. In Proceedings of the 24th International Conference on Machine Learning, Corvallis, OR, USA, 20–24 June 2007; pp. 935–942.
25. Akbani, R.; Kwek, S.; Japkowicz, N. Applying support vector machines to imbalanced datasets. In Proceedings of the European Conference on Machine Learning, Pisa, Italy, 20–24 September 2004; pp. 39–50.
26. Varma, S.; Simon, R. Bias in error estimation when using cross-validation for model selection. *BMC Bioinform.* **2006**, *7*, 1–8. [CrossRef]
27. Santos Santana, Í.V.; Silveira, A.C.; Sobrinho, Á.; e Silva, L.C.; da Silva, L.D.; Santos, D.F.; Gurjão, E.C.; Perkusich, A. Classification Models for COVID-19 Test Prioritization in Brazil: Machine Learning Approach. *J. Med. Internet Res.* **2021**, *23*, e27293. [CrossRef]
28. Sobrinho, A.; da Silva, L.D.; Perkusich, A.; Pinheiro, M.E.; Cunha, P. Design and evaluation of a mobile application to assist the self-monitoring of the chronic kidney disease in developing countries. *BMC Med. Informatics Decis. Mak.* **2018**, *18*, 1–14. [CrossRef] [PubMed]
29. Lamb, E.J.; Levey, A.S.; Stevens, P.E. The kidney disease improving global outcomes (KDIGO) guideline update for chronic kidney disease: Evolution not revolution. *Clin. Chem.* **2013**, *59*, 462–465. [CrossRef] [PubMed]
30. Forbes, A.; Gallagher, H. Chronic kidney disease in adults: Assessment and management. *Clin. Med.* **2020**, *2020*, 128–132. [CrossRef] [PubMed]
31. Inker, L.A.; Astor, B.C.; Fox, C.H.; Isakova, T.; Lash, J.P.; Peralta, C.A.; Tamura, M.K.; Feldman, H.I. KDOQI US commentary on the 2012 KDIGO clinical practice guideline for the evaluation and management of CKD. *Am. J. Kidney Dis.* **2014**, *63*, 713–735. [CrossRef] [PubMed]
32. Sobrinho, A.; da Silva, L.D.; Perkusich, A.; Queiroz, A.; Pinheiro, M.E. A Brazilian Dataset for Screening the Risk of the Chronic Kidney Disease. Available online: https://bit.ly/3rQxllg (accessed on 1 April 2022).
33. Lemaître, G.; Nogueira, F.; Aridas, C.K. Imbalanced-learn: Apython toolbox to tackle the curse of imbalanced datasets in machine learning. *J. Mach. Learn. Res.* **2017**, *18*, 1–5.
34. Chawla, N.V.; Bowyer, K.W.; Hall, L.O.; Kegelmeyer, W.P. SMOTE: Synthetic minority over-sampling technique. *J. Artif. Intell. Res.* **2002**, *16*, 321–357. [CrossRef]
35. Han, H.; Wang, W.-Y.; Mao, B.-H. Borderline-smote: A new over-sampling method in imbalanced datasets learning. In Proceedings of the International Conference on Intelligent Computing, Hefei, China, 23–26 August 2005; pp. 878–887.

36. Nguyen, H.M.; Cooper, E.W.; Kamei, K. Borderline over-sampling for imbalanced data classification. *J. Knowl. Eng. Soft Data Paradig.* **2011**, *3*, 4–21.
37. Bishop, C.M. *Pattern Recognition and Machine Learning*, 2nd ed.; Springer: Berlin/Heidelberg, Germany, 2011.
38. Langs, G.; Menze, B.H.; Lashkari, D.; Golland, P. Detecting stable distributed patterns of brain activation using gini contrast. *NeuroImage* **2011**, *56*, 497–507. [CrossRef]
39. Pedregosa, F.; Varoquaux, G.; Gramfort, A.; Michel, V.; Thirion, B.; Grisel, O.; Blon-del, M.; Prettenhofer, P.; Weiss, R.; Dubourg, V.; et al. Scikit-learn: Machine learning in Python. *J. Mach. Learn. Res.* **2011**, *12*, 2825–2830.
40. Boughorbel S.; Jarray, F.; El-Anbari, M. Optimal classifier for imbalanced data using Matthews Correlation Coefficient metric. *PLoS ONE* **2017**, *12*, e0177678. [CrossRef]
41. Fowlkes, E.B.; Mallows, C.L. A Method for Comparing Two Hierarchical Clusterings. *J. Am. Stat. Assoc.* **2012**, *78*, 553–569. [CrossRef]
42. Hand, D.J.; Till, R.J. A Simple Generalisation of the Area Under the ROC Curve for Multiple Class Classification Problems. *Mach. Learn.* **2001**, *45*, 171–186. [CrossRef]
43. Davis, J.; Goadrich, M. The relationship between Precision-Recall and ROC curves. In Proceedings of the 23rd International Conference on Machine Learning, Pittsburgh, PA, USA, 25–29 June 2006.
44. Wang, H.Y. Combination approach of SMOTE and biased-SVM for imbalanced datasets. In Proceedings of the IEEE International Joint Conference on Neural Networks (IEEE World Congress on Computational Intelligence), Hong Kong, China, 1–6 June 2008.
45. Chawla, N.V.; Lazarevic, A.; Hall, L.O.; Bowyer, K.W. SMOTEBoost: Improving Prediction of the Minority Class in Boosting. In Proceedings of the European Conference on Principles of Data Mining and Knowledge Discovery, Helsinki, Finland, 19–23 August 2003.
46. Das, B.; Krishnan, N.C.; Cook, D.J. RACOG and wRACOG: Two Probabilistic Oversampling Techniques. *IEEE Trans. Knowl. Data Eng.* **2015**, *27*, 222–234. [CrossRef] [PubMed]
47. Varoquaux, G. Cross-validation failure: Small sample sizes lead to large error bars. *NeuroImage* **2018**, *180*, 68–77. [CrossRef] [PubMed]
48. Krstajic, D.; Buturovic, L.J.; Leahy, D.E.; Thomas, S. Cross-validation pitfalls when selecting and assessing regression and classification models. *J. Cheminform.* **2014**, *6*, 1–15. [CrossRef]
49. Ilyas, H.; Ali, S.; Ponum, M.; Hasan, O.; Mahmood, M.T.; Iftikhar, M.; Malik, M.H. Chronic kidney disease diagnosis using decision tree algorithms. *BMC Nephrol.* **2021**, *22*, 1–11. [CrossRef]
50. Qin, J.; Chen, L.; Liu, Y.; Liu, C.; Feng, C.; Chen, B. A Machine Learning Methodology for Diagnosing Chronic Kidney Disease. *IEEE Access* **2020**, *8*, 20991–21002. [CrossRef]
51. Chittora, P.; Chaurasia, S.; Prasun, C.; Kumawat, G.; Chakrabarti, T.; Leonowicz, Z.; Jasiński, M.; Jasiński, Ł.; Gono, R.; Jasińska, E.; et al. Prediction of Chronic Kidney Disease—A Machine Learning Perspective. *IEEE Access* **2021**, **9**, 17312–17334. [CrossRef]
52. Chaurasia, V.; Pandey, M.K.; Pal, S. Chronic kidney disease: A prediction and comparison of ensemble and basic classifiers performance. *Hum. Intell. Syst. Integr.* **2022**, 1–10. [CrossRef]
53. Abdulaal, M.; Casson, A.; Gaydecki, P. Performance of Nested vs. Non-nested SVM Cross-validation Methods in Visual BCI: Validation Study. In Proceedings of the 2018 26rd European Signal Processing Conference (EUSIPCO), Rome, Italy, 3–7 September 2018.
54. CKD-Experiment. Available online: https://bit.ly/3BpnsOw (accessed on 1 April 2022).

applied sciences

Article

An Effective Approach to Detect and Identify Brain Tumors Using Transfer Learning

Naeem Ullah [1], Javed Ali Khan [2,*], Mohammad Sohail Khan [3], Wahab Khan [4], Izaz Hassan [2], Marwa Obayya [5], Noha Negm [6,*] and Ahmed S. Salama [7]

1 Department of Software Engineering, University of Engineering and Technology, Taxila 47050, Pakistan; naeemullahfeb1997@gmail.com
2 Department of Software Engineering, University of Science and Technology Bannu, Bannu 28100, Pakistan; izaz.hassan88@gmail.com
3 Department of Computer Software Engineering, University of Engineering and Technology Mardan, Mardan 23200, Pakistan; sohail.khan@uetmardan.edu.pk
4 Department of Electrical Engineering, University of Science and Technology Bannu, Bannu 28100, Pakistan; wahab487@yahoo.com
5 Department of Biomedical Engineering, College of Engineering, Princess Nourah bint Abdulrahman University, P.O. Box 84428, Riyadh 11671, Saudi Arabia; mobaya@pnu.edu.sa
6 Department of Computer Science, College of Science & Art at Mahayil, King Khalid University, Abha 62529, Saudi Arabia
7 Department of Electrical Engineering, Faculty of Engineering & Technology, Future University in Egypt, New Cairo 11845, Egypt; salama@fue.edu.eg
* Correspondence: engr_javed501@yahoo.com (J.A.K.); nohawesabi@gmail.com (N.N.)

Abstract: Brain tumors are considered one of the most serious, prominent and life-threatening diseases globally. Brain tumors cause thousands of deaths every year around the globe because of the rapid growth of tumor cells. Therefore, timely analysis and automatic detection of brain tumors are required to save the lives of thousands of people around the globe. Recently, deep transfer learning (TL) approaches are most widely used to detect and classify the three most prominent types of brain tumors, i.e., glioma, meningioma and pituitary. For this purpose, we employ state-of-the-art pre-trained TL techniques to identify and detect glioma, meningioma and pituitary brain tumors. The aim is to identify the performance of nine pre-trained TL classifiers, i.e., Inceptionresnetv2, Inceptionv3, Xception, Resnet18, Resnet50, Resnet101, Shufflenet, Densenet201 and Mobilenetv2, by automatically identifying and detecting brain tumors using a fine-grained classification approach. For this, the TL algorithms are evaluated on a baseline brain tumor classification (MRI) dataset, which is freely available on Kaggle. Additionally, all deep learning (DL) models are fine-tuned with their default values. The fine-grained classification experiment demonstrates that the inceptionresnetv2 TL algorithm performs better and achieves the highest accuracy in detecting and classifying glioma, meningioma and pituitary brain tumors, and hence it can be classified as the best classification algorithm. We achieve 98.91% accuracy, 98.28% precision, 99.75% recall and 99% F-measure values with the inceptionresnetv2 TL algorithm, which out-performs the other DL algorithms. Additionally, to ensure and validate the performance of TL classifiers, we compare the efficacy of the inceptionresnetv2 TL algorithm with hybrid approaches, in which we use convolutional neural networks (CNN) for deep feature extraction and a Support Vector Machine (SVM) for classification. Similarly, the experiment's results show that TL algorithms, and inceptionresnetv2 in particular, out-perform the state-of-the-art DL algorithms in classifying brain MRI images into glioma, meningioma, and pituitary. The hybrid DL approaches used in the experiments are Mobilnetv2, Densenet201, Squeeznet, Alexnet, Googlenet, Inceptionv3, Resnet50, Resnet18, Resnet101, Xception, Inceptionresnetv3, VGG19 and Shufflenet.

Keywords: brain tumor; deep learning; inceptionResNetv2; transfer learning; tumor detection

1. Introduction

The human brain is the management center and the central organ of the human nervous system, which is responsible for performing daily life activities. The brain receives stimuli or signals from sensory organs of the body, performs processing and sends final decisions and output information to the muscles. Uncontrolled cell division or mutations generate an abnormal group of cells in the brain, resulting in a brain tumor. This type of cell has the ability to affect normal brain function as well as damage healthy cells [1,2]. Headaches, cognitive issues, vomiting, personality changes, eyesight and speech are some of the most prevalent symptoms of brain tumors. The growth of a brain tumor affects the personality, way of thinking and all other essential functions of patients.

Usually, brain tumors are of two types: non-cancerous tumors, which are called benign, and cancerous tumors, which are called malignant. Benign tumors are non-progressive and originate in the brain. This kind of tumor is less aggressive and cannot expand in the body. On the other hand, malignant tumors are cancerous tumors that spread rapidly throughout the body. Furthermore, there are two categories of malignant tumors: primary malignant tumors that originate in the brain and transfer to other body parts, and secondary malignant tumors that initiate in other body regions and spread to the brain [3]. Meningioma, pituitary and glioma tumors are common types of brain tumors. Meningioma arises in the thin membranes, i.e., tissues surrounding the spinal cord and brain. Gliomas arise within the glial cells of the brain. Pituitary tumors grow when cells in the pituitary gland near the brain grow in an abnormal pattern. One of the most life-threatening disorders is a brain tumor. As a result, the timely treatment and identification of brain tumors are required to preserve patients' lives. One possible solution is to use machine learning (ML) algorithms to identify brain tumors and their types in patients automatically. However, because of brain tumors' wide range of sizes, shapes and intensities, classifying them into meningioma, pituitary and glioma tumors is a more difficult task [4]. Moreover, among all brain tumors, meningioma, pituitary and glioma tumors have the highest occurrence rate [5].

Furthermore, brain magnetic resonance imaging (MRI) provides detailed information about the brain's structure due to its high resolution. Hence, MRI images significantly impact automatic medical image analysis [6–9]. To detect and analyze brain tumors, researchers mostly rely on MRI techniques. Recently, many automated brain tumor detection and classification approaches have been proposed by researchers using MRI images. For the detection of brain tumors, traditional ML algorithms, particularly Multi-Layer Perceptron (MLP) and SVM classifiers, are widely used [10]. DL is a ML subfield in which low-level features aid in the construction of high-level features, producing a hierarchy of features [11]. The DL structure adds more hidden layers between the input and output layers to extend the traditional neural network framework. Researchers are now using DL techniques to solve various medical image analysis challenges, such as image denoising, segmentation, registration and classification [8,12–15]. CNNs, which use convolutional filters to accomplish complex tasks, have become the most extensively used DL framework in recent years. Feedforward layers with convolutional filters, pooling layers and fully connected (FC) layers make up the CNN framework. A CNN-based classifier can provide a fully automated classifier considered for brain tumor classification [11]. Pashaei et al. [16] suggested a CNN-based model to efficiently extract features from brain MRI. Since CNN-based models do not require manual feature extraction, they are faster than standard ML algorithms. However, training a CNN classifier from scratch is difficult and time-consuming and requires an extensive labeled dataset.

Additionally, there are a lot of irregularities in the sizes and positions of brain tumors, which makes the natural understanding of brain tumors problematic. Generally, for the classification of brain tumors, T1-weighted contrast-enhanced (with gadolinium-enhanced) MRI images (T1c) are used because tumors are considerably better visualized on T1c due to the stimulation of 0.150 mMol/kg of contrast material (gadolinium) in patients [17]. Diffusion-weighted imaging (DWI) is also considered vital for detecting brain tumors because it can visualize restrictions to the free diffusion of water caused by tissue microstructures [18].

The different features extracted from MRI images are key sources for tumor classification. DL makes predictions and decisions on data by learning data representation. DL practices are most widely used for medical imaging classification. However, DL-based methods have shown satisfactory results in various applications across a wide range of domains in various fields [19–22]. However, DL approaches are starving data approaches, i.e., they require a lot of training data. Recently, DL approaches, particularly the CNN model, have been attracting more and more attention. CNN outperforms other classifiers on larger datasets, such as ImageNet, consisting of millions of images. However, it is challenging to employ CNNs in the field of medical imaging. Firstly, medical image datasets contain limited data because expert radiologists are required to label the dataset's images, which is a tedious and time-consuming task. Secondly, CNN training is difficult for a small dataset because of overfitting. Thirdly, hyperparameters of CNN classifiers need to be adjusted to achieve better performance that requires domain expertise. Therefore, using pre-trained models on TL and fine tuning are viable solutions to address these challenges. In TL approaches, DL models are trained on a large dataset (base dataset) and transfer learned knowledge to the target dataset (small dataset) [23]. This paper proposes an automatic brain tumor classification approach intended for three-class classification. Several approaches utilize manually defined tumor regions to detect and classify brain tumors, preventing them from being fully automated [1,2,19]. However, the proposed new approach does not involve any segmentation or feature extraction and selection in the pre-processing step, in contrast to some previous methods [1,2,19], which require prior segmentation and feature extraction of tumors from MRI images. We use a standard Kaggle brain tumor classification (MRI) dataset, including three types of brain tumors: meningioma, pituitary and glioma. We perform extensive experiments based on this dataset to compare the performance of nine DL models for the classification of brain tumor MRI images using TL. We used Inceptionresnetv2, Inceptionv3, Xception, Resnet18, Resnet50, Resnet101, Shufflenet, Densenet201 and Mobilenetv2 for the automatic detection and classification of brain tumors using a fine-grained classification approach. Furthermore, several approaches utilize the manually defined tumor regions *to detect and classify* brain tumors that prevent them from being fully automated. The aim is to identify the most effective and efficient deep TL model for brain tumor classification. We report the overall accuracy, precision, recall, f-measure and elapsed time of the nine pre-trained frameworks in this paper.

The key contributions of our research include the following:

- Proposing a DL-based framework for automatically detecting and classifying brain tumors into meningioma, pituitary and glioma tumors.
- Analyzing and validating the TL concept for nine different deep neural networks.
- Analyzing the performance of each TL model in classifying brain MRI images correctly and efficiently.
- Comparing the performance of TL approaches with hybrid approaches (DL + SVM).

The remainder of the paper is organized into the following subsections. Section 2 provides details about the existing literature on brain MRI classification. Section 3 describes the proposed methodology and details of TL algorithms. Section 4 elaborates on the experimental work in comparison with existing state-of-the-art TL approaches and hybrid DL approaches. Finally, Section 5 concludes the research paper and discusses future directions.

2. Related Work

Recently, there has been a lot of work on brain tumor detection and classification [24–32]. For the detection and categorization of brain tumors, various techniques have been presented. These methods include traditional ML methods and DL methods. This section includes the investigation of existing brain tumor detection and classification approaches.

Ismael et al. introduced an approach that integrates statistical features and neural network techniques [24] to detect and classify brain tumor MRI images. Region of interest (ROI) is used in this method, defined as the tumor segment detected using any ROI segmentation technique. Moreover, 2D Discrete Wavelet Transform (DWT) and 2D Gabor filter techniques were used to determine features for the classifier. To create the feature set, they used many transform domain statistical features. For classification, a backpropagation neural network classifier was used. A Figshare dataset of 3064 slices of T1-weighted MRI images of three forms of brain tumors, meningioma, glioma, and pituitary, was used to evaluate the model. The authors achieved a maximum accuracy of 91.9%. A Deep Neural Network classifier, one of the DL frameworks, was used by Mohsen et al. to classify a dataset of 66 brain MRIs into four categories: normal, glioblastoma, sarcoma and metastatic bronchogenic carcinoma tumors [25]. The classifier was combined with the discrete wavelet transform (DWT), a powerful feature extraction approach, and principal component analysis (PCA), with promising results across all performance metrics. The authors achieved a maximum accuracy of 98.4% by combining DNN with DWT. Deepak et al. classified medical images using a combination of CNN features and SVM [26]. To analyze and validate their proposed approach, they used publicly available MRI images of brain tumors from Figshare that comprised three types of brain tumors. They extracted characteristics from MRI scans of the brain using the CNN classifier. For increased performance, a multiclass SVM was paired with CNN features. They also tested and evaluated an integrated system using a five-fold cross-validation technique. The proposed model surpassed the current techniques with respect to total classification accuracy by achieving a classification accuracy of 95.82%. When there is limited training data, the SVM classifier outperforms the softmax classifier for CNN feature extraction. They employed the CNN–SVM approach, which requires fewer computations and less memory than TL-based classification. For brain tumor identification, the authors of [27] presented a multi-level attention mechanism network (MANet). The suggested MANet incorporates both spatial and cross-channel attention, focusing on tumor region prioritization while also preserving cross-channel temporal relationships found in the Xception backbone's semantic feature sequence. The proposed method was tested using the Figshare and BraTS benchmark datasets. Experiments show that combining cross-channel and spatial attention blocks improves generalizations and results with improved performance with fewer model parameters. The suggested MANet outperforms various current models for tumor recognition, with a maximum accuracy of 96.51 percent on Figshare and 94.91 percent on BraTS'2018 datasets.

In image detection and recognition challenges, CNN plays a significant role. To extract features automatically from brain images, CNN filters are convolved with the input image. Most research methodologies use CNN-based approaches for brain tumor detection and classification. Afshar et al. used capsule networks for brain tumor classification and investigated the overfitting problem of CapsNets using a real collection of MRI data [28]. CapsNets require far less training data, making them perfect for medical imaging datasets such as brain MRI scans. They built a visualization paradigm for CapsNet's output to better illustrate the learned features. The achieved accuracy of 86.56% demonstrates that the presented method for brain tumor classification could successfully overcome CNNs. MR images are used to diagnose a brain tumor [29]. The use of CNN classification for automatic brain tumor detection was proposed by the authors. Small kernels were used to create deeper architecture. The neuron's weight is described as tiny. When compared to all other state-of-the-art methodologies, the experimental results demonstrate that CNN archives have a rate of 97.5% accuracy with little complexity.

Rai et al. adopted a Less Layered and Less Complex U-Net (LeU-Net) framework for brain tumor detection [30]. The LeU-Net idea was influenced by both the Le-Net and U-Net frameworks; however, it differs significantly from both architectural approaches. The performance of LeU-Net was compared to the existing basic CNN frameworks Le-Net, U-Net and VGG-16. Accuracy, precision, F-score, recall and specificity were used to assess CNN performance. The experiment was conducted on an MR dataset with cropped (removed unwanted area) and uncropped images. Moreover, the results were compared to all three models. The LeU-Net model has a much faster processing (simulation) time; training the network with 100 epochs achieved 98% accuracy on cropped images and achieved 94% accuracy on uncropped images, which took 252.36 s and 244.42 s, respectively. Kader et al. proposed a new hybrid model for brain tumor identification and classification based on MR brain images [31], intending to assist doctors in the early diagnosis and classification of brain tumors with maximum accuracy and performance. The approach was developed using a hybrid deep CNN and a deep watershed auto-encoder (CNN–DWA) model. The technique can be broken down into six steps: input MR images, preprocessing with a filter and morphological operation, generating a matrix that represents MR brain images, using the hybrid CNN–DWA framework, brain tumor detection and classification and model performance evaluation. The model was validated using five databases: BRATS2012, BRATS2013, BRATS2014, ISLES-SISS 2015 and BRATS2015. Based on the RCNN technique [32], Kesav et al. developed a new framework for brain tumor classification and tumor type object recognition, tested using two publicly available datasets from Figshare and Kaggle. The goal was to design a basic framework that would allow the classic RCNN framework to run faster. Glioma and healthy tumor MRI images were initially classified using a two-channel CNN. Later, a feature extractor in an RCNN was used to locate tumor locations in a glioma MRI sample categorized from a previous stage using the same framework. Bounding boxes were used to define the tumor region. Meningioma and pituitary tumors are two more malignancies that have been treated with this method. The proposed method achieved an average confidence level of 98.83% for two-class tumor classification, i.e., meningioma and pituitary tumors.

Existing works on brain tumor detection and classification have some limitations. Most of the approaches are validated with the figshare dataset, which is an imbalanced dataset and affects the performances of classification approaches. Hence, there is a need to validate brain tumor classification approaches on another balanced dataset. ML, in its traditional form, necessitates domain knowledge and experience. Manual feature extraction necessitates time and effort, reducing the system's efficiency. On the other hand, employing DL, particularly CNN, in medical imaging is challenging, as it requires a significant amount of data for training. In contrast, deep TL-based algorithms can avoid these drawbacks by using automatic feature extraction and robust classification applications based on convolutional layers. This study proposes an automatic classification system for multiclass brain tumor MR images, which is a more complex and difficult assignment than simple binary classification. However, our dataset is very small, and it is difficult to train CNN from scratch using small datasets without suffering from overfitting and with appropriate convergence. Inspired by the success of TL techniques [5,19,33,34], we adopted the concept of TL in this work. For this purpose, we employed various TL models in this research work, including Inceptionresnetv2, Inceptionv3, Xception, Resnet18, Resnet50, Resnet101, Shufflenet, Densenet201 and Mobilenetv2 to achieve brain tumor detection and classification on the target dataset. Furthermore, we compared the best model with other methods to show its efficacy in identifying brain tumors.

3. Research Methodology

This section elaborates on the proposed research methodology for fine-grained brain tumor classification. We thoroughly explain the proposed TL-based approach, its framework and the different pre-trained TL classifiers employed to detect and classify brain MRI images into meningioma, pituitary and glioma.

3.1. Proposed Approach

The proposed research methodology is depicted in Figure 1, which demonstrates an abstract view of the proposed TL-based approach for brain tumor classification using MRI images. The proposed TL-based brain tumor classification comprises the following steps. Firstly, we downloaded the freely available Kaggle MR image dataset [35], including glioma, meningioma and pituitary MR images, and we placed the dataset into the training directory. Secondly, we employed imageDataStore to read the MR images of the dataset from the training directory.

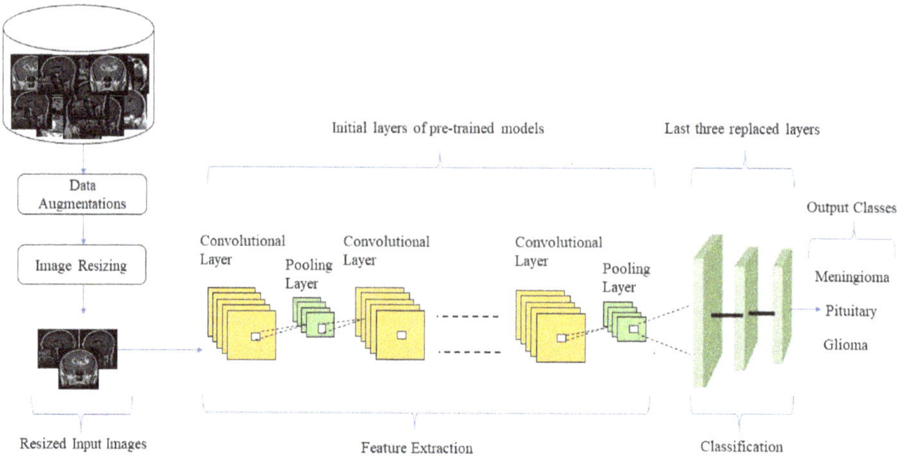

Figure 1. Overview of the proposed method for brain tumor classification.

In the third step, we applied a data augmentation technique to test the generalizability of the TL models. Data augmentation, or increasing the amount of available data without acquiring new data by applying multiple processes to the current data, has been proven to be advantageous in image classification. Due to the limited number of images in the dataset, we applied the data augmentation technique in this study. The images in the training set were rotated at a random angle between −20 and 20 degrees, and were arbitrarily translated up to thirty pixels vertically and horizontally to create additional images. It is also worth noting that the imageDataAugmenter function was utilized to dynamically create sets of augmented images during each training phase. The number of images in the training set was significantly expanded using this data augmentation method, enabling more effective use of our DL model by training with a much higher number of training images. Furthermore, the augmented images were only used to train the proposed framework, not to test it; hence, only real images from the dataset were utilized to test the learned framework.

In the fourth step, the input MRI images of the dataset were resized according to the pre-trained CNN model's input image requirements. The images in the dataset were of various sizes, and different models required input images of various sizes, such as the TL mobilenetv2 classifier, accepting 224 × 224 input images, and the inceptionv3 classifier, requiring 229 × 229 input images. Therefore, before being inserted into the DL network, the training and testing images were automatically scaled utilizing augmented image data stores of TL.

Next, we employed different pre-trained deep neural networks, i.e., Inceptionresnetv2, Inceptionv3, Xception, Resnet18, Resnet50, Resnet101, Shufflenet Densenet201 and Mobilenetv2, to identify their performance in identifying and classifying different kinds of brain tumors. The proposed TL models consisted of layers from the pre-trained networks and three new layers, i.e., the last three layers modified to suit the new image categories (meningioma, pituitary and glioma). The transfer learned models had a softmax layer, classifying images into meningioma, pituitary and glioma. For example, for "Inceptionv3" and "InceptionResNetV2", we replaced "predictions", "predictions_softmax" and "ClassificationLayer_predictions" with a "fully connected layer", a "softmax layer" and a "classification output" layer. We connected the additional layers to the network's last remaining transferred layer, i.e., "avg pool". We replaced the network's last three layers, i.e., "fc1000", "fc1000_softmax" and "ClassificationLayer_fc1000", with a "completely connected layer", a "softmax layer" and "classification output" layers for "ResNet50" and connected the additional layers to the network's last remaining transferred layer ("avg pool"). Similarly, we replaced the "fc1000", "prob" and "ClassificationLayer_predictions" layers of the network with a "fully connected layer", a "softmax layer" and a "classification output" layer for "ResNet101" and connected the new layers to the network's last remaining transferred layer ("pool5").

The detailed structure of the proposed DL framework is shown in Figure 2, extended from the concept of TL. Furthermore, we evaluated and validated each model to assess the performance of different pre-trained TL algorithms in identifying brain tumor types. For this purpose, we divided the dataset into training and testing sets to obtain accurate and reliable results; more specifically, we used 80% of the data for model training and the remaining 20% for testing. The overall process of pre-trained TL classification for brain tumor identification and classification is shown in Figure 1.

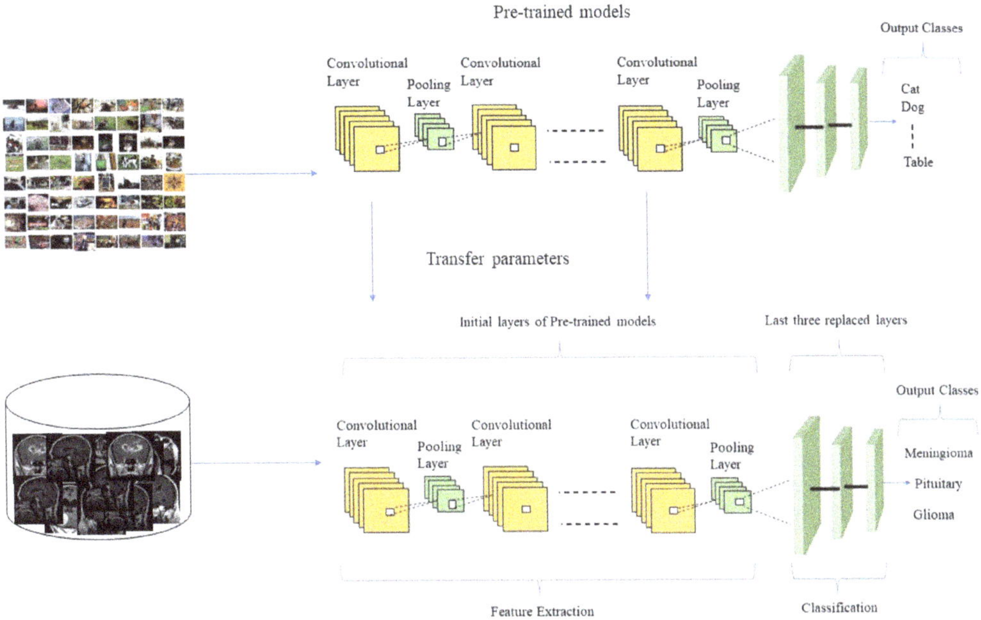

Figure 2. Transfer learning setting.

3.2. *Transfer Learning in an Inductive Setting*

To train and validate a classifier that can achieve accuracy on image classification tasks near or above the human level, a lot of training data, heavy computational power, time and resources are required. It becomes challenging to train and validate an image classifier from scratch until having a large data set. In contrast, TL is a method that uses the gained knowledge of a trained model and applies it to solve other related problems [19]. The aim is to employ a wide training dataset provided to the model with more image feature information before adapting it to a new data field. TL networks are intended to acquire spatial features using convolutional, pooling and FC layers. Moreover, traditional CNN requires a lot of training data, time and computation resources for training. Therefore, in the case of limited data (such as brain tumor recognition, where training image samples are scarce, then classifier performance suffers significantly) and computational resources, the TL of pre-trained deep neural networks is a faster and more cost-effective approach for classification tasks. When there are limited data to learn from, common information is transferred from old tasks to new ones, and some specialized knowledge is produced throughout the problem-solving process. The model learns high-level features specific to the target domain, e.g., brain tumor classification, whereas the pre-trained layers learns low-level features of the original networks. Depending on the type of task and the nature of the data accessible at the source and destination domains, several parameters for TL are offered [36]. The TL approach is known as inductive TL [37] when labeled data are available in the source and target domains for a classification task. TL algorithms enhance classification performance even with limited data available for training and validation. The key task in TL is selecting a pre-trained deep neural network among the available TL algorithms. This selection is based on the related problem relevant to the target problem. The chances of overfitting are high in the case of limited target data, similar to the source training dataset. In contrast, the chances of overfitting are low if the target dataset is larger and similar to the source dataset, and then it only needs fine tuning of the pre-trained deep neural network. For this purpose, we selected nine pre-trained TL algorithms to identify their performance in detecting and identifying meningioma, pituitary and glioma brain tumors. Figure 2 represents the basic framework of the TL method employed in our work. We changed the last three models' layers to adapt them to the brain tumor classification domain.

3.3. *Transfer-Learning-Based Networks*

This section provides in depth details about the nine TL algorithms, i.e., Inception-resnetv2, Inceptionv3, Xception, Resnet18, Resnet50, Resnet101, Shufflenet, Densenet201 and Mobilenetv2, selected for the purpose of brain tumor classification. The algorithms were selected based on their popularity and good performance for image classification. Below, we elaborate on each TL algorithm.

3.3.1. Inceptionresnetv2

Inceptionresnetv2 [37] is a deep CNN made from the family of Inception frameworks, and it incorporates residual connections. Inceptionresnetv2 uses inexpensive Inception blocks instead of the original Inception and a filter expansion layer after each Inception block, having 1×1 convolution without activation. Batch normalization (BN) is only employed on top of traditional layers, not on summations, to increase the number of inception blocks. This network takes a 299×299-pixel image as input for processing.

3.3.2. Inceptionv3

Inceptionv3 [38] is 48 layers deep, and it requires an input image of a size of 229×299. Inceptionv3 is a deep neural network that belongs to the Inception family, and it makes numerous improvements, such as Factorized 7×7 convolutions and label smoothing. The available pre-trained version of Inceptionv3 is trained on the ImageNet database and can classify images of 1000 objects into different categories.

3.3.3. Xception

The Xception [39] TL algorithm is 71 layers deep. The Xception network has 36 convolutional layers used as a base for feature extraction. Each convolutional layer has linear residual connections around it. Moreover, the Xception network is completely based on depth-wise separable convolutional layers. The framework of the Xception model can easily be modified. The pre-trained version of the Xception TL algorithm can classify new related tasks after being trained on millions of images from the ImageNet dataset.

3.3.4. Resnet101, Resnet50 and Resnet18

The residual networks [40] Resnet101, Resnet50 and Resnet18 are 101 layers, 50 layers and 18 layers deep, respectively. Residual deep neural networks use shortcut connections to skip some layers; skipping is used to compress the network, thus enabling faster learning. All three models are trained on the ImageNet database, and the pre-trained versions are available to classify new image-related tasks. Resnet101 provides more accurate results than Resnet18 and Resnet50 because of the increased depth of the TL algorithm.

3.3.5. Shufflenet

Shufflenet [41] is 50-layer-deep TL classifier. Shufflenet is computationally efficient and is designed for devices with limited computation power (i.e., mobile devices). Channel shuffle and pointwise group convolution are the core operations used by the Shufflenet model to reduce computational costs. Shufflenet accepts an input image of size 224 × 224. The pre-trained version of Shufflenet can be used to classify new image-related tasks.

3.3.6. Densenet201

Densenet201 [42] is 201-layer-deep TL classifier. In the Densenet201 model, all preceding layers' feature maps are utilized as inputs in subsequent layers; hence, the model encourages feature reuse and decreases feature redundancy. The Densenet's classifier reduces the vanishing gradient problem and boosts feature reuse. The Densenet's TL algorithm is a good feature extractor for numerous computer vision tasks because of its compact internal representations.

3.3.7. Mobilenetv2

The Mobilenetv2 [43] framework is a 53-layer-deep TL classifier used to classify image-related tasks. The image input size of Mobilenetv2 is 224 × 224. The Mobilenetv2 model is computationally efficient; therefore, this model is more suitable for real-time and mobile applications. The high speed of the Mobilenetv2 model is a result of point-wise and depth-wise convolution concepts used by the model. Residual connections between bottleneck layers are used in the network. An initial convolutional layer (with 32 filters) is followed by 19 residual bottleneck layers in the Mobilenetv2 network.

4. Results and Discussion

This section contains thorough information on the research dataset adopted for the fine-grained brain tumor classification experimental setup, i.e., the TL setting, and it provides an in-depth discussion of the findings of numerous experiments designed to assess the performance of our model. The experimental setup contains information regarding training the TL models and the software platform used in this study.

4.1. Dataset

For the proposed fine-grained classification approach, we employed the brain tumor classification (MRI) dataset [35] to test, train and validate the different TL-based approaches, with the intention of identifying the best DL classifier. The dataset is freely available as a standard Kaggle dataset. The dataset comprises two brain tumor MRI image collections, i.e., testing and training. Each collection contains four types of brain tumor MRI images, i.e., no tumor, meningioma tumors, pituitary tumors and glioma tumors. However, we only used the meningioma, pituitary and glioma tumor MRI images. The latest version of the research dataset contains 822 MRI images of meningioma, 827 MRI images of pituitary tumors and 826 MRI images of glioma brain tumors in the training folder. The samples from each brain tumor category are shown in Figure 3. Moreover, the testing folder contains 115 images of meningioma, 72 images of pituitary tumors and 100 images of glioma brain tumors. We combined images from both folders. Then, 80% of the data was used for training, and the remaining 20% was used for testing. The dataset comprises grayscale images of different resolutions. In the preprocessing stage, the MRI images of the dataset were resized by using the augmented image data store according to the image input size requirements of different DL models; for example, for mobilenetv2, MRI images were resized to 224 × 224, and for darknet19, images were resized to 256 × 256. The details of the research dataset adopted for brain image classification are shown in Table 1, which describes the number of images against each tumor type, image format and brain image type.

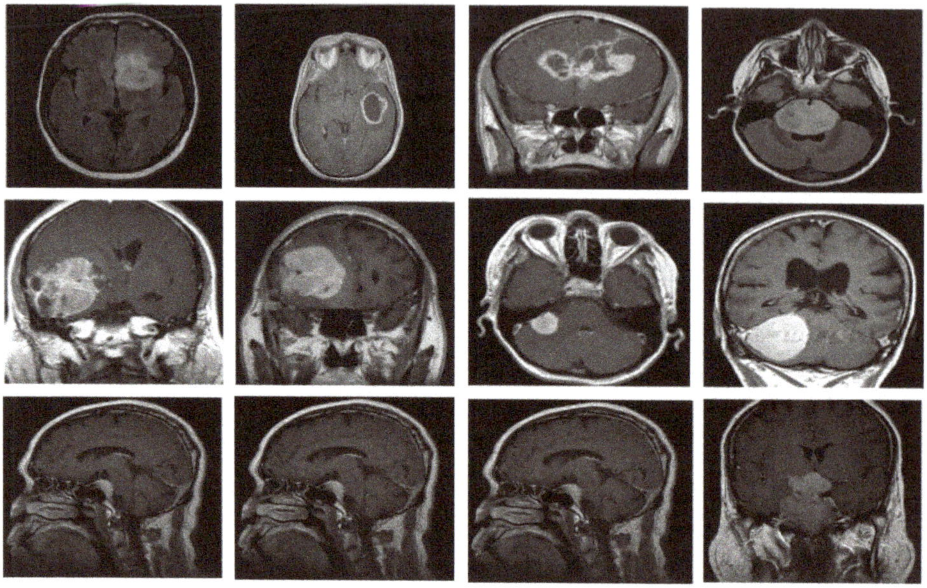

Figure 3. Samples of the brain tumor classification (MRI) dataset, upper row: Glioma tumor, middle row: meningioma tumor, and lower row: pituitary tumor.

Table 1. Brain tumor classification (MRI) dataset details.

Tumor Type	Number of Images	Format	Type
Meningioma	937		
Pituitary	898	JPG	Grayscale
Glioma	926		

4.2. *Transfer Learning Setting*

The pre-trained TL network classifiers adopted for this research study, i.e., Inception-resnetv2, Inceptionv3, Xception, Resnet18, Resnet50, Resnet101, Shufflenet, Densenet201 and Mobilenetv2, can categorize images into 1000 different item classes and are trained on 1.28 million images of ImageNet database. The focus of this study is a three-class classification of brain tumors using the brain tumor classification (MRI) dataset. Furthermore, we employed a trial-and-error strategy. Experiments were carried out by assigning different values to the parameters to determine the optimum values for each parameter. We used stochastic gradient descent (SGD) to train pre-trained DL models through TL. We utilized a 0.01 learning rate and a 10-image minibatch size. In addition, each DL model was trained for 14 epochs to conduct the TL experiments for detecting and categorizing brain tumor types, accounting for the possibility of overfitting. We performed all experimentations on a machine equipped with Intel (R) Core (TM) i5-5200U CPU and 8GB of RAM. For implementation, we used the R2020a version of MATLAB. The optimized parameters used for the classification experiment are shown in Table 2.

4.3. *Evaluation Metrics*

In this study, we employed the accuracy, precision, recall and $F1$-score [44] to assess the performance of all deep neural networks. All the performance metrics were computed as follows:

$$Accuracy = \frac{TP + TN}{TS} \tag{1}$$

$$Precision = \frac{TP}{TP + FP} \tag{2}$$

$$Sensitivity\ (Recall) = \frac{TP}{TP + FN} \tag{3}$$

$$F1\text{-}Score = 2 \cdot \frac{Precision \times Recall}{Precision + Recall} \tag{4}$$

TN stands for true negative, *TP* for true positive, *FP* for false positive and *FN* for false negative, and *TS* denotes the whole number of samples.

Table 2. Parameters of all transfer learning architectures.

Parameter	Value
Optimization algorithm	SGDM
Maximum Epochs	14
Learning rate	0.01
Verbose	False
Validation frequency	30
Shuffle	Every epoch

4.4. Results

This section discusses the performance of different pre-trained TL classifiers used to classify brain MRI images from the brain tumor classification (MRI) dataset into meningioma, pituitary and glioma. The main advantage of TL classifiers and fine tuning is decreasing overfitting issues that frequently occur in DL algorithms when experimenting with a smaller sample of training and testing images. All the TL models were trained and validated on the same TL settings indicated in Table 2 for the classification of brain tumors. We used 2762 brain tumor classification (MRI) images to classify brain tumors. Table 3 represents the detailed results of various TL algorithms in classifying brain tumor images and shows that each TL classifier achieved satisfactory results. We analyzed and evaluated the TL algorithms using accuracy, precision, recall and f-measure evaluation metrics. The results show that the inceptionresnetv2 DL model achieved the best average accuracy of 98.91%, and resnet50 achieved the lowest average accuracy of 67.03%. In contrast, the TL of the remaining seven deep neural networks achieved average classification accuracy. It is essential to mention that variants of the Resnet framework achieved different results. Resnet18 achieved a minimum accuracy of 67.03%, and Resnet50 attained an accuracy of 67.03%, whereas Resnet101 achieved an accuracy of 74.09%, which is the highest among all variants.

Table 3. Average classification accuracy.

Model	Accuracy	Precision	Recall	F-Measure	Elapsed Time
Inceptionresnetv2	98.91	98.28	99.75	99.00	1252 min 50 s
Inceptionv3	94.48	93.00	94.5	93.74	667 min 47 s
Xception	98.37	98.51	99.25	98.87	1730 min 25 s
Resnet101	74.09	73.19	67.23	70.08	801 min 36 s
Resnet18	63.04	64.63	52.09	57.68	187 min 47 s
Shufflenet	89.31	87.96	87.43	87.69	159 min 25 s
Densenet201	68.71	73.04	67.46	70.14	950 min 1 s
Resnet50	67.03	70.55	68.13	69.32	525 min 14 s
Mobilenetv2	82.61	81.11	80.32	80.71	318 min 15 s

The training and validation process of our best performing deep neural network, i.e., Inceptionresnetv2, is shown in Figure 4. The elapsed time returns the total CPU time used by the DL model since it was started, which is the time taken by the model to process (classify) all images of the dataset. Since we used the data augmentation technique, which significantly increased the dataset's size, all models took considerable time for classification. This time also depended on the depth and architectural design of the models. The elapsed time is expressed in seconds. The Shufflenet TL model was the most efficient elapsed time classifier, achieving satisfactory classification results and taking the shortest time, 159 min, for brain tumor classification. In contrast, the Xception TL model took a maximum time of 1730 min 25 sec to identify and classify brain tumor MRI images into different types. The Shufflenet model is fast because it uses two new operations, i.e., channel shuffle and pointwise group convolution, significantly reducing computation costs while retaining accuracy. It should be noted that the classification time for different variants of the Resnet TL classifiers increases with the number of framework layers. For example, Renset18 took a minimum time of 187 min 47 sec, and Resnet50 took 525 min 14 sec. Additionally, Resnet101 took the maximum time of 801 min 36 sec to classify brain tumors into meningioma, pituitary and glioma. Resnet18 achieved the lowest classification accuracy because of the ReLU activation function. The ReLU function outputs the positive input directly, whereas it outputs zero for negative inputs ($x < 0$). Therefore, the ReLU activation function fails to activate the neuron when it receives negative inputs, leaving no guarantee that all of the neurons would be active at all times, resulting in the dying ReLU problem. In this case, the network cannot learn using the optimization approach. The dying ReLU problem is undesirable because it causes a large percentage of the network to become idle over time. We can observe in Table 3 that, in the case of different variants of Resnet, accuracy improves with increasing depths of the networks because a deeper DL-based model captures more complicated and essential deep features and increases the network's classification performance. However, as the depth of the network expands, computational complexity increases, which ultimately affects the efficiency of the network. Furthermore, we can conclude from Table 3 that the inceptionresnetv2 TL algorithm is identified as the best classification method for detecting and classifying brain tumors.

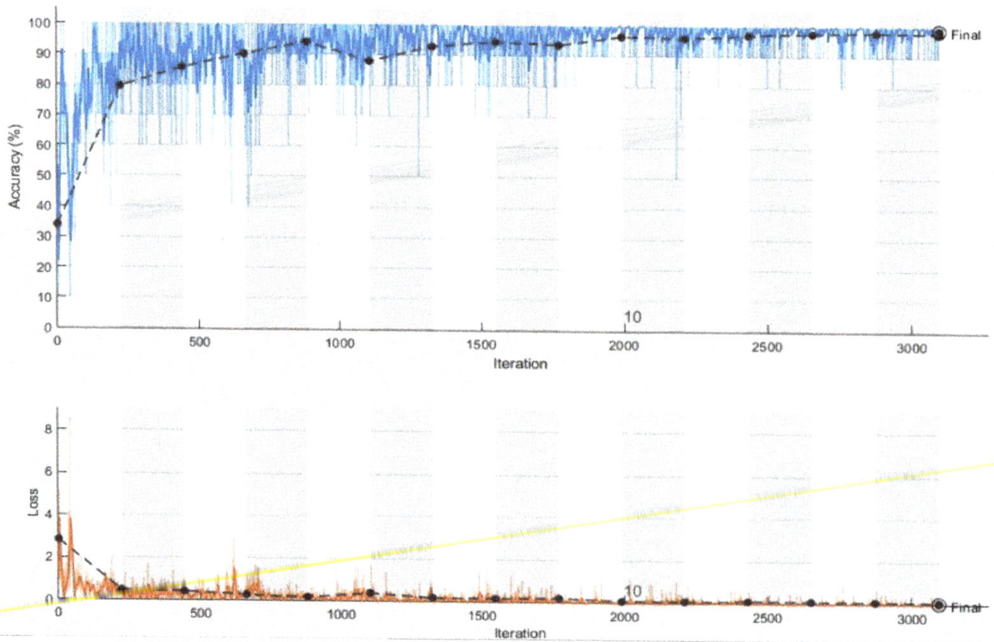

Figure 4. Training and validation accuracy and loss plots of Inceptionresnetv2 (black line shows the validation accuracy and loss. Also, the blue lines shows training accuracy and red line shows training loss).

Inceptionresnetv2 achieved effective results for several reasons. Inceptionresnetv2 achieved the best classification results because of its capability to extract more discriminative, detailed and robust deep features. Inceptionresnetv2 possesses the features of both Resnet and Inception such as wider networks, hyperparameters, kernel filters, etc. The two DL models, i.e., Inception and Resnet, were combined to achieve high-performance results at lower epochs. Each Inception block in Inceptionresnetv2 is followed by 1×1 convolution without activation, i.e., a filter expansion layer to compensate for the dimensionality reduction caused by the inception block. To better utilize computing resources for the classification experiment, the number of inception blocks was increased by adding BN only on top of traditional layers, not on summations.

The benefits of using pre-trained DL frameworks with TL for the detection and classification of brain tumors into meningioma, pituitary and glioma are numerous; for example, the classification method is completely automated, and it removes the traditional stages of noise filtering, ROI delineation, feature extraction and selection. Moreover, the results achieved by the pre-trained DL frameworks are reproducible, and, in contrast to [4–7], the highest level of accuracy is attained. Furthermore, running pre-trained frameworks with TL on a single CPU computer is computationally expensive. For all pre-trained frameworks, the computation times for the TLs are approximately 159 min, 187 min, 318 min s, 525 min, 667 min, 801 min, 950 min, 1252 min and 1730 min. Even the most efficient model, shufflenet, took 159 min for brain tumor classification. Longer computation times were a result of all models being developed using the MATLAB 2020a platform and running on a PC with an Intel (R) Core (TM) i5-5200U CPU and 8GB of RAM. The computation times were long because we ran the code in a MATLAB environment with a single CPU.

4.5. Comparison with the Hybrid Approach

In this section, another hybrid experiment is performed to classify brain tumors into meningioma, pituitary and glioma to assess the efficacy of the identified best TL model, i.e., Inceptionresnetv2. It has been claimed that using an SVM classifier instead of typical deep neural networks at the top of the net significantly improves classification performance [32]. Hence, we designed a hybrid approach in which we used the twelve most famous deep neural networks for in-depth feature extraction and used these features as inputs to train SVM with a linear kernel. We used Mobilnetv2, Densenet201, Squeeznet, Alexnet, Googlenet, Inceptionv3, Resnet50, Resnet18, Resnet101, Xception, Inceptionresnetv3, VGG19 and Shufflenet in the proposed work. The dataset images were resized differently according to the image input requirements of the deep neural networks by using augmented image data stores before inserting them into the DL network for feature extraction. We applied activations on the last global average pooling layer (a deeper layer) to extract high-level features. The classification results of deep features and the SVM approach are presented in Table 4. This experiment shows that the deep features of all twelve networks and the SVM approach achieved lower accuracy results compared to the TL of Inceptionresnetv2. An accuracy of 98.91% signifies the effectiveness of the Inceptionresnetv2 deep neural network for reliable tumor classification.

4.6. Comparison with State-of-the-Art Related Work

We compared the classification performance of the best deep neural network, i.e., Inceptionresnetv2, with existing methods for classifying brain tumors into meningioma, pituitary and glioma tumors. More specifically, we compared the proposed work with state-of-the-art DL approaches [4,11,16,17,24,26,28,45]. Deepak et al. and Swati et al. used the same TL techniques for brain tumor classification [17,26]. Deepak et al. suggested a three-class classification approach based on deep TL [26]. A pre-trained GoogLeNet model was used for the feature extraction of brain MRI scans to distinguish between glioma, meningioma and pituitary cancers. Proven classification models were employed to classify the collected features. The experiment used a five-fold cross-validation strategy on an MRI dataset from figshare. With an average accuracy of 98 %, the suggested method exceeds all current state-of the-art approaches. The performance metrics used were the area under the curve (AUC), precision, recall, F-score and specificity. According to the study results, TL appears to be a valuable method when the availability of medical images is limited.

Table 4. Accuracy comparison among the Inceptionresnetv2 and deep-features SVM approaches.

Model	Accuracy
Squeezenet	97.28
Alexnet	97.83
Inceptionresnetv2	98.01
Inceptionv3	97.86
Resnet101	98.01
Resnet18	96.38
Vgg19	97.46
Shufflenet	96.56
Googlenet	96.56
Densenet201	98.37
Resnet50	98.36
Mobilenetv2	98.5

Researchers have used TL techniques and have succeeded in achieving the best results. Using a pre-trained VGG19 deep CNN model, Swati et al. developed a block-wise fine-tuning technique based on TL [45]. A benchmark dataset of T1-weighted contrast-enhanced magnetic resonance imaging (CE-MRI) was used to test the proposed method. When validated in a five-fold cross-validation setting, the method achieved an average accuracy of 94.82% for the classification of meningioma, pituitary and glioma brain tumors. The proposed technique outperformed state-of-the-art classification on the CE-MRI dataset, according to experimental findings. Arshia Rehman et al. [17] proposed a framework and performed three studies to classify brain malignancies such as meningioma, glioma, and pituitary tumors utilizing three convolutional neural networks architectures (AlexNet, GoogLeNet, and VGGNet). Each study then investigated TL approaches, such as fine tuning and freezing, utilizing MRI slices from a brain tumor dataset (Figshare). Data augmentation techniques were used on MRI slices to help generalize results, increase dataset samples and reduce the risk of overfitting. In the presented studies, the fine-tuned VGG16 architecture achieved the greatest classification and detection accuracy of 98.69%.

Table 5 shows a comprehensive comparison of different approaches based on accuracy. Only accuracy is included in Table 5 as a performance parameter because it is the most prevalent metric used in all relevant studies. According to our current knowledge, Inceptionresnetv2's TL beats all current state-of-the-art approaches in the literature. The proposed approach attains the best results because of its capability to extract more robust and distinctive deep features for classification. Moreover, we used a balanced dataset (*brain tumor classification (MRI) dataset*). In contrast, the datasets (CE-MRI) used in previous approaches such as [17,26] and other approaches (mentioned in Table 5) were unbalanced, comprising 1426, 708, and 930 MRI images of glioma, meningioma, and pituitary brain tumors, respectively. The third column of Table 5 defines the percentage of the whole dataset used for training. We used 80% of the data for training all nine deep neural networks.

Table 5. Comparison with existing approaches.

Work	Method	Training Data	Accuracy
Deepak S et al. [26]	CNN features SVM classification	80%	95.82
Afshar et al. [28]	Capsnet	80%	86.56
El kader [31]	CNN–DWA	80%	98.00
Jun Cheng [4]	BoW–SVM	80%	91.28
Ismael [24]	DWT–Gabor NN	70%	91.90
Pashaei [16]	CNN–ELM	70%	93.68
Abiwinanda [11]	Proposed CNN	70%	84.19
Sawati [45]	Block-wise fine tuning	25–50–75%	94.82
Arshia Rehman [17]	Transfer Learning	70%	98.69
Proposed approach	Inceptionresnetv2	80%	98.91

5. Conclusions

This paper presents a comparative analysis of nine DL models for the classification of brain tumors through TL. The aim of this effort was to automate the process of detecting brain tumors by finding the best DL classifier for brain tumor classification. We applied TL to nine deep neural networks, i.e., Inceptionresnetv2, Inceptionv3, Xception, Resnet18, Resnet50, Resnet101, Shufflenet, Densenet201, and Mobilenetv2, and classified brain tumors into glioma, meningioma, and pituitary using a brain tumor classification (MRI) dataset. Our experimental findings validate that the Inceptionresnetv2 model achieved the most effective results for the classification of brain tumors. An accuracy of 98.71% signifies the effectiveness of Inceptionresnetv2 for reliable brain tumor classification. An accuracy of 98.91% for brain tumor classification has confirmed the superiority of the best model (Inceptionresnetv2) over other hybrid approaches in which we used DL models for deep features extraction and SVM for the classification of brain tumors. Although this paper explored TL of nine DL models for the classification of brain tumor MRI images, other models remain to be explored. Despite the limited data in our dataset, we have achieved satisfactory results. We applied data augmentation techniques to increase the size of the training dataset. However, the results can be further improved in the future by training the model with a larger dataset.

Moreover, despite the accomplishments of this study, some improvements are still possible: firstly, the comparatively weak performance of the pre-trained DL models as stand-alone classifiers; secondly, significant training time elapsed by the transfer of learned deep neural networks; and thirdly, because of limited training data, the phenomenon of overfitting was observed. Future exploration in this domain can address these issues, possibly utilizing larger datasets for training and further tuning the transfer of learned deep neural networks. In the future, we will explore the TL of the remaining powerful deep neural networks for brain tumor detection and classification with less time complexity. Furthermore, we will also apply image segmentation techniques to improve the performance of our best performing model.

Author Contributions: N.U. developed the method; N.U., M.S.K., W.K. and J.A.K. performed the experiments and analysis; I.H., M.O., N.N. and A.S.S. wrote the paper. All authors have read and agreed to the published version of the manuscript.

Funding: The authors extend their appreciation to the Deanship of Scientific Research at King Khalid University for funding this work under grant number (RGP2/46/43). Princess Nourah bint Abdulrahman University Researchers Supporting Project number (PNURSP2022R203), Princess Nourah bint Abdulrahman University, Riyadh, Saudi Arabia.

Data Availability Statement: The datasets used in this investigation are available on request from the corresponding author.

Conflicts of Interest: The authors declare no conflict of interest.

References

1. Kavitha, A.R.; Chitra, L.; Kanaga, R. Brain tumor segmentation using genetic algorithm with SVM classifier. *Int. J. Adv. Res. Electr. Electron. Instrum. Eng.* **2016**, *5*, 1468–1471.
2. Logeswari, T.; Karnan, M. An Improved Implementation of Brain Tumor Detection Using Segmentation Based on Hierarchical Self Organizing Map. *Int. J. Comput. Theory Eng.* **2010**, *2*, 591–595. [CrossRef]
3. Badran, E.F.; Mahmoud, E.G.; Hamdy, N. An algorithm for detecting brain tumors in MRI images. In Proceedings of the 2010 International Conference on Computer Engineering & Systems, Cairo, Egypt, 30 November 2010; pp. 368–373.
4. Cheng, J.; Huang, W.; Cao, S.; Yang, R.; Yang, W.; Yun, Z.; Feng, Q. Enhanced performance of brain tumor classification via tumor region augmentation and partition. *PLoS ONE* **2015**, *10*, e0140381. [CrossRef] [PubMed]
5. Swati, Z.N.K.; Zhao, Q.; Kabir, M.; Ali, F.; Ali, Z.; Ahmed, S.; Lu, J. Content-Based Brain Tumor Retrieval for MR Images Using Transfer Learning. *IEEE Access* **2019**, *7*, 17809–17822. [CrossRef]
6. Khambhata, K.G.; Panchal, S.R. Multiclass classification of brain tumor in MR images. *Int. J. Innov. Res. Comput. Commun. Eng.* **2016**, *4*, 8982–8992.
7. Zacharaki, E.I.; Wang, S.; Chawla, S.; Yoo, D.S.; Wolf, R.; Melhem, E.R.; Davatzikos, C. Classification of brain tumor type and grade using MRI texture and shape in a machine learning scheme. *Magn. Reson. Med.* **2009**, *62*, 1609–1618. [CrossRef] [PubMed]
8. Litjens, G.; Kooi, T.; Bejnordi, B.E.; Setio, A.A.A.; Ciompi, F.; Ghafoorian, M.; van der Laak, J.A.W.M.; van Ginneken, B.; Sánchez, C.I. A survey on deep learning in medical image analysis. *Med. Image Anal.* **2017**, *42*, 60–88. [CrossRef] [PubMed]
9. Singh, L.; Chetty, G.; Sharma, D. A Novel Machine Learning Approach for Detecting the Brain Abnormalities from MRI Structural Images. In *IAPR International Conference on Pattern Recognition in Bioinformatics*; Springer: Berlin/Heidelberg, Germany, 2012; pp. 94–105. [CrossRef]
10. Pan, Y.; Huang, W.; Lin, Z.; Zhu, W.; Zhou, J.; Wong, J.; Ding, Z. Brain tumor grading based on Neural Networks and Convolutional Neural Networks. In Proceedings of the 2015 37th Annual International Conference of the IEEE Engineering in Medicine and Biology Society (EMBC), Milan, Italy, 25–29 August 2015; Springer: Miami, FL, USA, 2015; pp. 699–702. [CrossRef]
11. Abiwinanda, N.; Hanif, M.; Hesaputra, S.T.; Handayani, A.; Mengko, T.R. Brain tumor classification using convolutional neural network. In Proceedings of the World Congress on Medical Physics and Biomedical Engineering 2018, Prague, Czech Republic, 3–8 June 2018; Springer: Singapore, 2019; pp. 183–189.
12. Tharani, S.; Yamini, C. Classification using convolutional neural network for heart and diabetics datasets. *Int. J. Adv. Res. Comp. Commun. Eng.* **2016**, *5*, 417–422.
13. Ravi, D.; Wong, C.; Deligianni, F.; Berthelot, M.; Andreu-Perez, J.; Lo, B.; Yang, G.-Z. Deep Learning for Health Informatics. *IEEE J. Biomed. Health Inform.* **2016**, *21*, 4–21. [CrossRef]
14. Le, Q.V.A. Tutorial on Deep Learning—Part 1: Nonlinear Classi-Fiers and the Backpropagation Algorithm. 2015. Available online: http://robotics.stanford.edu/$\sim$quocle/tutorial1.pdf (accessed on 10 March 2021).
15. Anuse, A.; Vyas, V. A novel training algorithm for convolutional neural network. *Complex. Intell. Syst.* **2016**, *2*, 221–234. [CrossRef]
16. Pashaei, A.; Sajedi, H.; Jazayeri, N. Brain Tumor Classification via Convolutional Neural Network and Extreme Learning Machines. In Proceedings of the 2018 8th International Conference on Computer and Knowledge Engineering (ICCKE), Mashhad, Iran, 25–26 October 2018; pp. 314–319.
17. Rehman, A.; Naz, S.; Razzak, M.I.; Akram, F.; Imran, M. A deep learning-based framework for automatic brain tumors classification using transfer learning. *Circuits Syst. Signal Process.* **2020**, *39*, 757–775. [CrossRef]
18. Kammer, N.N.; Coppenrath, E.; Treitl, K.M.; Kooijman, H.; Dietrich, O.; Saam, T. Comparison of contrast-enhanced modified T1-weighted 3D TSE black-blood and 3D MP-RAGE sequences for the detection of cerebral metastases and brain tumours. *Eur. Radiol.* **2016**, *26*, 1818–1825. [CrossRef] [PubMed]
19. Naseer, A.; Rani, M.; Naz, S.; Razzak, M.I.; Imran, M.; Xu, G. Refining Parkinson's neurological disorder identification through deep transfer learning. *Neural Comput. Appl.* **2020**, *32*, 839–854. [CrossRef]
20. Naz, S.; Umar, A.I.; Ahmad, R.; Siddiqi, I.; Ahmed, S.B.; Razzak, M.I.; Shafait, F. Urdu Nastaliq recognition using convolutional–recursive deep learning. *Neurocomputing* **2017**, *243*, 80–87. [CrossRef]
21. Razzak, M.I.; Imran, M.; Xu, G. Efficient brain tumor segmentation with multiscaleancer statistics twopathway-group conventional neural networks. *IEEE J. Biomed. Health Inf.* **2018**, *23*, 1911–1919. [CrossRef]
22. Razzak, M.I. Malarial parasite classification using recurrent neural network. *Int. J. Image Process.* **2015**, *9*, 69.
23. Rehman, A.; Naz, S.; Razzak, M.I.; Hameed, I.A. Automatic Visual Features for Writer Identification: A Deep Learning Approach. *IEEE Access* **2019**, *7*, 17149–17157. [CrossRef]
24. Ismael, M.R.; Abdel-Qader, I. Brain Tumor Classification via Statistical Features and Back-Propagation Neural Network. In Proceedings of the 2018 IEEE International Conference on Electro/Information Technology (EIT), Rochester, MI, USA, 3–5 May 2018; pp. 252–257. [CrossRef]
25. Mohsen, H.; El-Dahshan, E.S.A.; El-Horbaty, E.S.M.; Salem, A.B.M. Classification using deep learning neural networks for brain tumors. *Future Comput. Inform. J.* **2018**, *3*, 68–71. [CrossRef]
26. Deepak, S.; Ameer, P.M. Automated Categorization of Brain Tumor from MRI Using CNN features and SVM. *J. Ambient Intell. Humaniz. Comput.* **2020**, *12*, 8357–8369. [CrossRef]
27. Shaik, N.S.; Cherukuri, T.K. Multi-level attention network: Application to brain tumor classification. *Signal. Image Video Process.* **2021**, *16*, 817–824. [CrossRef]

28. Afshar, P.; Mohammadi, A.; Plataniotis, K.N. Brain tumor type classification via capsule networks. In Proceedings of the 2018 25th IEEE International Conference on Image Processing (ICIP), Athens, Greece, 7–10 October 2018; pp. 3129–3133.
29. Seetha, J.; Raja, S.S. Brain Tumor Classification Using Convolutional Neural Networks. *Biomed. Pharmacol. J.* **2018**, *11*, 1457–1461. [CrossRef]
30. Rai, H.M.; Chatterjee, K. 2D MRI image analysis and brain tumor detection using deep learning CNN model LeU-Net. *Multimed. Tools Appl.* **2021**, *80*, 36111–36141. [CrossRef]
31. El Kader, I.A.; Xu, G.; Shuai, Z.; Saminu, S. Brain tumor detection and classification by hybrid CNN-DWA model using MR images. *Curr. Med. Imaging* **2021**, *17*, 1248–1255. [CrossRef] [PubMed]
32. Kesav, N.; Jibukumar, M.G. Efficient and low complex architecture for detection and classification of Brain Tumor using RCNN with Two Channel CNN. *J. King Saud Univ. Comput. Inf. Sci.* **2021**, *33*, 1–14. [CrossRef]
33. Shao, L.; Zhu, F.; Li, X. Transfer learning for visual categorization: A survey. *IEEE Trans. Neural Netw. Learn. Syst.* **2014**, *26*, 1019–1034. [CrossRef]
34. Agarwal, N.; Sondhi, A.; Chopra, K.; Singh, G. Transfer learning: Survey and classification. In *Smart Innovations in Communication and Computational Sciences*; Springer: Singapore, 2021; pp. 145–155.
35. Sartaj, B.; Ankita, K.; Prajakta, B.; Sameer, D.; Swati, K. Brain Tumor Classification (MRI). *Kaggle* 2020. [CrossRef]
36. Pan, S.J.; Yang, Q. A survey on transfer learning. *IEEE Trans. Knowl. Data Eng.* **2010**, *22*, 1345–1359. [CrossRef]
37. Szegedy, C.; Ioffe, S.; Vanhoucke, V.; Alemi, A.A. Inception-v4, Inception-ResNet and the Impact of Residual Connections on Learning. In Proceedings of the Thirty-First AAAI Conference on Artificial Intelligence, San Francisco, CA, USA, 4–9 February 2017; pp. 1–12.
38. Szegedy, C.; Vanhoucke, V.; Ioffe, S.; Shlens, J.; Wojna, Z. Rethinking the inception architecture for computer vision. In Proceedings of the IEEE Conference on Computer Vision and Pattern Recognition, Washington, DC, USA, 19–24 June 2016; pp. 2818–2826.
39. Chollet, F. Xception: Deep Learning with Depthwise Separable Convolutions. In Proceedings of the IEEE Conference on Computer Vision and Pattern Recognition, Washington, DC, USA, 19–24 June 2016; p. 1610-02357.
40. He, K.; Zhang, X.; Ren, S.; Sun, J. Deep residual learning for image recognition. In Proceedings of the IEEE Conference on Computer Vision and Pattern Recognition, Washington, DC, USA, 19–24 June 2016; pp. 770–778.
41. Zhang, X.; Zhou, X.; Lin, M.; Sun, J. ShuffleNet: An Extremely Efficient Convolutional Neural Network for Mobile Devices. In Proceedings of the IEEE Conference on Computer Vision and Pattern Recognition, Washington, DC, USA, 19–24 June 2016; pp. 6848–6856.
42. Huang, G.; Zhuang, L.; Laurens, V.; Der, M.; Kilian, Q.W. Densely Connected Convolutional Networks. In Proceedings of the IEEE Conference on Computer Vision and Pattern Recognition, Washington, DC, USA, 19–24 June 2016; p. 3.
43. Sandler, M.; Howard, A.; Zhu, M.; Zhmoginov, A.; Chen, L.C. MobileNetV2: Inverted Residuals and Linear Bottlenecks. In Proceedings of the 2018 IEEE/CVF Conference on Computer Vision and Pattern Recognition, Salt Lake City, UT, USA, 18–23 June 2018; pp. 4510–4520.
44. Sokolova, M.; Japkowicz, N.; Szpakowicz, S. Beyond accuracy, F-score and ROC: A family of discriminant measures for performance evaluation. In Proceedings of the Australasian Joint Conference on Artificial Intelligence, Sydney, NSW, Australia, 2–4 February 2022; Springer: Berlin/Heidelberg, Germany, 4 December, 2016; pp. 1015–1021.
45. Swati, Z.N.K.; Zhao, Q.; Kabir, M.; Ali, F.; Ali, Z.; Ahmed, S.; Lu, J. Brain tumor classification for MR images using transfer learning and fine-tuning. *Comput. Med. Graph.* **2019**, *75*, 34–46. [CrossRef]

applied sciences

MDPI

Review

Molecular Techniques and Target Selection for the Identification of *Candida* spp. in Oral Samples

Joana Magalhães [1], Maria José Correia [1], Raquel M. Silva [1], Ana Cristina Esteves [2], Artur Alves [2] and Ana Sofia Duarte [1,*]

[1] Center for Interdisciplinary Research in Health (CIIS), Faculty of Dental Medicina (FMD), Universidade Católica Portuguesa, 3504-505 Viseu, Portugal
[2] CESAM, Department of Biology, Campus Universitário de Santiago, University of Aveiro, 3810-193 Aveiro, Portugal
* Correspondence: asduarte@ucp.pt; Tel.: +351-232-419-500

Abstract: *Candida* species are the causative agent of oral candidiasis, with medical devices being platforms for yeast anchoring and tissue colonization. Identifying the infectious agent involved in candidiasis avoids an empirical prescription of antifungal drugs. The application of high-throughput technologies to the diagnosis of yeast pathogens has clear advantages in sensitivity, accuracy, and speed. Yet, conventional techniques for the identification of *Candida* isolates are still routine in clinical and research settings. Molecular approaches are the focus of intensive research, but conversion into clinic settings requires overcoming important challenges. Several molecular approaches can accurately identify *Candida* spp.: Polymerase Chain Reaction, Microarray, High-Resolution Melting Analysis, Multi-Locus Sequence Typing, Restriction Fragment Length Polymorphism, Loop-mediated Isothermal Amplification, Matrix Assisted Laser Desorption Ionization-mass spectrometry, and Next Generation Sequencing. This review examines the advantages and disadvantages of the current molecular methods used for *Candida* spp. Identification, with a special focus on oral candidiasis. Discussion regarding their application for the diagnosis of oral infections aims to identify the most rapid, affordable, accurate, and easy-to-perform molecular techniques to be used as a point-of-care testing method. Special emphasis is given to the difficulties that health care professionals need to overcome to provide an accurate diagnosis.

Keywords: diagnosis; infection; oral candidiasis; oral health; species identification

1. Introduction

Candida albicans belongs to our normal mucosal surface's microbiota, from where it may emerge as a pathogen causing local infections, such as inflammation in the oral cavity and *Candida* vaginitis [1,2]. *Candida* species are still the most common cause of fungal diseases worldwide: these yeasts cause infections that range from superficial mucosal membranes to life-threatening invasive diseases, entailing extensive medical or surgical treatment [3–5]. *Candida* spp. exist as commensals, and as opportunist pathogens, being able to compromise various organs and cause diseases in immunocompromised or critically ill patients [6–9]. Therefore, for clinical purposes, the identification of *Candida albicans* per se does not have clinical relevance, especially in colonized environments such as the mouth.

Candida can lead to infection due to changes in the host environment. The infection process is dependent on the host tissue integrity and its ability to maintain normal microbiota, as well as on a healthy immune system. A change in the balance of the resident microbiota, such as the placement of dental implants [10,11], can result in favorable environmental conditions for the proliferation of organisms with the potential for host invasion [12].

Candidemia, a bloodstream infection, is a serious hazard to hospitalized patients, being considered the most clinically relevant form of *Candida* infection [13]. Candidemia is the most common invasive infection, with mortality rates reported in clinical settings ranging from 30 to 60% [14,15]. The species responsible for the infection has different susceptibility patterns to antifungal drugs, representing a serious challenge for patient treatment. Although oral candidiasis is also an important form of *Candida* infection occurring in the oral cavity, the amount of information available on candidemia is overwhelmingly more abundant.

Despite the clinical relevance of *Candida* spp., the distinction between different species causing oral candidiasis is often difficult. Although there are several molecular techniques currently available for the identification of *Candida* spp., the different strengths and weaknesses associated with these techniques mean it is difficult to reach a consensus on the adoption of an optimal identification method. Any diagnostic tool needs to combine a certain set of attributes in terms of accuracy, specificity, and cost, and at the same time, it must be user-friendly and as non-time-consuming as possible. Therefore, the purpose of this review is to analyze the molecular methods currently used for the detection of *Candida* spp. with a special focus on *Candida* involved in oral infections. A comparative analysis in terms of each method's accuracy, specificity, cost, time, and complexity will be formed. At the same time, we also describe currently used molecular targets as well as others with the potential to improve oral candidiasis diagnosis.

2. Epidemiology of *Candida* Infections

Several Candida species are commensal and colonize the human skin and mucosal surfaces either in a free cell form or in a biofilm. Biofilms, a dynamic community of surface-associated microbes, are protected by an extracellular polymeric matrix and are strongly related to Candida's infection [16–18].

Candida albicans is considered the most common Candida species associated with infection in humans, being often linked to life-threatening situations in elderly, immunocompromised, or critically ill patients [19–21]. The increasing number of invasive surgical procedures, the extensive use of broad-spectrum antimicrobials, and the prevalence of clinical illness, especially in infant and elderly populations, are some of the reasons for the globally increased incidence of candidemia [22]. The Centers for Disease Control and Prevention (CDC) estimate that approximately 25,000 cases of candidemia occur in the United States of America each year [23]. Non-C. albicans species cause approximately two-thirds of candidemia cases in the USA [24], with C. auris being considered a relevant emergent pathogen [15]. In 2019, an epidemiologic meta-analysis was performed in Europe, showing the increasing incidence rate of candidemia with a higher proportion of Candida spp. other than C. albicans [25].

Mortality among patients with invasive candidiasis is as high as 40%, even when receiving antifungal therapy [22,26]. High mortality rates in Candida infections are in part justified by diagnostic inaccuracy (i.e., incorrect identification at the species level and of the drug resistance profile), which may compromise the administration of adequate antifungal therapies and ultimately lead to the patient's death [27–29]. The criteria for initiating Candida antifungal therapy remains poorly specified and often contributes to the widespread prescription of antifungal drugs with no regard for toxicity risks, resistance selection, and unnecessarily high costs of antifungal treatments [30–33].

Oral candidiasis ("thrush") is an opportunist oral mucosa fungal infection [1] that can result in serious health complications and ultimately spread through the bloodstream and lead to candidemia. Furthermore, this infection is commonly associated with elderly patients, frequently leading to longer treatments and higher costs for the health systems. Regarding the diagnosis of oral candidiasis, saliva has been used as a target sample, being already used in the diagnosis of other oral and systemic diseases, such as oral cancer [34,35] and SARS-CoV-2 [36].

The antifungal agents in use for the treatment of oral candidiasis are polyenes (nystatin and amphotericin B), allylamines (terbinafine), and azoles (fluconazole, itraconazole, voriconazole, and ketaconazole). A major concern is the misuse of antimycotic agents contributing to antifungal resistance in Candida (Table S1). Miranda-Cadena and colleagues characterized Candida oral isolates and showed that most C. glabrata isolates are susceptible to miconazole and nystatin, but resistant to fluconazole and itraconazole. In the same study, Candida parapsilosis isolates were susceptible to fluconazole while azole cross-resistance to miconazole and itraconazole was noted [37]. Increased resistance to antifungal compounds, especially to azoles and to amphotericin B, was already reported [38–41]. All isolates investigated by Anjejo and colleagues (2011) were susceptible to amphotericin B, and 50% of the C. glabrata isolates were resistant to fluconazole [42]. The specific species of Candida responsible for candidemia and Candida spp. that cause oral candidiasis have different susceptibility patterns. Interestingly, Candida krusei susceptibility patterns show multidrug resistance patterns when they are isolated from both oral and blood samples (Table 1).

Table 1. Susceptibility patterns of *Candida* species from blood and oral samples. AmB amphotericin B, FLU fluconazole, ITRA itraconazole, VOR voriconazole, POS posaconazole, MICA micafungin; CAPS caspofungin, S-susceptible, I-intermediate, R-resistant [43–46].

	Blood Samples							Oral Samples		
		Azoles				Echinocandins			Azoles	
	AmB	FLU	ITRA	VOR	POS	MICA	CASP	AmB	FLU	VOR
C. albicans	S	R	S	I	I-R	S-I	S-I	S	S	S
C. tropicalis	S	R	S	S-I	I-R	S	S-I	S	S	S
C. parapsilosis	S	R	S	S-I	S	S	S	-	-	-
C. glabrata	S-I	R	I	S-I	I-R	S-I	S	S	S	S
C. krusei	S	R	S-I-R	S	S	S	S	S	R	S
C. lusitaniae	S	I	S	S	S	S	S	-	-	-
C. auris	S-I	R	R	R	-	R	R	-	-	-

3. Molecular Identification of *Candida* spp.

A definitive diagnosis of candidiasis does not rely merely on its detection in the oral cavity. Since Candida spp. are commensal organisms, a negative culture result, for example, has a greater diagnostic significance than a positive culture result. Conversely, a positive culture result for Candida does not mean that the patient has oral candidiasis. Furthermore, a negative result is only relevant if the techniques used can identify all members of the genus.

Several Polymerase Chain Reaction (PCR) and non-PCR-based methods are used for the molecular identification of Candida spp. The search for a precise, fast, and low-cost identification of fungal species is a great challenge in mycology [47], especially when dealing with species complexes. Phenotypic-based identification is frequently inconclusive.

Techniques based on PCR usually target fungal pathogens by using species–specific probes or primers [47–49]. Conventional PCR, semi-nested and nested PCR, PCR-enzyme immunoassay, various types of real-time PCR, and multiplex PCR have all been used for the in vitro detection of *Candida* species, both qualitative and quantitatively [50]. PCR-based methodologies are often applied in the diagnosis of fungal infections, although they can differ considerably in terms of the outcome. These techniques can be applied for the detection of antifungal resistance-inducing mutations, the quantification of fungal load, and the antifungal therapy surveillance and pathogenesis of *Candida* infection [51]. The PCR-based approaches rely on broad or genus-specific primers that amplify conserved rRNA regions that are sequenced afterwards [52,53] or subjected to other techniques such as analysis of polymorphic sequences (RFLP: Restriction Fragment Length Polymorphism; AFLP: Amplified Fragment Length Polymorphism; RAPD: Random Amplification of Polymorphic DNA; STR: Short Tandem Repeats) [54,55], high-resolution melting analysis (HRMA) [46,54,56,57], microarray-based detection [58,59], and capillary electrophoresis [60]. Capillary electrophoresis is better suited than classical electrophoresis for DNA separation due to its superior speed, efficiency, sensitivity, and simpler suitability for automation [61]. However, the use of this technique creates the need for complex equipment adding complexity to equipment maintenance and specialized personnel.

Existing PCR protocols require enhancements in sensitivity, standardization, and swiftness, as well as a decrease in complexity, in order to be applicable for routine clinical diagnostics [48]. There is a considerable lack of information related to protocols and techniques to identify Candida spp. from oral samples, especially when compared to blood.

3.1. Conventional PCR

Using conventional PCR, Tata and colleagues (2018) were able to identify different *Candida* species from oral samples [62]. *Candida albicans* was the most common (80.9%), followed by *C. tropicalis* (7.2%), and *C. glabrata* (5.3%). The region selected for the amplification was the *ITS2* (Internal Transcribed Spacer 2) of *C. albicans* and *C. dubliniensis* rDNA using fungal-specific primers (Table S1).

Shi (2016) used oral samples from 20 denture-wearing patients (10 with denture stomatitis and 10 healthy denture wearers) and used PCR (targeting *ITS*, Table S1) to assess each denture sample for the presence of *Candida* and other fungi and bacteria. In total, 90% of the samples from the stomatitis group had *Candida* while in only 50% of those from the healthy group was a positive identification found [63].

3.2. Real Time-PCR

Conventional PCR amplifies the DNA target that is later detected with an end-point analysis. In real-time PCR, the amplification product is assessed as the reaction evolves, in real time, which gives RT-PCR the possibility to track the amplification signals in real time. As for pitfalls, RT-PCR has the need for consistency with regard to reagents used [64], and careful consideration in the assay design, template preparation, and analytical methods [65].

Real-time PCR has been widely used for the identification of *Candida* spp. in blood and tissue samples [66], but the same does not apply for oral samples [67]. RT-PCR (using *ITS* as target) was used to identify *Candida* species in patients suffering from oral candidiasis, after piercing the tongue [68], with denture-induced stomatitis [69], and with diabetes mellitus [70].

3.3. Nested PCR

A nested polymerase chain reaction was designed to increase PCR sensitivity by re-amplifying PCR products. Two sets of primers are used in two successive reactions, where the second set intends to amplify a second target within the PCR product from the first run [71]. To limit the amplification of non-specific products, the first reaction allows amplification for a low number of cycles. The second primer set must amplify exclusively the target product from the first amplification and not non-specific products. Nested-PCR was used by Kanbe and colleagues to amplify the DNA topoisomerase II genes of *C. kefyr*, *C. krusei*, *C. tropicalis*, *C. dubliniensis*, *C. parapsilosis*, *C. guilliermondii* and *C. lusitaniae* [72]. The DNA topoisomerase II gene sequence includes highly conserved regions separated by species-specific regions [61]. Kanbe et al. [72] conducted a nested-PCR amplification, in which genomic DNA was amplified with a degenerated primer pair (Table S2), followed by the additional amplification using primer mixtures, to improve specificity.

Nested PCR requires more reagents than conventional PCR, an extra set of primers, and one extra round of agarose gel electrophoresis, becoming a costly and time-consuming method. Additionally, a second amplification reaction increases the risk of sample contamination.

3.4. Multiplex PCR

In Multiplex PCR, several pairs of primers are used to target simultaneously different DNA sequences. This technique takes advantage of the high copy number of rRNA genes, length, and sequence variability of the *ITS* regions of *Candida* spp. A comparison study between phenotypic methods and multiplex PCR portrayed this last one as a high-accuracy diagnostic tool [73]. Some authors used multiplex PCR to distinguish clinically important *Candida* species from oral samples [74–77] and blood [78]. A diagnostic strategy was created targeting approximately twenty clinically relevant yeast species, *Candida* included. The results were 100% consistent with the MALDI-TOF MS data [79].

Table S1 contains detailed information on primers' sequence and annealing temperature for *Candida* spp. Multiplex PCR provides rapid and effective results. In oral samples, the elimination of the DNA extraction step saves sample preparation time avoiding hazardous or expensive chemicals [80]. Although this method is used in some clinical laboratories, it requires proficiency in primer design and protocol optimization [81].

3.5. Restriction Fragment Length Polymorphism (RFLP)

RFLP uses unique patterns in DNA fragments after enzyme digestion (using restriction enzymes), to genetically differentiate organisms. The distance between these cleavage sites differs between each organism—the resulting restriction fragments—which can be separated by gel electrophoresis arranged by size [82].

RFLP can be used in combination with PCR. Williams and co-workers amplified, by PCR, a region of the *ITS* rRNA gene from 84 *Candida* isolates, including 29 from oral samples. The PCR was designed to amplify intergenic spacer regions of the rDNA with established primers (Table S3) [55]. Isolates of *C. albicans*, *C. tropicalis*, *C. stellatoidea*, *C. parapsilosis*, and *C. krusei* were identified following the restriction digestion of the PCR products.

The PCR-RFLP protocol used by Cirak and colleagues (2003) was successfully applied for the identification of five *Candida* species [83]. The choice of the specific and correct restriction enzyme is a pivotal point. Digestion with the restriction enzyme *Hae*II was effective to differentiate *C. albicans* from non-*Candida albicans*, while *Bfa*I digestion was useful to distinguish *C. parapsilosis* from *C. krusei*. The *Nla*III restriction enzyme was effective in differentiating the *C. parapsilosis* complex [84]. The predicted fragment sizes for different enzymes with the respective species are depicted in Table S4. Other studies were able to discriminate *Candida* species from clinical samples through RFLP, using the D1/D2 region of the 28S rDNA [84], the secondary alcohol dehydrogenase-encoding gene (*SADH*) [85], and the *ITS* region. RFLP analysis is considered a useful, rapid, and trustworthy method [9,86,87].

However, the additional steps of enzyme digestion add further complexity and time in comparison with assays that rely exclusively on PCR-based methods. The time necessary for PCR-RFLP assay can be similar to routine phenotypic conventional methods [87] but it is more sensitive. The storage (refrigeration) and use of restriction enzymes are considered expensive [88], adding to the resulting complex patterns which may be difficult to interpret.

3.6. Microarray

Microarrays consist of thousands of DNA sequences attached to a solid surface. They allow the detection of the presence of genomic DNA regions or the quantification of the expression of genes. The low number of studies using microarrays to identify *Candida* species is notable. The high cost per sample of a single experiment, when compared with sequencing, may be a factor that led to the disuse of microarray for species identification. On the other hand, microarrays depend on specific sequences, and therefore whole genome or RNA sequencing have clear advantages when compared to microarray technologies.

Microarrays can be applied not only to species identification but also to strain typing with high levels of specificity, sensitivity, and throughput capacity. In terms of molecular typing, microarrays were used to identify and obtain different sequence variants of specific

DNA sequences. Oligonucleotide probe sequences for the identification of different *Candida* spp. [89,90] are in Table S4.

Microarrays were used in the identification of *Candida* spp. from clinical samples, mostly blood [58,91]. Campa and colleagues used the arrayed-primer extension technique (APEX) in which the direct labeling of PCR products is not required. This technology combines the advantages of Sanger dideoxy sequencing with the high-throughput potential of microarrays [92]. The experiment led to the correct species identification, including of the highly related *C. parapsilosis* complex. The microarray was tested for its specificity with reference strains and blind clinical isolates [58].

The major advantages of gene chip technology are its miniature size, high performance, and process automation. The process of optimization is long to ensure stable, specific, sensitive, and reproducible results. The discrimination between specific and unspecific signals may be a challenge in a mixture analysis, as is the case, for instance, of cross-hybridization [93].

3.7. High-Resolution Melting Analysis (HRMA)

HRMA is a simple, rapid, and inexpensive tool useful in the identification of a broad range of clinically relevant *Candida* species. It is combined with RT-PCR, providing an alternative for directly analyzing genetic variations [94]. Alnuaimi and colleagues (2014) used HRMA using the *ITS* region of rDNA to classify relevant *Candida* spp. from oral samples [46]. The authors identified all species in their list and four different genotypes of *C. albicans* [46]. Another author suggests real-time PCR followed by HRMA directly in the biological samples as an efficient method that takes only 6 h to result [54]. HRMA followed by RT-PCR was more rapid and efficient than the classic biochemical methods used in the study [95].

HRMA has some advantages over other genotyping methods owing to the inexpensive single-step procedure, reducing the risk of contamination when compared to a multistep procedure (such as RFLP or nested PCR). Despite this, the technique does not distinguish between some *Candida* spp. due to Tm (Melting Temperature) ranges overlapping [54].

3.8. Multilocus Sequence Typing (MLST)

MLST is a sequencing-based method that analyses nucleotide polymorphisms in fragments from essential genes, the "housekeeping genes" [96,97]. MLST generates a molecular characterization with high discriminatory power and reproducibility. MLST can be used in the epidemiological differentiation of several clinical isolates from *Candida* species and polymorphism search [98–100]. MLST has been used to obtain information about allele diversity in *C. tropicalis* [101] and to access the evolution of virulence-associated mechanisms of the emergent pathogen *C. krusei* [102].

3.9. Loop-Mediated Isothermal Amplification (LAMP)

Amongst all of the currently available isothermal amplification techniques, only Nucleic Acid Sequence-based Amplification (NASBA) [103], Rolling Circle Amplification (RCA) [104], Transcription Mediated Amplification (TMA) [105], and LAMP have been used in the identification of *Candida* spp. Nonetheless, to the best of our knowledge, LAMP is the only technique that has been applied to oral samples.

LAMP is an isothermal one-step amplification method that uses two inner primers (FIP: Forward Inner Primers and BIP: Backward Inner Primer), and two loop primers creating a continuous loop structure during DNA amplification. LAMP uses a Bst DNA polymerase with increased activity, which can produce a high molecular weight DNA fragment within a short time. LAMP's exceptional specificity is due to a set of four primers with six binding sites that must hybridize correctly to the target sequence before DNA biosynthesis occurs. The detection methods include real-time turbidity, fluorescence probes, and others [106]. The use of LAMP to identify relevant fungi and yeasts has been reviewed by Niessen and colleagues [107]. LAMP has shown very good results in the identification of *Candida* spp. in clinical samples [108], dairy products [109], and oral samples [110]. When using oral samples, LAMP was executed by Noguchi and colleagues but only for the detection of *C. albicans* and not for non-*C. albicans* species.

The key elements for a good LAMP assay are primer design and concentration. A higher concentration of the loop primers, FIP and BIP, provides a faster amplification and therefore a quicker result.

Monitoring LAMP amplification can be performed with a water bath/heating block instead of an (expensive) thermocycler. It is real-time, fast, and has a higher amplification efficiency and sensitivity. Naked eye visual amplification monitoring is possible through the turbidity of magnesium pyrophosphate, a by-product of the reaction, color changes by fluorescent intercalating dyes using a UV lamp, and agarose gel analysis revealing patterns that are characterized by a ladder pattern [111]. A list of primers used for the identification of *Candida* spp. is available in Supplementary material—Table S5.

3.10. Next Generation Sequencing (NGS)

Next-generation sequencing, including Whole-Genome sequencing, can also be used for the identification of *Candida* species [112]. NGS can detect markers of antifungal drug resistance from pathogenic *Candida* strains [113,114], *ITS* variabilities in prevalent pathogenic *Candida* spp. [115] and provide insightful metagenomic studies [116]. NGS provided valuable input in the diagnosis of rare infections such as *Candida* meningitis [117] and pseudomembranous oral candidiasis [118].

Although discontinued, pyrosequencing was the first of the NGS technologies to be commercially available and has provided large amounts of sequence data [119], becoming a technology of historical interest. DNA pyrosequencing, or sequencing by synthesis, became possible in the late 1990s as a rapid, cost-effective alternative to Sanger (di-deoxy) DNA sequencing [120]. Third-generation sequencing, also known as next next-generation sequencing, refers to those technologies that do not depend on the PCR amplification of DNA.

The identification of yeasts, including *Candida* spp., has been performed by pyrosequencing using different targets like 18S rRNA gene [52], *ITS1*, and *ITS2* [63,121,122], with results consistent with classic biochemical tests [121,123,124]. Pyrosequencing has also been used for the identification of *Candida* pathogens in various clinical samples such as vaginal [125], blood [126], and oral samples [127]. Pyrosequencing is only able to read short-length sequences of nucleotides, providing a disadvantage for the technique when the target has a longer sequencer. Pyrosequencing data analysis can be complex and challenging. This approach has provided evidence about mutations, with no known previous association with phenotypic drug resistance of the *ERG* and *FKS* genes in *Candida* spp. [128].

The use of pyrosequencing has declined because of the rise of new methodologies of NGS such as Illumina [112], which are less expensive, provide longer sequences, higher sensitivity to detect low-frequency variants, have a faster turnaround time for high sample volumes, and a comprehensive genomic coverage [129].

3.11. Peptide Nucleic Acid Fluorescence In Situ Hybridization (PNA FISH)

Peptide Nucleic Acid molecules are synthetic DNA fragments in which the negatively charged sugar–phosphate backbone of DNA is replaced with a noncharged polyamide [130]. This grants probes to hybridize to their complementary DNA targets with higher affinity and specificity, which means this technique is perfect for targeting highly secondary structured rDNA molecules [131,132]. The technique has the capacity to identify *Candida* spp. within 2.5 h [133]. PNA confers very low background noise, showing it to have a high sensitivity [71].

The PNA FISH probe test was developed to evaluate multiple *Candida* spp. from blood cultures [134–136]. It encompasses three coverage colors: green, red, and yellow for *C. albicans* or *C. parapsilosis*, *C. glabrata* or *C. krusei*, and *C. tropicalis*, respectively [137]. An alternative multi-*Candida* probe was used by Reller and co-workers to identify all *Candida* species under study [138].

The PNA-FISH assay major throwback is that visualization implies the use of a fluorescence microscope, adding costs to the laboratory equipment. This method has proven to be expensive [139], reaching high economic costs per patient [140].

3.12. Matrix-Assisted Laser Desorption Ionization-Time of Flight Mass Spectrometry (MALDI-TOF MS)

MALDI-TOF MS is a molecular method broadly implemented in modern clinical microbiology laboratories [141]. This approach is a rapid and reliable alternative for yeast identification and consists of the generation of protein 'fingerprints' that are compared with reference spectra [142–144]. MALDI-TOF involves sample ionization with a laser striking a matrix of molecules to cause the analyte molecules to enter into a gas phase without fragmentation. It is coupled with the principle of Time-of-Flight analysis, in which ions of different mass/charge ratios are dispersed in time during their flight along a path of known length (the equipment analyzer) [145].

MALDI-TOF MS has been used for the speedy identification of *C. albicans* and non-*albicans* species on blood [146,147] and oral samples [148–150], with shorter turn-around times and higher accuracy compared to conventional biochemical methods [151]. MALDI-TOF MS was performed on a library composed of clinical and reference strains with an accuracy of 94% when compared with *ITS* sequence analysis [142,152]. This method provided results of genus-specific proteins within 24 h of *Candida* causing bloodstream infections [50,143,153].

MALDI-TOF is a promising technique, but the lack of spectra characterization for microorganisms still needs to be addressed. Without available reference spectra, results cannot be achieved. This availability of spectra seems to be changing through the emergence of new studies, building information about *Candida* spp. [147,154–156]. The equipment cost is one of the strongest disadvantages of a clinical and routine setting.

Figure 1 provides a qualitative comparison of the molecular techniques used for the identification of *Candida* spp. Table 2 presents advantages and disadvantages for each molecular technique.

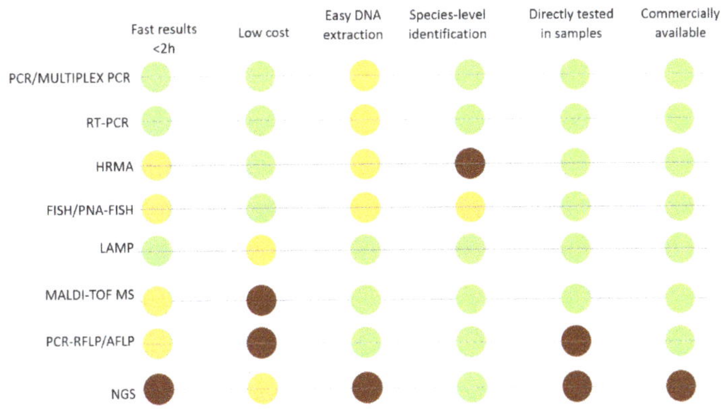

Figure 1. Qualitative analysis of the main molecular approaches for *Candida* species detection. RT-PCR: Real-Time - Polymerase Chain Reaction; NGS: Next Generation Sequencing; HRMA: High-Resolution Melting Analysis; FISH/PNA-FISH: Fluorescent In Situ Hybridization/Peptide Nucleic Acids-FISH; PCR-RFLP/AFLP: Polymerase Chain Reaction - Restriction Fragment Length Amplification/Amplified Fragment Length Polymorphism; LAMP: Loop-Mediated isothermal amplification; PCR-ESI-MS: Electrospray Ionization Mass Spectrometry coupled with broad-spectrum PCR; MALDI-TOF MS: Matrix-Assisted Laser Desorption IonizationTime of Flight Mass Spectrometry; [95,157]. Brown: Low; Yellow: Medium; Green: Good.

Table 2. Resume of advantages and disadvantages for currently used molecular techniques in the identification of *Candida* spp.

Molecular Technique	Advantages	Disadvantages
Conventional PCR	Low cost compared with other PCR-based techniques, low in complexity	Requires an additional amplification detection step
RT-PCR	Real-time detection and quantification, no additional step of detection	Expensive equipment
Nested PCR	Sequence primers available for different gene targets	Requires more reagents than other PCR-based techniques and an additional set of primers. Prone to contamination
Multiplex PCR	Detection of multiple gene targets	Requires an additional amplification detection step
RFLP	High specificity, Sequence primers available for different gene targets	High-cost enzymes and storage, requires an additional amplification detection step.
HRMA	Low risk of contamination when compared to RFLP or nested PCR	Not capable of distinguishing between some *Candida* spp.
MLST	High discriminatory power, useful for epidemiological studies, and evolution of virulence-associated mechanisms	High cost
LAMP	High specificity, high sensitivity, high-speed, low-cost equipment. Several methods for amplification detection	Requires attention in optimization and primer design
NGS	High discriminatory power, large dataset allows for additional analysis	High cost, complex results which require specialized analysis
PNA FISH	Rapid identification of *Candida* spp. in blood cultures	Results visualization adds a cost to equipment
MALDI-TOF MS	High specificity, rapid identification	High cost of equipment, lack of spectra characterization for comparison

3.13. *Promising Molecular Techniques: ddPCR*

Droplet digital PCR (ddPCR) is a new technology based on water–oil emulsion droplets which provides accurate DNA quantification [158]. ddPCR shows a higher quantitative range in comparison to qPCR for the identification of clinical *Candida* spp. in blood samples, providing an early diagnosis as well as a prognostic value for candidemia [159]. ddPCR has yet to be used with oral samples.

4. DNA Target Selection for the Identification of *Candida* spp.

The selection of a suitable molecular target in the diagnosis of any infectious disease is of pivotal importance. Regardless of the molecular technique, an accurate diagnostic strongly depends on the molecular target specificity and its discriminatory capacity. *ITS* has been selected as the barcode of choice for the identification of fungal species [160]. The same happens for *Candida* spp., with *ITS1* and *ITS2* being widely used. Nonetheless, there are some alternatives available. The *MP65* gene plays a role in maintaining cell wall integrity, adherence to epithelia, and biofilm formation in *C. albicans* [57,161]. DNA topoisomerase II coding gene is used due to its highly conserved regions, separated by species-specific regions [72].

Other molecular targets related to virulence, pathogenesis, and antifungal resistance can also be useful as a complement in the identification of *Candida* spp. The ergosterol biosynthetic genes, *ERG3*, *ERG5*, *ERG6*, and *ERG11*, are common targets for the detection of antifungal drug resistance to amphotericin B (AMB) [17,162]. A study also showed that potential mutations in the *ERG5* gene confer resistance against AMB [163].

Several genes are useful for MLST, although their use is not widespread. Sequencing can contribute to improving and simplifying current MLST strategies, as recently described for *C. glabrata* and *C. albicans* [164,165]. Additionally, as mentioned in the NGS Section 3.10, sequencing is relevant for metagenomics studies, the identification of drug resistance, and the diagnosis of rare infections. This is crucial for difficult-to-identify or emerging pathogens, such as *C. auris* [166], or for adequate therapeutic directions in drug-resistant species [161].

5. Conclusions

The oral mycobiome is intricate, dynamic and involves extensive biofilm formation. *Candida* is frequently found in the human mouth and, as with several other pathogenic fungi, appears to be an oral resident in some individuals. Because of the similarity between species, the correct identification is difficult but crucial to the success of the therapy outcome. When choosing a technique for *Candida* identification in clinic settings, material costs, the use of trained professionals, the complexity of the technique, the specificity of the results, and time should be taken into consideration.

We focused on a broad range of molecular techniques that have been used for the identification of *Candida* species in oral samples, having in mind that a timely and accurate diagnosis of *Candida* infection is indispensable for timely intervention with appropriate antifungal therapy. To overcome this challenge, a fast, reliable, inexpensive, and uncomplicated point-of-care diagnosis is needed. For *Candida* spp. identification, only a few techniques fit this criterion: from the necessary sample treatment to time-to-result, only LAMP and Multiplex PCR seem to look promising.

LAMP is considered by many authors to be a highly useful diagnostic technique, especially in areas where access to complex healthcare facilities is limited. However, the amount of data and results on the efficiency of this technique when applied to the diagnosis of *Candida* infections are still scarce when compared to other techniques. Furthermore, the clinical application of LAMP on a larger scale has yet to be achieved. LAMP requires the least amount of time out of all the techniques to reach a diagnosis and does not require costly equipment. Using the *ITS* sequence as a target, it is possible to design primers to identify *Candida* spp. sampled from the area of infection. Taken together, LAMP specificities and requirements seem to be the most adequate for the simplest and most time-efficient diagnostic of oral candidiasis. It is worth highlighting that the exponential growth of gene sequence databases has provided the ideal conditions to develop more efficient and reliable primer designs, enhancing target specificity and the accuracy of diagnosis.

Ultimately, the pros and cons of each molecular technique detailed in this review can hopefully help dentists who deal with patients with inflammatory conditions to choose the most appropriate diagnostic method. Nevertheless, novel developments within this field of research may lead to improvements in currently available techniques and to the development of new ones.

Supplementary Materials: The following supporting information can be downloaded at: https://www.mdpi.com/article/10.3390/app12189204/s1, Table S1: Primers (Universal and species-specific) used for *Candida* species detection and size of fragments separated by agarose gel electrophoresis; Table S2: List of primers used for Nested PCR; Table S3: Restriction Fragment Length Polymorphism (RFLP) fragment patterns in oral *Candida* spp. isolates with restriction enzymes; Table S4: Oligonucleotide probes used for *Candida* spp. in non-oral isolates; Table S5: Primers used in Kasahara (2014) for the detection of *Candida* spp. with LAMP.

Author Contributions: Conceptualization, A.S.D., M.J.C., and A.A.; methodology, J.M., A.S.D. and R.M.S.; validation, J.M., M.J.C., R.M.S., A.C.E., A.A. and A.S.D.; formal analysis, J.M.; investigation, J.M., R.M.S. and A.S.D.; resources, A.S.D.; data curation, R.M.S., A.C.E., A.A. and A.S.D.; writing—original draft preparation, J.M.; writing—review and editing, J.M., M.J.C., R.M.S., A.C.E., A.A. and A.S.D.; supervision, A.S.D. and A.A.; project administration, A.S.D. All authors have read and agreed to the published version of the manuscript.

Funding: This research was funded by the Portuguese Foundation for Science and Technology (FCT) through national funds to the Center for Interdisciplinary Research in Health (CIIS) (UIDB/04279/2020+UIDP/04279/2020) and the Centre for Environmental and Marine Studies CESAM (UIDP/50017/2020+UIDB/50017/2020+LA/P/0094/2020). Thanks, are also due to FCT and UCP for the CEEC institutional financing of AS Duarte (CEEC-INST/00137/2018/CP1520/CT0013), and RM Silva (CEECINST/00137/2018/CP1520/CT0012).

Institutional Review Board Statement: Not applicable.

Informed Consent Statement: Not applicable.

Data Availability Statement: Not applicable.

Conflicts of Interest: The authors declare no conflict of interest.

References

1. Baumgardner, D.J. Oral Fungal Microbiota: To Thrush and Beyond. *J. Patient-Centered Res. Rev.* **2019**, *6*, 11. [CrossRef] [PubMed]
2. Harriott, M.M.; Lilly, E.A.; Rodriguez, T.E.; Fidel, P.L.; Noverr, M.C. *Candida albicans* Forms Biofilms on the Vaginal Mucosa. *Microbiology* **2010**, *156*, 3635–3644. [CrossRef] [PubMed]
3. Koehler, P.; Stecher, M.; Cornely, O.A.; Koehler, D.; Vehreschild, M.J.G.T.; Bohlius, J.; Wisplinghoff, H.; Vehreschild, J.J. Morbidity and Mortality of Candidaemia in Europe: An Epidemiologic Meta-Analysis. *Clin. Microbiol. Infect.* **2019**, *25*, 1200–1212. [CrossRef] [PubMed]
4. Lamoth, F.; Lockhart, S.R.; Berkow, E.L.; Calandra, T. Changes in the Epidemiological Landscape of Invasive Candidiasis. *J. Antimicrob. Chemother.* **2018**, *73*, i4–i13. [CrossRef]
5. Yapar, N. Epidemiology and Risk Factors for Invasive Candidiasis. *Ther. Clin. Risk Manag.* **2014**, *10*, 95–105. [CrossRef]
6. Alam, M.Z.; Alam, Q.; Jiman-Fatani, A.; Kamal, M.A.; Abuzenadah, A.M.; Chaudhary, A.G.; Akram, M.; Haque, A. *Candida* Identification: A Journey from Conventional to Molecular Methods in Medical Mycology. *World J. Microbiol. Biotechnol.* **2014**, *30*, 1437–1451. [CrossRef]
7. Silva, D.B.d.S.; de Oliveira, K.M.P.; Grisolia, A.B. Molecular Methods Developed for the Identification and Characterization of *Candida* Species. *Int. J. Genet. Sci.* **2017**, *4*, 1–6. [CrossRef]
8. Małek, M.; Paluchowska, P.; Bogusz, B.; Budak, A. Molecular Characterization of *Candida* Isolates from Intensive Care Unit Patients, Krakow, Poland. *Rev. Iberoam. Micol.* **2017**, *34*, 10–16. [CrossRef]
9. Hamzeh, S.; Kalantar-Neyestanaki, D.; Ali Mohammadi, M.; Nasibi, S.; Ayatollahi Mousavi, S.A. Identification of *Candida* spp. Isolated from Oral Mucosa in Patients with Leukemias and Lymphomas in Iran. *Iran. J. Microbiol.* **2019**, *11*, 114–119. [CrossRef]
10. Butera, A.; Pascadopoli, M.; Pellegrini, M.; Gallo, S.; Zampetti, P.; Scribante, A. Oral Microbiota in Patients with Peri-Implant Disease: A Narrative Review. *Appl. Sci.* **2022**, *12*, 3250. [CrossRef]
11. Slazhneva, E.; Orekhova, L.; Tikhomirova, E.; Tsarev, V.; Loboda, E.; Atrushkevich, V. Candida Species Detection in Patients with Chronic Periodontitis: A Systematic Review and Meta-Analysis Review Questions. *Clin. Exp. Dent. Res.* **2022**, 1–22. [CrossRef] [PubMed]
12. Henriques, M.; Azeredo, J.; Oliveira, R. *Candida* Species Adhesion to Oral Epithelium: Factors Involved and Experimental Methodology Used. *Crit. Rev. Microbiol.* **2006**, *32*, 217–226. [CrossRef] [PubMed]
13. McCarty, T.P.; White, C.M.; Pappas, P.G. Candidemia and Invasive Candidiasis. *Infect. Dis. Clin. North Am.* **2021**, *35*, 389–413. [CrossRef] [PubMed]
14. Hirano, R.; Sakamoto, Y.; Kudo, K.; Ohnishi, M. Retrospective Analysis of Mortality and *Candida* Isolates of 75 Patients with Candidemia: A Single Hospital Experience. *Infect. Drug Resist.* **2015**, *8*, 199–205. [CrossRef] [PubMed]
15. Spivak, E.S.; Hanson, K.E. *Candida auris*: An Emerging Fungal Pathogen. *J. Clin. Microbiol.* **2018**, *56*, 1–10. [CrossRef]
16. Hasan, F.; Xess, I.; Wang, X.; Jain, N.; Fries, B.C. Biofilm Formation in Clinical *Candida* Isolates and Its Association with Virulence. *Microbes Infect.* **2009**, *11*, 753–761. [CrossRef]
17. Lopes, J.P.; Lionakis, M.S. Pathogenesis and Virulence of *Candida albicans*. *Virulence* **2022**, *13*, 89–121. [CrossRef]
18. Sardi, J.C.O.; Scorzoni, L.; Bernardi, T.; Fusco-Almeida, A.M.; Mendes Giannini, M.J.S. *Candida* Species: Current Epidemiology, Pathogenicity, Biofilm Formation, Natural Antifungal Products and New Therapeutic Options. *J. Med. Microbiol.* **2013**, *62*, 10–24. [CrossRef]
19. Ho, J.; Camilli, G.; Griffiths, J.S.; Richardson, J.P.; Kichik, N.; Naglik, J.R. *Candida albicans* and Candidalysin in Inflammatory Disorders and Cancer. *Immunology* **2021**, *162*, 11–16. [CrossRef]

20. Jenks, J.D.; Cornely, O.A.; Chen, S.C.A.; Thompson, G.R.; Hoenigl, M. Breakthrough Invasive Fungal Infections: Who Is at Risk? *Mycoses* **2020**, *63*, 1021–1032. [CrossRef]
21. Zakaria, M.N.; Furuta, M.; Takeshita, T.; Shibata, Y.; Sundari, R.; Eshima, N.; Ninomiya, T.; Yamashita, Y. Oral Mycobiome in Community-Dwelling Elderly and Its Relation to Oral and General Health Conditions. *Oral Dis.* **2017**, *23*, 973–982. [CrossRef] [PubMed]
22. Mathur, P.; Hasan, F.; Singh, P.K.; Malhotra, R.; Walia, K.; Chowdhary, A. Five-Year Profile of Candidaemia at an Indian Trauma Centre: High Rates of *Candida auris* Blood Stream Infections. *Mycoses* **2018**, *61*, 674–680. [CrossRef] [PubMed]
23. Ricotta, E.; Lai, Y.L.; Sameer, K.S.; Lionakis, M.; Prevots, R.; Adjemian, J. Species Distribution and Trends of Invasive Candidiasis in the United States. *Abstr. • OFID* **2018**, *362*, 2016–2017.
24. Cleveland, A.A.; Harrison, L.H.; Farley, M.M.; Hollick, R.; Stein, B.; Chiller, T.M.; Lockhart, S.R.; Park, B.J. Declining Incidence of Candidemia and the Shifting Epidemiology of *Candida* Resistance in Two US Metropolitan Areas, 2008-2013: Results from Population-Based Surveillance. *PLoS One* **2015**, *10*, 2008–2013. [CrossRef]
25. Campion, E.W.; Kullberg, B.J.; Arendrup, M.C. Invasive Candidiasis. *N. Engl. J. Med.* **2015**, *373*, 1445–1456. [CrossRef]
26. Alexander, B.D.; Pfaller, M.A. Contemporary Tools for the Diagnosis and Management of Invasive Mycoses. *Clin. Infect. Dis.* **2006**, *43* (Supplement article), S15–S27. [CrossRef]
27. Garey, K.W.; Rege, M.; Pai, M.P.; Mingo, D.E.; Suda, K.J.; Turpin, R.S.; Bearden, D.T. Time to Initiation of Fluconazole Therapy Impacts Mortality in Patients with Candidemia: A Multi-Institutional Study. *Clin. Infect. Dis.* **2006**, *43*, 25–31. [CrossRef]
28. Parkins, M.D.; Sabuda, D.M.; Elsayed, S.; Laupland, K.B. Adequacy of Empirical Antifungal Therapy and Effect on Outcome among Patients with Invasive *Candida* Species Infections. *J. Antimicrob. Chemother.* **2007**, *60*, 613–618. [CrossRef]
29. Clancy, C.J.; Nguyen, M.H. Diagnosing Invasive Candidiasis. *J. Clin. Microbiol.* **2018**, *56*. [CrossRef]
30. Dadar, M.; Tiwari, R.; Karthik, K.; Chakraborty, S.; Shahali, Y.; Dhama, K. *Candida albicans* - Biology, Molecular Characterization, Pathogenicity, and Advances in Diagnosis and Control – An Update. *Microb. Pathog.* **2018**, *117*, 128–138. [CrossRef]
31. Lewis, M.A.O.; Williams, D.W. Diagnosis and Management of Oral Candidosis. *Br. Dent. J.* **2017**, *223*, 675–681. [CrossRef] [PubMed]
32. Pfaller, M.A.; Castanheira, M. Nosocomial Candidiasis: Antifungal Stewardship and the Importance of Rapid Diagnosis. *Med. Mycol.* **2016**, *54*, 1–22. [CrossRef] [PubMed]
33. Buzalaf, M.A.R.; Ortiz, A.d.C.; Carvalho, T.S.; Fideles, S.O.M.; Araújo, T.T.; Moraes, S.M.; Buzalaf, N.R.; Reis, F.N. Saliva as a Diagnostic Tool for Dental Caries, Periodontal Disease and Cancer: Is There a Need for More Biomarkers? *Expert Rev. Mol. Diagn.* **2020**, *20*, 543–555. [CrossRef] [PubMed]
34. Khurshid, Z.; Zafar, M.S.; Khan, R.S.; Najeeb, S.; Slowey, P.D.; Rehman, I.U. *Role of Salivary Biomarkers in Oral Cancer Detection;* Elsevier Ltd.: Amsterdam, The Netherlands, 2018. [CrossRef]
35. Fernandes, L.L.; Pacheco, V.B.; Borges, L.; Athwal, H.K.; de Paula Eduardo, F.; Bezinelli, L.; Correa, L.; Jimenez, M.; Dame-Teixeira, N.; Lombaert, I.M.A.; et al. Saliva in the Diagnosis of COVID-19: A Review and New Research Directions. *J. Dent. Res.* **2020**, *99*, 1435–1443. [CrossRef] [PubMed]
36. Miranda-Cadena, K.; Marcos-Arias, C.; Mateo, E.; Aguirre, J.M.; Quindós, G.; Eraso, E. Prevalence and Antifungal Susceptibility Profiles of *Candida glabrata, Candida parapsilosis* and Their Close-Related Species in Oral Candidiasis. *Arch. Oral Biol.* **2018**, *95*, 100–107. [CrossRef]
37. d'Enfert, C. Biofilms and Their Role in the Resistance of Pathogenic *Candida* to Antifungal Agents. *Curr. Drug Targets* **2006**, *7*, 465–670. [CrossRef] [PubMed]
38. Gold, J.A.W.; Seagle, E.E.; Nadle, J.; Barter, D.M.; Czaja, C.A.; Johnston, H.; Farley, M.M.; Thomas, S.; Harrison, L.H.; Fischer, J.; et al. Treatment Practices for Adults with Candidemia at 9 Active Surveillance Sites-United States, 2017–2018. *Clin. Infect. Dis.* **2021**, *73*, 1609–1616. [CrossRef]
39. Robbins, N.; Uppuluri, P.; Nett, J.; Rajendran, R.; Ramage, G.; Lopez-Ribot, J.L.; Andes, D.; Cowen, L.E. Hsp90 Governs Dispersion and Drug Resistance of Fungal Biofilms. *PLoS Pathog.* **2011**, *7*, e1002257. [CrossRef]
40. Zarrinfar, H.; Kord, Z.; Fata, A. High Incidence of Azole Resistance among *Candida albicans* and *C. glabrata* Isolates in Northeastern Iran. *Curr. Med. Mycol.* **2021**, *17*, 18–21. [CrossRef]
41. Ajenjo, M.C.; Aquevedo, A.; Guzmán, A.M.; Poggi, H.; Calvo, M.; Castillo, C.; León, E.; Andresen, M.; Labarca, J. Perfil Epidemiológico de La Candidiasis Invasora En Unidades de Pacientes Críticos En Un Hospital Universitario. *Rev. Chill. Infecttiologia* **2011**, *28*, 118–122. [CrossRef]
42. Cernáková, L.; Anna, L.; Lengyelová, L.; ROdrigues, C.F. Prevalence and Antifungal Susceptibility Profile of Oral *Candida* spp. Isolates from a Hospital in Slovakia. *Medicina (B. Aires)* **2022**, *58*, 576. [CrossRef] [PubMed]
43. Jeffery-Smith, A.; Taori, S.K.; Schelenz, S.; Jeffery, K.; Johnson, E.M.; Borman, A.; Manuel, R.; Browna, C.S. *Candida auris*: A Review of the Literature. *Clin. Microbiol. Rev.* **2018**, *31*, 1–18. [CrossRef]
44. Terças, A.L.G.; Marques, S.G.; Moffa, E.B.; Alves, M.B.; de Azevedo, C.M.P.S.; Siqueira, W.L.; Monteiro, C.A. Antifungal Drug Susceptibility of *Candida* Species Isolated from HIV-Positive Patients Recruited at a Public Hospital in São Luís, Maranhão, Brazil. *Front. Microbiol.* **2017**, *8*, 1–8. [CrossRef] [PubMed]
45. Willinger, B. What Is the Target? Clinical Mycology and Diagnostics. In *Clinically Relevant Mycoses;* Springer: Berlin/Heidelberg, Germany, 2019. [CrossRef]

46. Alnuaimi, A.D.; Wiesenfeld, D.; O'Brien-Simpson, N.M.; Reynolds, E.C.; Peng, B.; Mccullough, M.J. The Development and Validation of a Rapid Genetic Method for Species Identification and Genotyping of Medically Important Fungal Pathogens Using High-Resolution Melting Curve Analysis. *Mol. Oral Microbiol.* **2014**, *29*, 117–130. [CrossRef] [PubMed]
47. Dunyach, C.; Bertout, S.; Phelipeau, C.; Drakulovski, P.; Reynes, J.; Mallié, M. Detection and Identification of *Candida* spp. in Human Serum by LightCycler® Real-Time Polymerase Chain Reaction. *Diagn. Microbiol. Infect. Dis.* **2008**, *60*, 263–271. [CrossRef]
48. Fricke, S.; Fricke, C.; Schimmelpfennig, C.; Oelkrug, C.; Schönfelder, U.; Blatz, R.; Zilch, C.; Faber, S.; Hilger, N.; Ruhnke, M.; et al. A Real-Time PCR Assay for the Differentiation of *Candida* Species. *J. Appl. Microbiol.* **2010**, *109*, 1150–1158. [CrossRef] [PubMed]
49. Guiver, M.; Levi, K.; Oppenheim, B.A. Rapid Identification of *Candida* Species by TaqMan PCR. *J. Clin. Pathol.* **2001**, *54*, 362–366. [CrossRef]
50. Neppelenbroek, K.H.; Seó, R.S.; Urban, V.M.; Silva, S.; Dovigo, L.N.; Jorge, J.H.; Campanha, N.H. Identification of *Candida* Species in the Clinical Laboratory: A Review of Conventional, Commercial, and Molecular Techniques. *Oral Dis.* **2014**, *20*, 329–344. [CrossRef]
51. Deorukhkar, S.C.; Saini, S. Laboratory Approach for Diagnosis of Candidiasis through Ages. *Int. J. Curr. Microbiol.App. Sci* **2014**, *3*, 206–218.
52. Gharizadeh, B.; Norberg, E.; Löffler, J.; Jalal, S.; Tollemar, J.; Einsele, H.; Klingspor, L.; Nyrén, P. Identification of Medically Important Fungi by the Pyrosequencing^{TM} Technology. *Mycoses* **2004**, *47*, 29–33. [CrossRef]
53. Leaw, S.N.; Chang, H.C.; Sun, H.F.; Barton, R.; Bouchara, J.; Chang, T.C. Identification of Medically Important Yeast Species by Sequence Analysis of the Internal Transribed Spacer Regions. *J. Clin. Microbiol.* **2006**, *44*, 693–699. [CrossRef] [PubMed]
54. Nemcova, E.; Cernochova, M.; Ruzicka, F.; Malisova, B.; Freiberger, T.; Nemec, P. Rapid Identification of Medically Important *Candida* Isolates Using High Resolution Melting Analysis. *PLoS ONE* **2015**, *10*, 1–15. [CrossRef]
55. Williams, D.W.; Wilson, M.J.; Lewis, M.A.O.; Potts, A.J.C. Identification of *Candida* Species by PCR and Restriction Fragment Length Polymorphism Analysis of Intergenic Spacer Regions of Ribosomal DNA. *J. Clin. Microbiol.* **1995**, *33*, 2476–2479. [CrossRef] [PubMed]
56. Arancia, S.; Sandini, S.; De Bernardis, F.; Fortini, D. Rapid, Simple, and Low-Cost Identification of *Candida* Species Using High-Resolution Melting Analysis. *Diagn. Microbiol. Infect. Dis.* **2011**, *69*, 283–285. [CrossRef]
57. Arancia, S.; Sandini, S.; Cassone, A.; De Bernardis, F. Use of 65 KDa Mannoprotein Gene Primers in PCR Methods for the Identification of Five Medically Important *Candida* Species. *Mol. Cell. Probes* **2009**, *23*, 218–226. [CrossRef]
58. Campa, D.; Tavanti, A.; Gemignani, F.; Mogavero, C.S.; Bellini, I.; Bottari, F.; Barale, R.; Landi, S.; Senesi, S. DNA Microarray Based on Arrayed-Primer Extension Technique for Identification of Pathogenic Fungi Responsible for Invasive and Superficial Mycoses. *J. Clin. Microbiol.* **2008**, *46*, 909–915. [CrossRef]
59. Spiess, B.; Seifarth, W.; Hummel, M.; Frank, O.; Fabarius, A.; Zheng, C.; Mörz, H.; Hehlmann, R.; Buchheidt, D. DNA Microarray-Based Detection and Identification of Fungal Pathogens in Clinical Samples from Neutropenic Patients. *J. Clin. Microbiol.* **2007**, *45*, 3743–3753. [CrossRef]
60. Obručová, H.; Tihelková, R.; Kotásková, I.; Růžička, F.; Holá, V.; Němcová, E.; Freiberger, T. Evaluation of Fluorescent Capillary Electrophoresis for Rapid Identification of *Candida* Fungal Infections. *J. Clin. Microbiol.* **2016**, *54*, 1295–1303. [CrossRef]
61. Liu, D. *Molecular Detection of Human Fungal Pathogen*; CRC Press; Taylor & Francis Group: London, UK, 2011. [CrossRef]
62. Tata, W.; Viraporn, P.; Chatsri, T.; Kuansuwan, K. Distribution of *Candida* Species in Oral Candidiasis Patients: Association between Sites of Isolation, Ability to Form Biofilm, and Susceptibility to Antifungal Drugs. *J. Assoc. Med. Sci.* **2018**, *51*, 32–37. [CrossRef]
63. Shi, B.; Wu, T.; Mclean, J.; Edlund, A.; Young, Y. The Denture-Associated Oral Microbiome. *Clininal Sci. Epidemiol.* **2016**, *1*, 1–13. [CrossRef]
64. Wolffs, P.; Grage, H.; Hagberg, O.; Rådström, P. Impact of DNA Polymerases and Their Buffer Systems on Quantitative Real-Time PCR. *J. Clin. Microbiol.* **2004**, *42*, 408–411. [CrossRef] [PubMed]
65. Ginzinger, D.G. Gene Quantification Using Real-Time Quantitative PCR: An Emerging Technology Hits the Mainstream. *Exp. Hematol.* **2002**, *30*, 503–512. [CrossRef]
66. Metwally, L.; Fairley, D.J.; Coyle, P.V.; Hay, R.J.; Hedderwick, S.; McCloskey, B.; O'Neill, H.J.; Webb, C.H.; Elbaz, W.; McMullan, R. Improving Molecular Detection of *Candida* DNA in Whole Blood: Comparison of Seven Fungal DNA Extraction Protocols Using Real-Time PCR. *J. Med. Microbiol.* **2008**, *57*, 296–303. [CrossRef] [PubMed]
67. White, P.L.; Williams, D.W.; Kuriyama, T.; Samad, S.A.; Lewis, M.A.O.; Barnes, R.A. Detection of *Candida* in Concentrated Oral Rinse Cultures by Real-Time PCR. *J. Clin. Microbiol.* **2004**, *42*, 2101–2107. [CrossRef]
68. Tomov, G.; Stamenov, N.; Neychev, D.; Atliev, K. *Candida* Carriers among Individuals with Tongue Piercing—A Real-Time PCR Study. *Antibiotics* **2022**, *11*, 742. [CrossRef]
69. Amarasinghe, A.A.P.B.N.; Muhandiram, M.R.S.; Kodithuwakku, S.P.; Thilakumara, I.P.; Jayatilake, J.A.M.S. Identification, Genotyping and Invasive Enzyme Production of Oral *Candida* Species from Denture Induced Stomatitis Patients and Healthy Careers. *J. Oral Maxillofac. Surgery Med. Pathol.* **2021**, *33*, 467–474. [CrossRef]
70. Zarei, N.; Roudbary, M.; Roudbar Mohammadi, S.; dos Santos, A.S.; Nikoomanesh, F.; Mohammadi, R.; Shirvan, B.; Yaalimadad, S. Prevalence, Molecular Identification, and Genotyping of *Candida* Species Recovered from Oral Cavity among Patients with Diabetes Mellitus from Tehran, Iran. *Adv. Biomed. Res.* **2022**, *11*, 29. [CrossRef]

71. Tang, Y.-W.; Stratton, C.W. *Advanced Techniques in Diagnostic Microbiology*, 2nd ed.; Yi-Wei, Stratton, C.Y., Eds., Springer: New York, NY, USA; Heidelberg Germany; Dordracht, The Netherlands; London, UK, 2017; Volume 53. [CrossRef]
72. Kanbe, T.; Horii, T.; Arishima, T.; Ozeki, M.; Kikuchi, A. PCR-Based Identification of Pathogenic *Candida* Species Using Primer Mixes Specific to *Candida* DNA Topoisomerase II Genes. *Yeast* **2002**, *19*, 973–989. [CrossRef]
73. Coronado-castellote, L.; Jiménez-soriano, Y. Clinical and Microbiological Diagnosis of Oral Candidiasis. *Oral Med. Pathol.* **2013**, *5*, 279–286. [CrossRef]
74. Liguori, G.; Di Onofrio, V.; Lucariello, A.; Gallé, F.; Signoriello, G.; Colella, G.; D'Amora, M.; Rossano, F. Oral Candidiasis: A Comparison between Conventional Methods and Multiplex Polymerase Chain Reaction for Species Identification. *Oral Microbiol. Immunol.* **2009**, *24*, 76–78. [CrossRef]
75. Luo, G.; Mitchell, T.G. Rapid Identification of Pathogenic Fungi Directly from Cultures by Using Multiplex PCR. *J. Clin. Microbiol.* **2002**, *40*, 2860–2865. [CrossRef]
76. Romeo, O.; Scordino, F.; Pernice, I.; Lo Passo, C.; Criseo, G. A Multiplex PCR Protocol for Rapid Identification of *Candida glabrata* and Its Phylogenetically Related Species *Candida nivariensis* and Candida Bracarensis. *J. Microbiol. Methods* **2009**, *79*, 117–120. [CrossRef]
77. Sampath, A.; Weerasekera, M.; Gunasekara, C.; Dilhari, A.; Bulugahapitiya, U.; Fernando, N. A Sensitive and a Rapid Multiplex Polymerase Chain Reaction for the Identification of *Candida* Species in Concentrated Oral Rinse Specimens in Patients with Diabetes. *Acta Odontol. Scand.* **2017**, *75*, 113–122. [CrossRef]
78. Carvalho, A.; Costa-De-Oliveira, S.; Martins, M.L.; Pina-Vaz, C.; Rodrigues, A.G.; Ludovico, P.; Rodrigues, F. Multiplex PCR Identification of Eight Clinically Relevant *Candida* Species. *Med. Mycol.* **2007**, *45*, 619–627. [CrossRef]
79. Arastehfar, A.; Fang, W.; Pan, W.; Lackner, M.; Liao, W.; Badiee, P.; Zomorodian, K.; Badali, H.; Hagen, F.; Lass-Flörl, C.; et al. YEAST PANEL Multiplex PCR for Identification of Clinically Important Yeast Species: Stepwise Diagnostic Strategy, Useful for Developing Countries. *Diagn. Microbiol. Infect. Dis.* **2019**, *93*, 112–119. [CrossRef]
80. Liguori, G.; Lucariello, A.; Colella, G.; De Luca, A.; Marinelli, P. Rapid Identification of *Candida* Species in Oral Rinse Solutions by PCR. *J. Clin. Pathol.* **2007**, *60*, 1035–1039. [CrossRef]
81. Hajia, M. Limitations of Different PCR Protocols Used in Diagnostic Laboratories: A Short Review. *Mod. Med. Lab. J.* **2017**, *1*, 1–6. [CrossRef]
82. Teasdale, B.; West, A.; Taylor, H.; Klein, A. A Simple Restriction Fragment Length Polymorphism (RFLP) Assay to Discriminate Common Porphyra (Bangiophyceae, Rhodophyta) Taxa from the Northwest Atlantic. *J. Appl. Phycol.* **2002**, *14*, 293–298. [CrossRef]
83. Cirak, M.Y.; Kalkanci, A.; Kustimur, S. Use of Molecular Methods in Identification of *Candida* Species and Evaluation of Fluconazole Resistance. *Mem. Inst. Oswaldo Cruz* **2003**, *98*, 1027–1032. [CrossRef]
84. Barbedo, L.S.; Figueiredo-Carvalho, M.H.G.; de Medeiros Muniz, M.; Zancopé-Oliveira, R.M. The Identification and Differentiation of the *Candida parapsilosis* Complex Species by Polymerase Chain Reaction-Restriction Fragment Length Polymorphism of the Internal Transcribed Spacer Region of the RDNA. *Mem. Inst. Oswaldo Cruz* **2016**, *111*, 267–270. [CrossRef]
85. Mirhendi, H.; Bruun, B.; Schønheyder, H.C.; Christensen, J.J.; Fuursted, K.; Gahrn-hansen, B.; Johansen, H.K.; Nielsen, L.; Knudsen, J.D.; Arendrup, M.C. Molecular Screening for *Candida orthopsilosis* and *Candida metapsilosis* among Danish *Candida parapsilosis* Group Blood Culture Isolates: Proposal of a New RFLP Profile for Differentiation. *J. Med. Microbiol.* **2010**, *59*, 414–420. [CrossRef] [PubMed]
86. Aslani, N.; Abastabar, M.; Hedayati, M.T.; Shokohi, T.; Aghili, S.R.; Diba, K.; Hosseini, T.; Bahrami, B.; Ebrahimpour, A.; Salehi, M.; et al. Molecular Identification and Antifungal Susceptibility Testing of *Candida* Species Isolated from Dental Plaques. *J. Mycol. Med.* **2018**, *28*, 433–436. [CrossRef] [PubMed]
87. Fatima, A.; Bashir, G.; Wani, T.; Jan, A.; Kohli, A.; Khan, M.S. Molecular Identification of *Candida* Species Isolated from Cases of Neonatal Candidemia Using Polymerase Chain Reaction-Restriction Fragment Length Polymorphism in a Tertiary Care Hospital. *Indian J. Pathol. Microbiol.* **2017**, *60*, 61–65. [CrossRef] [PubMed]
88. Jafari, Z.; Motamedi, M.; Jalalizand, N.; Shokoohi, G.R.; Charsizadeh, A.; Mirhendi, H. A Comparison between CHROMagar, PCR-RFLP and PCR-FSP for Identification of *Candida* Species. *Curr. Med. Mycol.* **2017**, *3*, 10–15. [CrossRef] [PubMed]
89. Huang, A.; Li, J.W.; Shen, Z.Q.; Wang, X.W.; Jin, M. High-Throughput Identification of Clinical Pathogenic Fungi by Hybridization to an Oligonucleotide Microarray. *J. Clin. Microbiol.* **2006**, *44*, 3299–3305. [CrossRef]
90. Nett, J.E.; Lepak, A.J.; Marchillo, K.; Andes, D.R. Time Course Global Gene Expression Analysis of an in vivo *Candida* Biofilm. *J. Infect. Dis.* **2009**, *200*, 307–313. [CrossRef]
91. Leinberger, D.M.; Schumacher, U.; Autenrieth, I.B.; Bachmann, T.T. Development of a DNA Microarray for Detection and Identification of Fungal Pathogens Involved in Invasive Mycoses. *J. Clin. Microbiol.* **2005**, *43*, 4943–4953. [CrossRef]
92. Kurg, A.; Tõnisson, N.; Georgiou, I.; Shumaker, J.; Tollett, J.; Metspalu, A. Arrayed Primer Extension: Solid-Phase Four-Color DNA Resequencing and Mutation Detection Technology. *Genet. Test.* **2000**, *4*, 1–7. [CrossRef]
93. Volokhov, D.; Rasooly, A.; Chumakov, K.; Chizhikov, V. Identification of Listeria Species by Microarray-Based Assay. *J. Clin. Microbiol.* **2002**, *40*, 4720–4728. [CrossRef]
94. Reed, G.H.; Kent, J.O.; Wittwer, C.T. High-Resolution DNA Melting Analysis for Simple and Efficient Molecular Diagnostics. *Pharmacogenomics* **2007**, *8*, 597–608. [CrossRef]

95. Arastehfar, A.; Boekhout, T.; Butler, G.; Buda De Cesare, G.; Dolk, E.; Gabaldón, T.; Hafez, A.; Hube, B.; Hagen, F.; Hovhannisyan, H.; et al. Recent Trends in Molecular Diagnostics of Yeast Infections: From PCR to NGS. *FEMS Microbiol. Rev.* **2019**, *43*, 517–547. [CrossRef]
96. Bougnoux, M.E.; Morand, S.; D'Enfert, C. Usefulness of Multilocus Sequence Typing for Characterization of Clinical Isolates of *Candida albicans*. *J. Clin. Microbiol.* **2002**, *40*, 1290–1297. [CrossRef] [PubMed]
97. Odds, F.C.; Jacobsen, M.D. Multilocus Sequence Typing of Pathogenic *Candida* Species. *Eukaryot. Cell* **2008**, *7*, 1075–1084. [CrossRef] [PubMed]
98. Choo, K.H.; Lee, H.J.; Knight, N.J.; Holmes, A.R.; Cannon, R.D. Multilocus Sequence Typing (MLST) Analysis of *Candida albicans* Isolates Colonizing Acrylic Dentures before and after Denture Replacement. *Med. Mycol.* **2017**, *55*, 673–679. [CrossRef]
99. Odds, F.C. Molecular Phylogenetics and Epidemiology of *Candida albicans*. *Rev. Futur. Microbiol.* **2010**, 67–79. [CrossRef]
100. Tavanti, A.; Gow, N.A.R.; Senesi, S.; Maiden, M.C.J.; Odds, F.C. Optimization and Validation of Multilocus Sequence Typing for *Candida albicans*. *J. Clin. Microbiol.* **2003**, *41*, 3765–3776. [CrossRef]
101. Dougue, A.N.; El-Kholy, M.A.; Giuffrè, L.; Galeano, G.; D'Aleo, F.; Kountchou, C.L.; Nangwat, C.; Paul, D.J.; Giosa, D.; Pernice, I.; et al. Multilocus Sequence Typing (MLST) Analysis Reveals Many Novel Genotypes and a High Level of Genetic Diversity in *Candida tropicalis* Isolates from Italy and Africa. *Mycoses* **2022**, 1–12. [CrossRef]
102. Domán, M.; Makrai, L.; Bányai, K. Molecular Phylogenetic Analysis of *Candida krusei*. *Mycopathologia* **2022**, *0123456789*. [CrossRef]
103. Widjojoatmodjo, M.N.; Borst, A.; Schukkink, R.A.F.; Box, A.T.A.; Tacken, N.M.M.; Van Gemen, B.; Verhoef, J.; Top, B.; Fluit, A.C. Nucleic Acid Sequence-Based Amplification (NASBA) Detection of Medically Important *Candida* Species. *J. Microbiol. Methods* **1999**, *38*, 81–90. [CrossRef]
104. Zhou, X.; Kong, F.; Sorrell, T.C.; Wang, H.; Duan, Y.; Chen, S.C.A. Practical Method for Detection and Identification of *Candida*, *Aspergillus*, and *Scedosporium* spp. by Use of Rolling-Circle Amplification. *J. Clin. Microbiol.* **2008**, *46*, 2423–2427. [CrossRef]
105. Richter, S.S.; Otiso, J.; Goje, O.J.; Vogel, S.; Aebly, J.; Keller, G.; van Heule, H.; Wehn, D.; Stephens, A.L.; Zanotti, S.; et al. Prospective Evaluation of Molecular Assays for Diagnosis of Vaginitis. *J. Clin. Microbiol.* **2020**, *58*, 6–10. [CrossRef] [PubMed]
106. Zhang, X.; Lowe, S.B.; Gooding, J.J. Brief Review of Monitoring Methods for Loop-Mediated Isothermal Amplification (LAMP). *Biosens. Bioelectron.* **2014**, *61*, 491–499. [CrossRef] [PubMed]
107. Niessen, L. Current State and Future Perspectives of Loop-Mediated Isothermal Amplification (LAMP)-Based Diagnosis of Filamentous Fungi and Yeasts. *Appl. Microbiol. Biotechnol.* **2015**, *99*, 553–574. [CrossRef] [PubMed]
108. Fallahi, S.; Babaei, M.; Rostami, A.; Mirahmadi, H.; Arab-Mazar, Z.; Sepahvand, A. Diagnosis of *Candida albicans*: Conventional Diagnostic Methods Compared to the Loop-Mediated Isothermal Amplification (LAMP) Assay. *Arch. Microbiol.* **2019**, 0123456789. [CrossRef]
109. Kasahara, K.; Ishikawa, H.; Sato, S.; Shimakawa, Y.; Watanabe, K. Development of Multiplex Loop-Mediated Isothermal Amplification Assays to Detect Medically Important Yeasts in Dairy Products. *FEMS Microbiol. Lett.* **2014**, *357*, 208–216. [CrossRef]
110. Noguchi, H.; Nakamura, R.; Ueki, K.; Iwase, T.; Omagari, D.; Asano, M.; Shinozuka, K.; Kaneko, T.; Tonogi, M.; Ohki, H. Rapid Detection of *Candida albicans* in Oral Exfoliative Cytology Samples by Loop-Mediated Isothermal Amplification. *J. Oral Sci.* **2017**, *59*, 541–547. [CrossRef]
111. Soroka, M.; Wasowicz, B.; Rymaszewska, A. Loop-Mediated Isothermal Amplification (Lamp): The Better Sibling of PCR? *Cells* **2021**, *10*, 1931. [CrossRef]
112. Robinson, S.; Peterson, C.B.; Sahasrabhojane, P.; Ajami, N.J.; Shelburne, S.A.; Kontoyiannis, D.P.; Galloway-Peña, J.R. Observational Cohort Study of Oral Mycobiome and Interkingdom Interactions over the Course of Induction Therapy for Leukemia. *mSphere* **2020**, *5*, e00048-20. [CrossRef]
113. Biswas, C.; Chen, S.C.A.; Halliday, C.; Martinez, E.; Rockett, R.J.; Wang, Q.; Timms, V.J.; Dhakal, R.; Sadsad, R.; Kennedy, K.J.; et al. Whole Genome Sequencing of *Candida glabrata* for Detection of Markers of Antifungal Drug Resistance. *J. Vis. Exp.* **2017**, *2017*, 1–13. [CrossRef]
114. Garnaud, C.; Botterel, F.; Sertour, N.; Bougnoux, M.E.; Dannaoui, E.; Larrat, S.; Hennequin, C.; Guinea, J.; Cornet, M.; Maubon, D. Next-Generation Sequencing Offers New Insights into the Resistance of *Candida* spp. To Echinocandins and Azoles. *J. Antimicrob. Chemother.* **2015**, *70*, 2556–2565. [CrossRef]
115. Colabella, C.; Pierantoni, D.C.; Corte, L.; Roscini, L.; Conti, A.; Bassetti, M.; Tascini, C.; Robert, V.; Cardinali, G. Single Strain High-Depth Ngs Reveals High Rdna (Its-Lsu) Variability in the Four Prevalent Pathogenic Species of the Genus *Candida*. *Microorganisms* **2021**, *9*, 302. [CrossRef] [PubMed]
116. Colabella, C.; Corte, L.; Roscini, L.; Bassetti, M.; Tascini, C.; Mellor, J.C.; Meyer, W.; Robert, V.; Vu, D.; Cardinali, G. NGS Barcode Sequencing in Taxonomy and Diagnostics, an Application in "*Candida*" Pathogenic Yeasts with a Metagenomic Perspective. *IMA Fungus* **2018**, *9*, 91–105. [CrossRef] [PubMed]
117. Cuo, X.G.; Yu, C.W.; Zhou, S.S.; Huang, Y.; Wang, C.Y. Case Report: A *Candida* Meningitis in an Immunocompetent Patient Detected Through the Next-Generation Sequencing. *Front. Med.* **2021**, *8*, 1–7. [CrossRef] [PubMed]
118. Imabayashi, Y.; Moriyama, M.; Takeshita, T.; Ieda, S.; Hayashida, J.N.; Tanaka, A.; Maehara, T.; Furukawa, S.; Ohta, M.; Kubota, K.; et al. Molecular Analysis of Fungal Populations in Patients with Oral Candidiasis Using Next-Generation Sequencing. *Sci. Rep.* **2016**, *6*, 1–8. [CrossRef] [PubMed]

119. Fakruddin, M.; Chowdhury, A.; Hossain, N.; Mahajan, S.; Islam, S. Pyrosequencing-A next Generation Sequencing Technology. *World Appl. Sci. J.* **2013**, *24*, 1558–1571. [CrossRef]
120. Ronaghi, M.; Karamohamed, S.; Pettersson, B.; Uhlén, M.; Nyrén, P. Real-Time DNA Sequencing Using Detection of Pyrophosphate Release. *Anal. Biochem.* **1996**, *242*, 84–89. [CrossRef]
121. Boyanton, B.L.; Luna, R.A.; Fasciano, L.R.; Menne, K.G.; Versalovic, J. DNA Pyrosequencing–Based Identification of Pathogenic *Candida* Species by Using the Internal Transcribed Spacer 2 Region. *Arch. Pathol. Lab. Med.* **2008**, *132*, 667–674. [CrossRef]
122. Ghannoum, M.A.; Jurevic, R.J.; Mukherjee, P.K.; Cui, F.; Sikaroodi, M.; Naqvi, A.; Gillevet, P.M. Characterization of the Oral Fungal Microbiome (Mycobiome) in Healthy Individuals. *PLoS Pathog.* **2010**, *6*. [CrossRef]
123. Borman, A.M.; Linton, C.J.; Miles, S.; Johnson, E.M. Molecular Identification of Pathogenic Fungi. *J. Antimicrob. Chemother.* **2008**, *61*, 7–12. [CrossRef]
124. Criseo, G.; Scordino, F.; Romeo, O. Current Methods for Identifying Clinically Important Cryptic *Candida* Species. *J. Microbiol. Methods* **2015**, *111*, 50–56. [CrossRef]
125. Trama, J.P.; Mordechai, E.; Adelson, M.E. Detection and Identification of *Candida* Species Associated with *Candida* Vaginitis by Real-Time PCR and Pyrosequencing. *Mol. Cell. Probes* **2005**, *19*, 145–152. [CrossRef] [PubMed]
126. Quiles-Melero, I.; García-Rodríguez, J.; Gómez-López, A.; Mingorance, J. Evaluation of Matrix-Assisted Laser Desorption/Ionisation Time-of-Flight (MALDI-TOF) Mass Spectrometry for Identification of *Candida parapsilosis*, *C. orthopsilosis* and *C. metapsilosis*. *Eur. J. Clin. Microbiol. Infect. Dis.* **2012**, *31*, 67–71. [CrossRef]
127. Siqueira, J.F.; Fouad, A.F.; Rôças, I.N. Pyrosequencing as a Tool for Better Understanding of Human Microbiomes. *J. Oral Microbiol.* **2012**, *4*. [CrossRef] [PubMed]
128. Chew, K.L.; Octavia, S.; Jureen, R.; Lin, R.T.P.; Teo, J.W.P. Targeted Amplification and MinION Nanopore Sequencing of Key Azole and Echinocandin Resistance Determinants of Clinically Relevant *Candida* spp. from Blood Culture Bottles. *Lett. Appl. Microbiol.* **2021**, *73*, 286–293. [CrossRef] [PubMed]
129. Fan, Y.; Gale, A.N.; Bailey, A.; Barnes, K.; Colotti, K.; Mass, M.; Morina, L.B.; Robertson, B.; Schwab, R.; Tselepidakis, N.; et al. Genome and Transcriptome of a Pathogenic Yeast, *Candida nivariensis*. *G3 Genes Genomes Genet.* **2021**, *11*, jkab137. [CrossRef] [PubMed]
130. Sandhu, G.S.; Kline, B.C.; Stockman, L.; Roberts, G.D. Molecular Probes for Diagnosis of Fungal Infections. *J. Clin. Microbiol.* **1995**, *33*, 2913–2919. [CrossRef] [PubMed]
131. Egholm, M.; Buchardt, O.; Christensen, L.; Behrens, C.; Freier, S.M.; Driver, D.A.; Berg, R.H.; Kim, S.K.; Norden, B.; Nielsen, P.E. PNA Hybridizes to Complementary Oligonucleotides Obeying the Watson-Crick Hydrogen-Bonding Rules. *Nature* **1993**, *365*, 566–568. [CrossRef]
132. Stender, H.; Fiandaca, M.; Hyldig-Nielsen, J.J.; Coull, J. PNA for Rapid Microbiology. *J. Microbiol. Methods* **2002**, *48*, 1–17. [CrossRef]
133. Rigby, S.; Procop, G.W.; Haase, G.; Wilson, D.; Hall, G.; Kurtzman, C.; Oliveira, K.; Von Oy, S.; Hyldig-Nielsen, J.J.; Coull, J.; et al. Fluorescence in Situ Hybridization with Peptide Nucleic Acid Probes for Rapid Identification of *Candida albicans* Directly from Blood Culture Bottles. *J. Clin. Microbiol.* **2002**, *40*, 2182–2186. [CrossRef]
134. Harris, D.M.; Hata, D.J. Rapid Identification of Bacteria and *Candida* Using Pna-Fish from Blood and Peritoneal Fluid Cultures: A Retrospective Clinical Study. *Ann. Clin. Microbiol. Antimicrob.* **2013**, *12*, 1. [CrossRef]
135. Lau, A.; Chen, S.; Sleiman, S.; Sorrell, T. Current Status and Future Perspectives on Molecular and Serological Methods in Diagnostic Mycology. *Future Microbiol.* **2009**, *4*, 1185–1222. [CrossRef] [PubMed]
136. Shepard, J.R.; Addison, R.M.; Alexander, B.D.; Della-Latta, P.; Gherna, M.; Haase, G.; Hall, G.; Johnson, J.K.; Merz, W.G.; Peltroche-Llacsahuanga, H.; et al. Multicenter Evaluation of the *Candida albicans/Candida glabrata* Peptide Nucleic Acid Fluorescent *in situ* Hybridization Method for Simultaneous Dual-Color Identification of *C. albicans* and *C. glabrata* Directly from Blood Culture Bottles. *J. Clin. Microbiol.* **2008**, *46*, 50–55. [CrossRef] [PubMed]
137. Ibáñez-Martínez, E.; Ruiz-Gaitán, A.; Pemán-García, J. Update on the Diagnosis of Invasive Fungal Infection. *Rev. Españhola Quimioter.* **2017**, *30*, 16–21. [CrossRef]
138. Reller, M.E.; Mallonee, A.B.; Kwiatkowski, N.P.; Merz, W.G. Use of Peptide Nucleic Acid-Fluorescence in Situ Hybridization for Definitive, Rapid Identification of Five Common *Candida* Species. *J. Clin. Microbiol.* **2007**, *45*, 3802–3803. [CrossRef] [PubMed]
139. Alexander, B.D.; Ashley, E.D.; Reller, L.B.; Reed, S.D. Cost Savings with Implementation of PNA FISH Testing for Identification of *Candida albicans* in Blood Cultures. *Diagn. Microbiol. Infect. Dis.* **2006**, *54*, 277–282. [CrossRef]
140. Forrest, G.N.; Mankes, K.; Jabra-Rizk, M.A.; Weekes, E.; Johnson, J.K.; Lincalis, D.P.; Venezia, R.A. Peptide Nucleic Acid Fluorescence *in situ* Hybridization-Based Identification of *Candida albicans* and Its Impact on Mortality and Antifungal Therapy Costs. *J. Clin. Microbiol.* **2006**, *44*, 3381–3383. [CrossRef]
141. Tsuchida, S.; Umemura, H.; Nakayama, T. Current Status of Matrix-Assisted Laser. *Molecules* **2020**, *25*, 4775. [CrossRef]
142. Clark, A.E.; Kaleta, E.J.; Arora, A.; Wolk, D.M. Matrix-Assisted Laser Desorption Ionization-Time of Flight Mass Spectrometry: A Fundamental Shift in the Routine Practice of Clinical Microbiology. *Clin. Microbiol. Rev.* **2013**, *26*, 547–603. [CrossRef]
143. Dhiman, N.; Hall, L.; Wohlfiel, S.L.; Buckwalter, S.P.; Wengenack, N.L. Performance and Cost Analysis of Matrix-Assisted Laser Desorption Ionization-Time of Flight Mass Spectrometry for Routine Identification of Yeast. *J. Clin. Microbiol.* **2011**, *49*, 1614–1616. [CrossRef]

144. Hamprecht, A.; Christ, S.; Oestreicher, T.; Plum, G.; Kempf, V.A.J.; Göttig, S. Performance of Two MALDI-TOF MS Systems for the Identification of Yeasts Isolated from Bloodstream Infections and Cerebrospinal Fluids Using a Time-Saving Direct Transfer Protocol. *Med. Microbiol. Immunol.* **2014**, *203*, 93–99. [CrossRef]
145. Singhal, N.; Kumar, M.; Kanaujia, P.K.; Virdi, J.S. MALDI-TOF Mass Spectrometry: An Emerging Technology for Microbial Identification and Diagnosis. *Front. Microbiol.* **2015**, *6*, 1–16. [CrossRef] [PubMed]
146. De Carolis, E.; Hensgens, L.A.M.; Vella, A.; Posteraro, B.; Sanguinetti, M.; Senesi, S.; Tavanti, A. Identification and Typing of the *Candida parapsilosis* Complex: MALDI-TOF MS vs. AFLP. *Med. Mycol.* **2014**, *52*, 123–130. [CrossRef] [PubMed]
147. Oviaño, M.; Rodríguez-Sánchez, B. MALDI-TOF Mass Spectrometry in the 21st Century Clinical Microbiology Laboratory. *Enferm. Infecc. Microbiol. Clin.* **2021**, *39*, 192–200. [CrossRef]
148. Molkenthin, F.; Hertel, M.; Neumann, K.; Schmidt-Westhausen, A.M. Factors Influencing the Presence of *Candida dubliniensis* and Other Non-*albicans* Species in Patients with Oral Lichen Planus: A Retrospective Observational Study. *Clin. Oral Investig.* **2022**, *26*, 333–342. [CrossRef] [PubMed]
149. Pawlak, Z.; Andrusiów, S.; Pajączkowska, M.; Janczura, A. Identification of Fungi Isolated from Oral Cavity of Patients with HIV Using MALDI-TOF MS. *J. Clin. Med.* **2021**, *10*, 1570. [CrossRef] [PubMed]
150. Wei, P.; Fu, J.-Y.; Zahng, Y.-F.; Lyu, X.; Guan, X.-B.; Yan, Z.-M.; Chen, F.; Hua, H. Diagnostic Accuracy of MALDI-TOF Mass Spectrum in Identification of Oral Candidiasis Isolates. *Shanghai Kou Qiang Yi Xue* **2020**, *29*, 567–572. [PubMed]
151. Pinto, A.; Halliday, C.; Zahra, M.; Van Hal, S.; Olma, T.; Maszewska, K.; Iredell, J.R.; Meyer, W.; Chen, S.C. Matrix-Assisted Laser Desorption Ionization-Time of Flight Mass Spectrometry Identification of Yeasts Is Contingent on Robust Reference Spectra. *PLoS One* **2011**, *6*, e25712. [CrossRef]
152. Marklein, G.; Josten, M.; Klanke, U.; Müller, E.; Horré, R.; Maier, T.; Wenzel, T.; Kostrzewa, M.; Bierbaum, G.; Hoerauf, A.; et al. Matrix-Assisted Laser Desorption Ionization-Time of Flight Mass Spectrometry for Fast and Reliable Identification of Clinical Yeast Isolates. *J. Clin. Microbiol.* **2009**, *47*, 2912–2917. [CrossRef]
153. Spanu, T.; Posteraro, B.; Fiori, B.; D'Inzeo, T.; Campoli, S.; Ruggeri, A.; Tumbarello, M.; Canu, G.; Trecarichi, E.M.; Parisi, G.; et al. Direct MALDI-TOF Mass Spectrometry Assay of Blood Culture Broths for Rapid Identification of *Candida* Species Causing Bloodstream Infections: An Observational Study in Two Large Microbiology Laboratories. *J. Clin. Microbiol.* **2011**, *50*, 176–179. [CrossRef]
154. Montoya, A.M.; Luna-Rodríguez, C.E.; Bonifaz, A.; Treviño-Rangel, R.d.J.; Rojas, O.C.; González, G.M. Physiological Characterization and Molecular Identification of Some Rare Yeast Species Causing Onychomycosis. *J. Med. Mycol.* **2021**, *31*, 101121. [CrossRef]
155. Oliver, J.C.; Laghi, L.; Parolin, C.; Foschi, C.; Marangoni, A.; Liberatore, A.; Dias, A.L.T.; Cricca, M.; Vitali, B. Metabolic Profiling of *Candida* Clinical Isolates of Different Species and Infection Sources. *Sci. Rep.* **2020**, *10*, 16716. [CrossRef] [PubMed]
156. Scapaticci, M.; Bartolini, A.; Del Chierico, F.; Accardi, C.; Di Girolamo, F.; Masotti, A.; Muraca, M.; Putignani, L. Phenotypic Typing and Epidemiological Survey of Antifungal Resistance of *Candida* Species Detected in Clinical Samples of Italian Patients in a 17 Months' Period. *GERMS* **2018**, *8*, 58–66. [CrossRef] [PubMed]
157. Schell, W.A.; Johnson, M.D.; Alexander, B.D.; Perfect, J.R.; Smith, P.B.; Benjamin, D.K.; Mitchell, T.G.; Benton, J.L.; Poore, M.; Rouse, J.L.; et al. Evaluation of a Digital Microfluidic Real-Time PCR Platform to Detect DNA of *Candida albicans* in Blood. *Eur. J. Clin. Microbiol. Infect. Dis.* **2012**, *31*, 2237–2245. [CrossRef] [PubMed]
158. Chen, B.; Xie, Y.; Zhang, N.; Li, W.; Liu, C.; Li, D.; Bian, S.; Jiang, Y.; Yang, Z.; Li, R.; et al. Evaluation of Droplet Digital PCR Assay for the Diagnosis of Candidemia in Blood Samples. *Front. Microbiol.* **2021**, *12*, 700008. [CrossRef]
159. Fajarningsih, N.D. Internal Transcribed Spacer (ITS) as DNA Barcoding to Identify Fungal Species: A Review. *Squalen Bull. Mar. Fish. Postharvest Biotechnol.* **2016**, *11*, 37. [CrossRef]
160. Sandini, S.; Stringaro, A.; Arancia, S.; Colone, M.; Mondello, F.; Murtas, S.; Girolamo, A.; Mastrangelo, N.; De Bernardis, F. The *MP65* Gene Is Required for Cell Wall Integrity, Adherence to Epithelial Cells and Biofilm Formation in *Candida albicans*. *BMC Microbiol.* **2011**, *11*, 106. [CrossRef]
161. Branco, J.; Fonseca, E.; Gomes, N.C.; Martins-Cruz, C.; Silva, A.P.; Silva-Dias, A.; Pina-Vaz, C.; Rodrigues, A.G.; Miranda, I.M.; Erraught, C.; et al. Impact of *ERG3* Mutations and Expression of Ergosterol Genes Controlled by *UPC2* and *NDT80* in *Candida parapsilosis* Azole Resistance. *Clin. Microbiol. Infect.* **2017**, *23*, 575.e1–575.e8. [CrossRef]
162. Martel, C.M.; Parker, J.E.; Bader, O.; Weig, M.; Gross, U.; Warrilow, A.G.S.; Kelly, D.E.; Kelly, S.L. A Clinical Isolate of *Candida albicans* with Mutations in *ERG11* (Encoding Sterol 14α-Demethylase) and *ERG5* (Encoding C22 Desaturase) Is Cross Resistant to Azoles and Amphotericin B. *Antimicrob. Agents Chemother.* **2010**, *54*, 3578–3583. [CrossRef]
163. Arastehfar, A.; Marcet-Houben, M.; Daneshnia, F.; Taj-Aldeen, S.J.; Batra, D.; Lockhart, S.R.; Shor, E.; Gabaldón, T.; Perlin, D.S. Comparative Genomic Analysis of Clinical *Candida glabrata* Isolates Identifies Multiple Polymorphic Loci That Can Improve Existing Multilocus Sequence Typing Strategy. *Stud. Mycol.* **2021**, *100*, 1–15. [CrossRef]
164. Muñoz, M.; Wintaco, L.M.; Muñoz, S.A.; Ramírez, J.D. Dissecting the Heterogeneous Population Genetic Structure of *Candida albicans*: Limitations and Constraints of the Multilocus Sequence Typing Scheme. *Front. Microbiol.* **2019**, *10*, 1–16. [CrossRef]

165. Huang, X.; Welsh, R.M.; Deming, C.; Proctor, D.M.; Thomas, P.J.; Gussin, G.M.; Huang, S.S.; Kong, H.H.; Bentz, M.L.; Vallabhaneni, S.; et al. Skin Metagenomic Sequence Analysis of Early *Candida auris* Outbreaks in U.S. Nursing Homes. *mSphere* **2021**, *6*, 1–10. [CrossRef] [PubMed]
166. Abharian, P.H.; Dehghan, P.; Abharian, P.H.; Tolouei, S. Molecular Characterization of *Candida dubliniensis* and *Candida albicans* in the Oral Cavity of Drug Abusers Using Duplex Polymerase Chain Reaction. *Curr. Med. Mycol.* **2018**, *4*, 12–17. [CrossRef] [PubMed]

applied sciences

MDPI

Article

Soft Sets Extensions: Innovating Healthcare Claims Analysis

Daniela Gifu

Institute of Computer Science, Romanian Academy-Iași Branch, Codrescu 2, 700481 Iași, Romania; daniela.gifu@iit.academiaromana-is.ro; Tel.: +40-742050673

Abstract: In the dynamic arena of healthcare research, where the complexities of data often rival the intricacies of biological systems, the ability to model and analyze such multifaceted datasets is crucial. This comprehensive review delves into the evolution and application of soft sets and their extensions, including HyperSoft Sets, SuperHyperSoft Sets, IndetermSoft Sets, IndetermHyperSoft Sets, and TreeSoft Sets, in healthcare claims data analysis. These extensions address intricate challenges in data analysis, offering versatile frameworks for managing the uncertainty and indeterminacy inherent in healthcare claims data. By exploring their definitions and applications, this review elucidates how these mathematical tools have evolved and their significance in advancing healthcare research and enhancing data analysis methodologies. Real-world examples underscore the implications of these tools, emphasizing their pivotal role in facilitating informed decision-making and knowledge discovery in healthcare. The review systematically examines various case studies and research findings to illustrate the practical utility of soft set extensions. Detailed analyses of real-world scenarios highlight advancements in processing complex healthcare data. The conclusions drawn from this analysis indicate that the adoption of soft sets and their extensions can significantly improve the accuracy and efficiency of healthcare data analysis, ultimately contributing to better healthcare outcomes and more informed policy-making. Future research directions are also discussed, suggesting further potential applications and developments in this field.

Keywords: soft sets; healthcare data analysis; hypersoft sets; data modeling; healthcare claims data; decision-making; advanced data methodologies

1. Introduction

In the fast-evolving field of healthcare research [1,2], the complexity of data, particularly within healthcare claims, mirrors the intricacies of biological systems. The ability to model and analyze this vast, multifaceted data is crucial for making informed decisions about patient care, diagnostics, and treatment pathways. Soft sets and their numerous extensions provide a valuable toolkit for addressing the uncertainty and variability prevalent in healthcare claims data, which encompasses details about treatments, providers, costs, and prescriptions [3].

These mathematical constructs, first introduced by Molodtsov in 1999 [4], offer a flexible framework for tackling imprecision. Healthcare claims data, where uncertainty is intrinsic, benefits from soft set theory, which models this uncertainty more effectively than classical statistical methods [5,6]. Since their inception, soft sets have evolved significantly. Extensions like HyperSoft Sets, introduced by Smarandache in 2018 [7], and more recent advancements such as SuperHyperSoft Sets, IndetermSoft Sets, IndetermHyperSoft Sets, and TreeSoft Sets [8–11] have been developed to address specific challenges in handling intricate relationships within healthcare data. Furthermore, the contributions of Alkhazaleh in 2010 with MultiSoft Sets have further enriched these mathematical tools [12].

While the evolution of soft sets has been robust, with applications spreading across diverse fields, including bioinformatics, chemistry, and public health, healthcare remains a relatively underexplored area for these models. The paucity of studies applying soft set theory to healthcare claims data presents an opportunity for significant advancements.

A legitimate question arises: *How can the application of soft set theory and its recent extensions in analyzing and modeling healthcare claims data contribute to improving diagnostics and personalized treatments?*

Recent works have examined the fusion of soft set theory with fuzzy logic, yielding combinations like neutrosophic, picture fuzzy, and plithogenic soft sets, each contributing unique perspectives on handling uncertainty. TreeSoft Sets, for instance, offer promise for improving healthcare analytics in the era of Industry 4.0 [13], while IndetermSoft Sets are increasingly applied to real-world challenges in healthcare [14,15]. However, further research is needed to explore how these methodologies can be combined with modern computational techniques to address complex real-world problems.

Future research should focus on refining these applications and addressing existing limitations, ensuring that soft set methodologies can be fully leveraged to enhance healthcare decision-making and improve patient outcomes.

2. Evolving Impact of Soft Sets in Healthcare Data Analysis

The ongoing exploration and application of soft sets and their extensions represent a significant advancement in the realm of data analysis, particularly for addressing real-world challenges within healthcare. Soft sets, with their ability to handle uncertainty, imprecision, and indeterminacy, offer a versatile framework for analyzing complex healthcare claims data. This evolving methodology has the potential to transform how we interpret and utilize healthcare information for improved diagnostics, treatment decisions, and resource allocation.

The fusion of soft set theory with complementary mathematical frameworks, such as fuzzy logic, paves the way for deeper insights into healthcare datasets. This convergence not only enhances our understanding of complex data patterns but also provides a foundation for the development of innovative tools and techniques that address the specific needs of healthcare researchers and practitioners.

Current Survey Mission

This paper seeks to explore and assess the evolution and application of soft sets and their extensions within the domain of healthcare claims data analysis. Our study addresses the inherent complexities, uncertainties, and interrelationships present in such datasets. The key contributions of our research are outlined as follows:

- **Comprehensive Review of Soft Sets:**

  We provide a thorough examination of the development of soft sets and their extensions—such as HyperSoft Sets, SuperHyperSoft Sets, IndetermSoft Sets, IndetermHyperSoft Sets, and TreeSoft Sets—highlighting their relevance and utility in healthcare claims analysis. This review offers an in-depth understanding of how these extensions have evolved to handle complex, multi-attribute data in healthcare scenarios.

- **Real-World Applications:**

  We present practical examples and case studies from healthcare claims data to demonstrate the real-world applicability of these soft set frameworks. These examples illustrate how soft set-based methodologies can be leveraged to improve decision-making, optimize treatment strategies, and enhance the analysis of healthcare claims by capturing uncertainties often overlooked by traditional statistical methods.

- **Methodological Advancements:**

  Our review emphasizes key methodological advancements made possible through the use of soft sets and their extensions. We show how these tools can improve the accuracy and efficiency of healthcare data analysis by addressing challenges such as missing information, imprecise relationships, and multi-dimensional dependencies. This study contrasts soft set-based methods with classical approaches to highlight their benefits.

- **Future Research Directions:**

Building on the advancements reviewed in this paper, we propose future research directions aimed at further enhancing data analysis in healthcare. Specifically, we suggest exploring the integration of soft sets with fuzzy logic and other computational techniques to improve predictive accuracy and develop personalized treatment models. We also identify opportunities for expanding soft set applications to other complex, data-intensive domains beyond healthcare.

The data discussed in this paper are made available as open-source collections (Browse by Research Unit, Center, or Department | UNM Digital Repository, https://digitalrepository.unm.edu/communities.html, accessed on 2 August 2024), with the aim of fostering further research and development in this field, along with the demonstrations of soft sets and their multifarious extensions (available at https://fs.unm.edu/NSS/ExtensionOfSoftSetToHypersoftSet.pdf; https://fs.unm.edu/NSS/IndetermSoftIndetermHyperSoft38.pdf, accessed on 2 August 2024).

3. Related Work

In this section, we provide a comprehensive overview of the contributions in the field, emphasizing their impact and relevance to the application of soft set theory in healthcare claims data analysis. In fact, soft set theory, applied to healthcare claims data, provides a flexible framework for analyzing the uncertainty and imprecision inherent in medical records. Consider a scenario where a patient's diagnosis is uncertain due to incomplete information or conflicting test results. Traditional methods may struggle to handle such ambiguity, leading to inaccurate assessments or diagnoses.

However, by employing soft set theory, we can represent the uncertainty associated with each diagnosis or treatment option using membership functions. These membership functions assign degrees of certainty to various outcomes based on available evidence, allowing healthcare practitioners to make informed decisions despite incomplete or conflicting data.

For example, a soft set approach could be used to determine the likelihood of a patient having a particular condition based on their symptoms, medical history, and test results, even when some information is missing or contradictory. This flexibility makes soft set theory a valuable tool for analyzing healthcare claims data, improving diagnostic accuracy, and ultimately enhancing patient care.

The most notable contributions in this field are mentioned below.

1. Molodtsov's seminal work laid the foundation for soft set theory, offering a novel approach to handling uncertainty and vagueness in data analysis [3]. This foundational work has been pivotal in subsequent research exploring various extensions and applications of soft sets in different domains, including healthcare claims data analysis.

2. In 2018, Smarandache introduced HyperSoft Sets, an extension designed to better handle multi-attribute decision-making processes. This extension has shown promise in dealing with the complex and multi-dimensional nature of healthcare claims datasets, providing a more nuanced framework for analysis [7].

3. The MultiSoft Set, introduced by Alkhazaleh and his team, expanded the versatility of soft sets by accommodating multiple parameters, making it particularly useful for applications in healthcare claims data where multiple factors need to be considered simultaneously. This work has significantly enriched the toolkit available for researchers and specialists in healthcare [10].

4. In 2022, Smarandache introduced IndetermSoft Sets and IndetermHyperSoft Sets, which address indeterminacy in data analysis. These extensions have been applied to real-world scenarios in healthcare, demonstrating their utility in dealing with uncertain and incomplete healthcare claims data [6,9]. The next year, Smarandache proposed SuperHyperSoft Sets [15].

5. Convergence with Fuzzy Logic and its Extensions

The integration of soft set theory with fuzzy logic and its various extensions has formed a robust framework for managing the inherent fuzziness and uncertainty in healthcare claims data. P. K. Maji's seminal work, exemplified by "Intuitionistic Fuzzy Soft Sets", has played a pivotal role in this domain [16].

Furthermore, the foundational contributions of Lotfi A. Zadeh and other collaborators in fuzzy logic have paved the way for the amalgamation of fuzzy logic with soft set theory, notably documented in fuzzy set applications to pattern classification and clustering analysis [17] or decision analysis [18].

S. K. Samanta's research on neutrosophic soft sets and their applications has significantly bolstered this convergence, offering invaluable insights into managing uncertainty in biomedical data analysis [19,20].

Additionally, Florentin Smarandache's exploration of neutrosophic sets, particularly showcased in 2020 [21] alongside collaborative endeavors with K. Atanassov on intuitionistic fuzzy sets [22], have greatly propelled the methodologies for extracting actionable insights from complex datasets [23]. The research conducted by M. Shabir and M. Naz on bipolar soft sets [24] and their fusion with fuzzy logic has contributed substantial insights into multi-criteria decision-making problems, further enhancing the analytical capabilities in healthcare contexts.

These advancements underscore the potential of integrating soft set theory and its extensions into healthcare data analysis, offering avenues for enhancing diagnostics and personalized treatments.

The adeptness of these mathematical constructs in handling uncertainty, multidimensionality, and indeterminacy aligns seamlessly with the intricacies inherent in healthcare claims datasets.

Consequently, delving into systematic applications of these tools to improve medical outcomes stands as an imperative avenue for future research.

Collectively, these studies underscore the dynamic evolution of soft set theory and its extensions, emphasizing their growing significance and versatility in the domain of healthcare claims data analysis. The ongoing research and development in this sphere hold the promise of unlocking novel possibilities for advancing diagnostics, therapeutics, and personalized medicine.

6. Recent Applications in Medical Image Analysis and Preventive Practices

Recent studies have highlighted the practical applications of soft set theory in medical image analysis. For instance, Dhanalakshmi and Bhaskaran explore the application of soft set methodologies to evaluate the degree of evidence in medical recommendations and assess factors influencing preventive practices in clinical images with indeterminate features [25].

Similarly, Yang and Zhao provide insights into the advantages and specific methods used in employing soft set theory for similar purposes [26]. Additionally, Khan and Gupta offer a detailed examination of soft set-based approaches in medical image analysis, focusing on their role in evaluating evidence in medical recommendations and analyzing factors influencing preventive practices in clinical images [27].

These applications underscore the relevance and adaptability of soft sets in contemporary healthcare research, particularly in the domain of medical image analysis and preventive practices.

7. The innovative work by Alqazzaz and Sallam explored the use of TreeSoft Sets combined with interval-valued neutrosophic sets, providing novel insights into data analysis within the context of Industry 4.0. [13]. This study demonstrates the evolving nature of soft set applications and their potential to address modern data challenges.

Given these advancements, it becomes evident that the integration of soft set theory and its extensions into healthcare claims data analysis holds significant potential for enhancing diagnostics and personalized treatments. The ability of these mathematical constructs to handle uncertainty, multi-dimensionality, and indeterminacy aligns well with the complexities inherent in healthcare claims datasets. Therefore, exploring how these tools can be systematically applied to improve medical outcomes is a compelling avenue for future research.

These studies collectively highlight the dynamic evolution of soft set theory and its extensions, showcasing their growing importance and versatility in the realm of healthcare claims data analysis.

The ongoing research and development in this field promise to unlock new possibilities for improving diagnostics, therapeutics, and personalized medicine.

4. Soft Sets Extensions

In this section, we delve into the various extensions of soft sets, each offering unique capabilities and applications within the realm of healthcare claims data analysis.

These extensions include the HyperSoft Set, SuperHyperSoft Set, Fuzzy-Extension-SuperHyperSoft Set, IndetermSoft Set, IndetermHyperSoft Set, and TreeSoft Set.

Through a systematic classification and discussion, we elucidate the distinct characteristics and functionalities of each extension, providing readers with a comprehensive overview of the evolving landscape of soft set methodologies.

We recall the definitions of soft set, HyperSoft Set, IndetermSoft Set, IndetermHyperSoft Set, and TreeSoft Set, including a few suggestive examples applied to healthcare claims data.

4.1. *Soft Set*

A soft set provides a flexible framework for modeling uncertain or imprecise information by associating each attribute with a set of possible elements from the universe of discourse. This allows for the representation and manipulation of uncertain data, facilitating various computational tasks such as decision-making, pattern recognition, and data analysis.

4.1.1. Definition

A soft set is a mathematical abstraction designed to encapsulate uncertainty and fuzziness inherent in data within a specific domain of discourse. Let us break down this definition:

Firstly, we define a universe of discourse, denoted as U, which encompasses all conceivable elements or entities relevant to the context under consideration. The power set of U, represented as $P(U)$, comprises all possible subsets derived from the elements within the universe of discourse. Essentially, it represents the complete range of potential combinations or groupings of elements from U.

Next, we introduce a set of attributes, denoted as A, which serves to characterize the properties or features associated with the elements within the universe U. These attributes could represent any discernible traits, qualities, or characteristics relevant to the domain being studied.

Now, a soft set is formally defined as a pair (F, U), where $F: A \rightarrow P(U)$.

F represents a mapping function that associates each attribute in A with a subset of elements from the universe U. In other words, for every attribute within set A, there exists a corresponding subset of elements from the universe of discourse U, as determined by the mapping function F.

In summary, a soft set provides a structured framework for capturing and managing uncertainty by linking attributes to subsets of elements within a given universe of discourse. This enables the representation and manipulation of imprecise or indeterminate data, facilitating various computational tasks such as decision-making, pattern recognition, and data analysis within the specified domain.

4.1.2. Example

Let us define the universe of discourse U as a set of patients.

U = {Patient1, Patient2, Patient3, Patient4} and a subset included in U representing patients with specific conditions:

$$M = \{\text{Patient1, Patient3, Patient4}\}.$$

Now, let us consider an attribute related to medical conditions:

$$a = \text{condition},$$

with attribute values representing different medical conditions:

$$\text{Condition} = A_1 = \{\text{diabetes, hypertension, asthma}\}.$$

$$\text{We define a function: } F\text{: } A_1 \rightarrow P(U),$$

where $P(U)$ represents the power set of U.

Then, for example,

$$F(asthma) = \{\text{Patient2, Patient3}\},$$

This means that both Patient2 and Patient3 have been diagnosed with asthma.

This representation (Figure 1) allows us to capture complex relationships between patients and their conditions. It is particularly useful in healthcare claims data analysis because

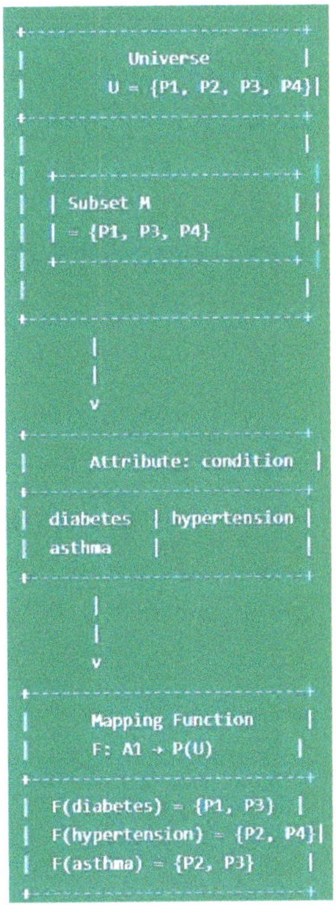

Figure 1. Soft set representation of patient conditions.

It can handle uncertainty: if a patient's diagnosis is uncertain, we could represent it by associating the attribute with multiple patients or using fuzzy sets within the mapping.

It accommodates missing data: if we do not know whether a patient has a particular condition, we simply would not include them in the corresponding subset.

It facilitates pattern recognition: by looking at the mappings, we can easily see patterns like comorbidities (e.g., Patient 2 has both hypertension and asthma).

This soft set representation provides a flexible framework for analyzing healthcare claims data, allowing us to capture and manipulate uncertain or imprecise information effectively.

4.2. *IndetermSoft Set*

An IndetermSoft Set provides a flexible framework for modeling uncertain or imprecise information by associating each attribute with a set of possible elements from the universe of discourse. This enables the representation and manipulation of uncertain data, facilitating various computational tasks such as decision-making, pattern recognition, and data analysis.

4.2.1. Definition

An IndetermSoft Set expands upon the foundational principles of the classical soft set by accommodating indeterminate data, reflecting the inherent uncertainty and ambiguity prevalent in real-world scenarios. Let us dissect this definition:

We begin with the establishment of a universe of discourse, denoted as U, which encompasses all relevant elements or entities under consideration. Additionally, we identify a non-empty subset of U, denoted as H, and its corresponding powerset, $P(H)$, which comprises all possible subsets derived from the elements within H.

Furthermore, we introduce an attribute, denoted as 'a', and a set of attribute-values, denoted as A.

The mapping function $F: A \rightarrow P(H)$ is designated as an IndetermSoft Set if one or more of the following conditions are met:

(i) The set A exhibits some level of indeterminacy.
(ii) The sets H or $P(H)$ demonstrate indeterminacy.
(iii) The function F itself contains elements of indeterminacy, indicating the presence of attribute-values for which the mapping is unclear, incomplete, conflicting, or non-unique.

IndetermSoft Sets, characterized by their capacity to handle indeterminate data, arise from real-world situations where information sources may provide approximate, uncertain, incomplete, or conflicting data. Rather than introducing indeterminacy artificially, such as in the classical soft set framework, the indeterminacy is identified within the data itself, reflecting the limitations and nuances of our world.

The term "Indeterm" signifies "Indeterminate", encompassing attributes of uncertainty, conflict, incompleteness, or lack of uniqueness within the outcomes. This distinction prompts the consideration of determinate versus indeterminate operators, leading to the development of an IndetermSoft Algebra.

Smarandache's contributions extend the concept further with the introduction of HyperSoft Sets, which involve multi-attribute functions, and subsequently, the hybridization of various soft set variants. These hybrids incorporate elements from crisp, fuzzy, intuitionistic fuzzy, neutrosophic, and other fuzzy extensions, as well as the plithogenic HyperSoft Set.

While the classical soft set relies on determinate functions with certain and unique values, the reality of our world often involves sources that provide indeterminate information due to a lack of knowledge or precision. Consequently, operators with varying degrees of indeterminacy are utilized to model such scenarios, acknowledging the inherent imprecision of our environment.

4.2.2. Example

Consider a dataset comprising healthcare claims from various patients.

I. Indeterminacy with respect to the function:

(1a) You inquire from a source:
—"Which patients have been diagnosed with diabetes?"
The source responds:
—"I'm uncertain; it could be patients Patient1 or Patient2".
Thus, F(diabetes) = Patient1 or Patient2 (an indeterminate/uncertain response).
(1b) Another query:
—"And which patients have undergone surgery?"
The source replies:
—"I'm not certain; all I can confirm is that Patient5 has not had surgery because I have their records".
Thus, F(surgery) = not Patient5 (again, an indeterminate/uncertain response).
(1c) Further inquiry:
—"Then, which patients have high blood pressure?"
The source asserts:
—"It's either Patient8 or Patient9 for sure".
Thus, F(high blood pressure) = either Patient8 or Patient9 (yet another indeterminate/uncertain response).

II. Indeterminacy with respect to the set P of patients:

You ask the source:
—"How many patients are included in the dataset?"
The source replies:
—"I haven't counted them, but I estimate the number to be between 100–120 patients".

III. Indeterminacy with respect to the set C of medical conditions:

You inquire:
—"What are all the medical conditions diagnosed in the patients?"
The source states:
—"I'm certain there are patients diagnosed with diabetes, high blood pressure, and heart disease, but I'm unsure if there are patients with other conditions".

The IndetermSoft Set addresses the inherent indeterminacy present in healthcare claims data by introducing a flexible framework that accommodates varying degrees of uncertainty. Through the incorporation of indeterminacy measures, the IndetermSoft Set offers researchers the ability to effectively manage and quantify uncertainty, facilitating more robust decision-making processes and knowledge discovery.

4.3. *Hypersoft Set*

A HyperSoft Set provides a robust framework for modeling uncertain or imprecise information by associating each attribute with a collection of potential elements from the universe of discourse. This framework is designed to handle a wide range of data uncertainties, enabling effective decision-making, pattern recognition, and comprehensive data analysis.

4.3.1. Definition

The extension from soft sets to HyperSoft Sets (HS Sets) marks a significant advancement in modeling complex relationships by expanding the mapping function to accommodate multiple attributes.

Here is a breakdown.

Initially, the soft set concept is broadened into the realm of HyperSoft Sets by transitioning the mapping function F into a multi-attribute function. This transformation enables the representation of intricate relationships between elements within the universe of discourse.

Let us delve into the formal definition.

We begin with the universe of discourse, denoted as U, along with its powerset, $P(U)$, which encompasses all conceivable elements or entities.

Next, we introduce n distinct attributes, denoted as $a_1, a_2, \ldots, a_n$, for $n \geq 1$. Each attribute is associated with a set of attribute values, denoted, respectively, as $A_1, A_2, \ldots, A_n$, with $A_i \cap A_j = \Phi$, for $i \neq j$, and i, j in $\{1, 2, \ldots, n\}$.

Notably, these attribute sets are pairwise disjoint, ensuring no overlap between them.

The pair $(F, A_1 \times A_2 \times \ldots \times A_n)$ represent a HyperSoft Set over U, where F is a mapping function defined on the Cartesian product of the attribute sets where $A_1 \times A_2 \times \ldots \times A_n$.

Formally,

$$F: A_1 \times A_2 \times \ldots \times A_n \rightarrow P(U), \text{ is called a} \rightarrow P(U),$$

signifies that for each combination of attribute values, there exists a corresponding subset of elements from U.

The introduction of HyperSoft Sets facilitates the exploration of complex relationships and interactions among multiple attributes within the universe of discourse. This extension opens avenues for the comprehensive analysis and modeling of intricate systems, spanning various domains and applications.

Moreover, Smarandache's contributions have led to the hybridization of HyperSoft Sets with diverse frameworks, including crisp, fuzzy, intuitionistic fuzzy, neutrosophic, and other fuzzy extensions, as well as the plithogenic set. These hybrid models integrate elements from different mathematical paradigms, enhancing their adaptability and utility in addressing real-world complexities.

In essence, HyperSoft Sets offer a versatile and robust framework for modeling and analyzing complex systems characterized by multiple attributes, thereby facilitating informed decision-making and knowledge discovery across diverse domains.

4.3.2. Example

Let the attributes be
a_1 = diagnosis,
a_2 = treatment,
a_3 = cost,
a_4 = duration,
and their attributes' values, respectively,
Diagnosis = A_1 = {diabetes, heart condition, respiratory issue},
Treatment = A_2 = {medication, surgery, therapy},
Cost = A_3 = {low, medium, high},
Duration = A_4 = {short-term, medium-term, long-term}.
Let the function be F: $A_1 \times A_2 \times A_3 \times A_4 \rightarrow$ P(U).

Then, for example, consider a healthcare claims dataset with the following attributes:

- Diagnosis: {Diabetes, Hypertension}
- Treatment: {Medication, Therapy}
- Cost: {Low, High}
- Duration: {Short-term, Long-term}

We want to analyze claims that involve a diagnosis of diabetes, treatment with medication, low cost, and short-term duration.

Soft Set Representation:

In a soft set, we might represent the data as follows: F(Diagnosis, Treatment, Cost, Duration) where F(Diabetes, Medication, Low, Short-term) = {Claim1,Claim2}

This means that both Claim1 and Claim2 involve

- A diagnosis of diabetes,
- Medication as treatment,
- Low cost,
- Short-term duration.

HyperSoft Set Extension:

The HyperSoft Set extends this by incorporating hyperparameters to refine the analysis. Let us introduce two hyperparameters:

1. Hyperparameter 1: Interaction Weight for Diagnosis and Treatment
    - Description: Adjusts the significance of the interaction between diagnosis and treatment. For example, a higher weight might indicate that the combination of diabetes and medication is more significant in the analysis.
    - Value: $w_{Diabetes,Medication}$
2. Hyperparameter 2: Interaction Weight for Cost and Duration
    - Description: Adjusts the importance of the relationship between cost and duration. For instance, a higher weight might emphasize the impact of low cost and short-term duration on the overall analysis.
    - Value: $w_{Low,Short\text{-}term}$

Enhanced Representation:

With these hyperparameters, the HyperSoft Set can be expressed as: FHyper(Diagnosis, Treatment, Cost, Duration)

Using the hyperparameters, we refine our dataset representation: Enhanced $Score_{Diabetes,Medication,Low,Short\text{-}term} = w_{Diabetes,Medication} \times Frequency_{Diabetes,Medication} + w_{Low,Short\text{-}term} \times Frequency_{Low,Short\text{-}term}$

Where

- Frequency is the count of claims matching the respective attributes.
- Enhanced Score combines these weights to provide a more nuanced view of how often and significantly these attributes co-occur in the dataset.

Practical Implication:

By integrating hyperparameters, the HyperSoft Set allows for a more detailed and flexible analysis of healthcare claims data:

- It captures complex relationships between attributes.
- It adjusts the influence of these relationships based on predefined weights, leading to a more accurate and reliable representation of uncertainty.
- It improves the decision-making process by providing insights into the significance of various attribute combinations.

Comparison to Classical Methods:

In classical statistical analysis, relationships are often considered in isolation or through basic frequency counts, which may not capture nuanced interactions. The HyperSoft Set, with its hyperparameters, offers a more sophisticated approach by incorporating these interactions into the analysis, enhancing the overall accuracy and interpretability of the results.

Basically, this is an extension of the previous real example of soft set use.

The HyperSoft Set extends the foundational principles of soft sets by incorporating hyperparameters that capture complex relationships and interactions within healthcare claims datasets.

By integrating hyperparameters, the HyperSoft Set enables a more nuanced representation of uncertainty, thereby enhancing the accuracy and reliability of data analysis and interpretation within the healthcare domain.

4.4. *SuperHypersoft Set*

A SuperHyperSoft Set introduces an innovative framework for modeling complex and uncertain information, where each attribute is associated with an expansive set of potential elements from the universe of discourse. This advanced approach enables the comprehensive representation and manipulation of intricate data, facilitating advanced computational tasks including decision-making, pattern recognition, and data analysis at a highly refined level.

4.4.1. Definition

The SuperHyperSoft Set (SHS Set) is an extension of the HyperSoft Set. As for the SuperHyperAlgebra, SuperHyperGraph, SuperHyperTopology, and, in general, for Super-HyperStructure and neutrosophic SuperHyperStructure (that includes indeterminacy) in any field of knowledge, "Super" stands for working on the powersets (instead of sets) of the attribute value sets.

Let $\mathcal{U}$ be a universe of discourse, $\mathcal{P}(\mathcal{U})$ the powerset of $\mathcal{U}$.

Let $a_1, a_2, \ldots, a_n$, for $n \geq 1$, be n distinct attributes, whose corresponding attribute values are, respectively, the sets $A_1, A_2, \ldots, A_n$, with $A_i \cap A_j = \emptyset$, for $i \neq j$, and $i, j \in \{1,2, \ldots, n\}$.

Let $\mathcal{P}(A_1), \mathcal{P}(A_2), \ldots, \mathcal{P}(A_n)$ be the powersets of the sets $A_1, A_2, \ldots, A_n$, respectively. Then, the pair

$(F, \mathcal{P}(A_1) \times \mathcal{P}(A_2) \times \ldots \times \mathcal{P}(A_n))$, where $\times$ meaning Cartesian product, or

F: $\mathcal{P}(A_1) \times \mathcal{P}(A_2) \times \ldots \times \mathcal{P}(A_n) \rightarrow \mathcal{P}(\mathcal{U})$

is called a SuperHyperSoft Set.

4.4.2. Example

If we define the function

F: $\mathcal{P}(A_1) \times \mathcal{P}(A_2) \times \mathcal{P}(A_3) \times \mathcal{P}(A_4) \rightarrow \mathcal{P}(\mathcal{U})$.

we get a SuperHyperSoft Set.

Let us consider a scenario involving healthcare claim data, extending the previous examples. Assume we have a dataset comprising healthcare claims, and we want to categorize them based on various attributes.

Let us define the attributes and their possible values as follows:

Attribute A_1: Type of Treatment (e.g., Surgery, Medication, Therapy)

A_1: {Surgery, Medication, Therapy}

Attribute A_2: Diagnosis Code (e.g., Injury, Illness, Chronic Condition)

A_2: {Injury, Illness, Chronic Condition}

Attribute A_3: Patient Age Group (e.g., Child, Adult, Senior)

A_3: {Child, Adult, Senior}

Attribute A_4: Insurance Provider (e.g., Company A, Company B, Company C)

A_4: {Company A, Company B, Company C}

Let the function F:$A_1 \times A_2 \times A_3 \times A_4 \rightarrow P(U)$ map combinations of these attributes to subsets of the set of healthcare claims U.

$$F(\{Surgery,Medication\}, \{Injury,Illness\}, \{Adult\}, \{CompanyA,CompanyB\}) = \{claim_1,claim_2\},$$

this means that claims $claim_1$ and $claim_2$ involve either surgery or medication, are related to either injury or illness, are for adult patients, and are covered by either CompanyA or CompanyB insurance providers.

This SuperHyperSoft Set approach allows for a flexible categorization of healthcare claims, accommodating various combinations of treatment types, diagnoses, patient age groups, and insurance providers, reflecting the complexity and diversity of real-world healthcare scenarios.

In fact, we assume a new theorem: the SuperHyperSoft Set is equivalent to a union of HyperSoft Sets.

4.4.3. Demonstration

Let us consider the SuperHyperSoft:

F: $\mathcal{P}(A_1) \times \mathcal{P}(A_2) \times \ldots \times \mathcal{P}(A_n) \rightarrow \mathcal{P}(\mathcal{U})$

Assume that the non-empty sets

$B_1 \subseteq A_1, B_2 \subseteq A_2, \ldots, B_n \subseteq A_n$ and

$F(B_1, B_2, \ldots, B_n) \in P(U)$

$B_1 = \{b_{11}, b_{12}, \ldots\}, B_2 = \{b_{21}, b_{22}, \ldots\}, \ldots, B_n = \{b_{n1}, b_{n2}, \ldots\}$, therefore

$F(\{\{b_{11}, b_{12}, \ldots\}, \{b_{21}, b_{22}, \ldots\}, \ldots, \{b_{n1}, b_{n2}, \ldots\})$ can be composed in many $F(b_{1k_1}, b_{2k_2}, \ldots, b_{nk_n})P(U)$, which are actually HS Sets.

Considering the attributes diagnosis, treatment, cost, and duration, we can derive the following 12 possibilities:

1. Diagnosis: diabetes, Treatment: medication, Cost: low, Duration: short-term;
2. Diagnosis: diabetes, Treatment: medication, Cost: low, Duration: medium-term;
3. Diagnosis: diabetes, Treatment: medication, Cost: low, Duration: long-term;
4. Diagnosis: diabetes, Treatment: medication, Cost: medium, Duration: short-term;
5. Diagnosis: diabetes, Treatment: medication, Cost: medium, Duration: medium-term;
6. Diagnosis: diabetes, Treatment: medication, Cost: medium, Duration: long-term;
7. Diagnosis: diabetes, Treatment: medication, Cost: high, Duration: short-term;
8. Diagnosis: diabetes, Treatment: medication, Cost: high, Duration: medium-term;
9. Diagnosis: diabetes, Treatment: medication, Cost: high, Duration: long-term;
10. Diagnosis: diabetes, Treatment: surgery, Cost: low, Duration: short-term;
11. Diagnosis: diabetes, Treatment: surgery, Cost: low, Duration: medium-term;
12. Diagnosis: diabetes, Treatment: surgery, Cost: low, Duration: long-term.

For each of these combinations, the function F yields the set of patients who meet these criteria, represented by $\{x_1, x_2\}$. In total, 12 are HyperSoft Sets.

4.5. *Fuzzy-Extension-SuperHyperSoft Set*

A Fuzzy-Extension-SuperHyperSoft Set introduces an advanced framework that combines fuzzy logic with HyperSoft Set theory, providing a robust approach for modeling highly complex and uncertain information. Each attribute is associated with an expansive set of potential elements from the universe of discourse, allowing for nuanced representation and manipulation of uncertain data. This innovative approach empowers advanced computational tasks such as decision-making, pattern recognition, and data analysis with enhanced adaptability, precision, and the ability to handle fuzzy boundaries effectively.

4.5.1. Definition

F: $\mathcal{P}(A_1) \times \mathcal{P}(A_2) \times \ldots \times \mathcal{P}(A_n) \rightarrow \mathcal{P}(\mathcal{U}(x(d_0)))$ where $x(d_0)$ is the fuzzy or any fuzzy extension degree of appurtenance of the element x to the set $\mathcal{U}$.

Fuzzy-Extensions mean all types of fuzzy sets [14], such as: suzzy sets, intuitionistic fuzzy sets, inconsistent intuitionistic fuzzy sets (picture fuzzy sets, ternary fuzzy sets), Pythagorean fuzzy sets (Atanassov's intuitionistic fuzzy set of second type), Fermatean fuzzy sets, q-Rung Orthopair fuzzy sets, spherical fuzzy sets, n-HyperSpherical fuzzy sets, neutrosophic sets, spherical neutrosophic sets, refined fuzzy/intuitionistic fuzzy/neutrosophic/other fuzzy extension sets, plithogenic sets, etc.

4.5.2. Example

In the previous example, considering the attributes diagnosis, treatment, cost, and duration, we can envision a neutrosophic SuperHyperSoft Set.

Let us assume

({diabetes},{medication},{low},{short-term}) = $x_1(0.7, 0.4, 0.1)$

F({diabetes},{medication},{low},{medium-term}) = $x_2(0.9, 0.2, 0.3)$.

This would mean that x_1, corresponding to the values ({diabetes}, {medication}, {low}, {short-term}), holds an appurtenance degree of 0.7, an indeterminate degree of 0.4, and a non-appurtenance degree of 0.1.

Similarly, x_2, associated with the values ({diabetes}, {medication}, {low}, {medium-term}), exhibits an appurtenance degree of 0.9, an indeterminate degree of 0.2, and a non-appurtenance degree of 0.3.

4.6. *IndetermHyperSoft Set*

An IndetermHyperSoft Set builds upon the HyperSoft Set framework by incorporating advanced mechanisms for dealing with indeterminacy in data. Each attribute in this model is linked to a set of potential elements, similar to HyperSoft Sets, but with enhanced capabilities to manage and represent varying degrees of uncertainty. This extension facilitates more nuanced decision-making, pattern recognition, and data analysis, providing greater adaptability and precision in complex scenarios.

4.6.1. Definition

The IndetermHyperSoft Set represents an extension of the HyperSoft Set to accommodate indeterminate data, functions, or sets. Here is a refined explanation:

We start with the universe of discourse, denoted as U, along with a non-empty subset H of U, and its powerset, $P(H)$, which encompasses all possible subsets of H.

Next, we introduce n distinct attributes, denoted as $a_1, a_2, \ldots, a_n$, for $n \geq 1$.

Each attribute is associated with a set of attribute values, denoted, respectively, as A_1, $A_2, \ldots, A_n$, with $A_i \cap A_j = \Phi$ for $i \neq j$, and i, j in $\{1, 2, \ldots, n\}$.

Notably, these attribute sets are pairwise disjoint, ensuring no overlap between them.

Then, the pair $(F, A_1 \times A_2 \times \ldots \times A_n)$, where $F: A_1 \times A_2 \times \ldots \times A_n \rightarrow P(H)$ represents an IndetermHyperSoft Set over U if at least one of the following conditions holds true:

(i). At least one of the attribute sets $A_1, A_2, \ldots, A_n$ has some indeterminacy;
(ii). The sets H or $P(H)$ exhibit indeterminacy;
(iii). There exists at least one n-tuple $(e_1, e_2, \ldots, e_n)$ ε $A_1 \times A_2 \times \ldots \times A_n$ such that the function $F(e_1, a_2, \ldots, e_n)$ = indeterminate (unclear, uncertain, conflicting, or not unique). In other words, F yields an indeterminate outcome for that tuple.

In essence, the IndetermHyperSoft Set extends the HyperSoft Set framework to accommodate situations where uncertainty or vagueness is present in the attribute sets, subsets, or the mapping function itself.

Moreover, the IndetermHyperSoft Set provides a flexible and adaptable approach for modeling and analyzing complex systems in which precise information may be lacking or uncertain. By incorporating indeterminate elements, functions, or sets, this extension enhances the applicability of the HyperSoft Set framework in real-world scenarios characterized by inherent uncertainty or ambiguity.

4.6.2. Example

Assume there are many patients in a hospital database.

1. Indeterminacy with respect to the function.

(1a) You ask a source:

—What patients have been diagnosed with diabetes and prescribed medication?

The source:

—I am not sure, I think it is either Patient1 or Patient2. Therefore, F(diabetes, medication) = Patient1 or Patient2 (indeterminate/uncertain answer).

(1b) You ask again:

—But what patients have hypertension and are undergoing surgery?

The source:

—I do not know, the only thing I know is that Patient5 does not have hypertension and did not undergo surgery because I have checked their records.

Therefore, F(hypertension, surgery) = not Patient5 (again indeterminate/uncertain answer).

(1c) Another question you ask:

—Then what patients have asthma and are being treated with therapy?

The source:

—For sure, either Patient8 or Patient9.

Therefore, F(asthma, therapy) = either Patient8 or Patient9 (again indeterminate/uncertain answer).

2. Indeterminacy with respect to the set P of patients.

   You ask the source:
   —How many patients are in the database?
   The source:
   —I never counted them, but I estimate their number to be between 100 and 120 patients.

3. Indeterminacy with respect to the product set $A_1 \times A_2 \times \ldots \times A_n$ of attributes.

   You ask the source:
   —What are all diagnoses and treatments of the patients?
   The source:
   —I know for sure that there are patients diagnosed with diabetes, hypertension, and asthma, but I do not know if there are patients with other diagnoses (?) About the treatments, I recall seeing many patients receiving medication, but I do not remember seeing patients undergoing surgery or therapy.

Combining the strengths of both the IndetermSoft Set and the HyperSoft Set, the IndetermHyperSoft Set provides a comprehensive framework for analyzing complex healthcare claims datasets characterized by both uncertainty and hyperparameters.

By synergistically integrating indeterminacy measures and hyperparameters, this extension empowers researchers to unravel intricate relationships and patterns within biological data, thereby advancing our understanding of biological systems.

4.7. TreeSoft Set

A TreeSoft Set introduces a structured framework for modeling uncertain or imprecise information, where each attribute is organized in a hierarchical tree-like structure, associating each node with a set of potential elements from the universe of discourse. This hierarchical approach enables the systematic representation and manipulation of uncertain data, facilitating various computational tasks such as decision-making, pattern recognition, and data analysis with a focus on hierarchical relationships and dependencies.

Definition

The TreeSoft Set is an innovative extension that introduces a hierarchical structure to soft sets, providing a comprehensive framework for modeling complex systems with multiple levels of attributes. Here is a refined explanation:

We begin with a universe of discourse, denoted as U, and a non-empty subset H of U, along with its powerset, $P(H)$, which encompasses all possible subsets of H.

Next, we define a set of attributes, denoted as A, which consists of parameters, factors, and other relevant characteristics. This set is organized hierarchically into levels: first-level attributes $A = \{A_1, A_2, \ldots, A_n\}$, for integer $n \geq 1$, where $A_1, A_2, \ldots, A_n$ are considered attributes of first level (since they have one-digit indexes).

Each attribute A_i, $1 \leq i \leq n$, is formed by sub-attributes:

$$A_1=\{A_{1,1}, A_{1,2}, \ldots\}$$

$$A_2= \{A_{2,1}, A_{2,2}, \ldots\}$$

$$\ldots\ldots\ldots\ldots$$

$$A_n = \{A_{n,1}, A_{n,2}, \ldots\}$$

where the above $A_{i,j}$ are sub-attributes (or attributes of second level) (since they have two-digit indexes).

Again, each sub-attribute $A_{i,j}$ is formed by sub-sub-attributes (or attributes of third level):

$$A_{i,j,k}$$

And so on, with as much refinement as needed going into each application, up to sub-sub-. . .-sub-attributes (or attributes of m-level (or having m digits into the indexes):

$$A_{i1,i2,\cdots,im}$$

This hierarchical structure forms a graph-tree, denoted as $Tree(A)$, with A as the root node (level zero), followed by nodes at levels 1 to m, where m represents the maximum level of refinement. The leaves of this graph-tree are terminal nodes that have no descendants.

The TreeSoft Set, denoted as

$$F: P(Tree(A)) \to P(H),$$

maps subsets of the graph-tree Tree(A) to subsets of H. The powerset P(Tree(A)) encompasses all possible subsets of the graph-tree.

All node sets of the TreeSoft Set of level m are

$$Tree(A) = \{A_{i1} \mid {}_{i1}= 1, 2,\ldots\}$$

The sets within the TreeSoft Set correspond to nodes at each level of the graph-tree: the first set consists of nodes at level 1, the second set consists of nodes at level 2, and so on, up to the last set comprising nodes at level m. If the graph-tree has only two levels (m = 2), then the TreeSoft Set simplifies to a MultiSoft Set [7].

In summary, the TreeSoft Set provides a structured approach for representing and analyzing complex systems with hierarchical attributes.

By incorporating a hierarchical organization, it enhances the flexibility and expressiveness of soft set-based methodologies, enabling more nuanced modeling and analysis of multi-level systems across various domains.

An illustrative example of a classical tree is shown in Figure 2.

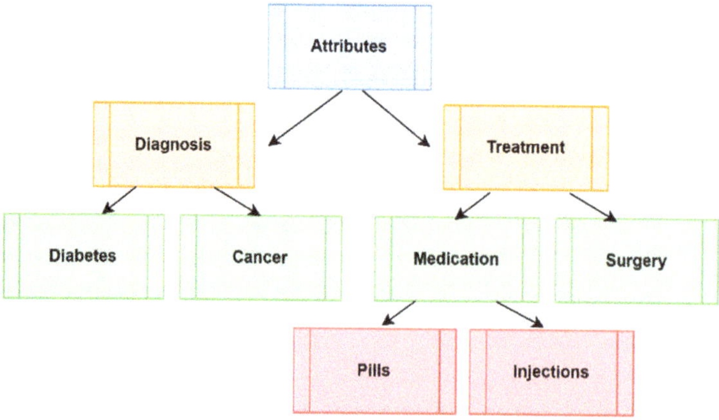

Figure 2. Schematic representation of a TreeSoft Set of level 3 framework, illustrating the incorporation of hyperparameters to capture complex relationships within healthcare claims datasets.

This tree contains three levels as followed:

Level 0 (the root) is the node Attributes;

Level 1 is formed by the nodes: Diagnosis, Treatment;

Level 2 is formed by the nodes Diabetes, Cancer, Medication, and Surgery;

Level 3 is formed by the nodes Pills, Injections.

Let us consider p = $\{patient_1, patient_2, \ldots, patient_{10}\}$ to be a set of patients, and $P(p)$ to be the power set of p.

The attributes are defined as follows: $A = \{A_1, A_2\}$

where

$$A_1 = \text{Diagnosis}$$

and

$$A_2 = \text{Treatment}$$

Then,

$$A_1 = \{A_{11}, A_{12}\} = \{\text{Diabetes}, \text{Cancer}\}$$

and $A_2 = \{A_{21}, A_{22}\} = \{\text{Medication}, \text{Surgery}\}$.

Let us further break down A_{22} into A_{221} and A_{222}, representing specific treatments:

A_{221} = {Pills,Injections} for medication and A_{222} = {Chemotherapy,Radiation} for surgery.

Now, let us assume the function F has the following values:

1. F(Diabetes,Medication,Pills) = $\{p1, p2, p3, p4\}$;
2. F(Diabetes,Medication,Injections) = $\{p5, p6\}$;
3. F(Diabetes,Surgery,Chemotherapy) = $\{p7, p8\}$;
4. F(Cancer,Surgery,Radiation) = $\{p9, p10\}$.

The TreeSoft Set introduces a hierarchical structure to soft set methodologies, enabling the representation and analysis of complex biological data in a hierarchical manner.

By organizing data into hierarchical trees, the TreeSoft Set facilitates the exploration of nested relationships and dependencies within healthcare claims datasets, offering insights into the hierarchical organization of biological systems.

5. Discussion

While the application of soft sets and their extensions in healthcare claims data analysis offers numerous advantages, it is essential to address the limitations and challenges associated with these methods:

- Complexity in Integration: The integration of soft sets with fuzzy logic and its extensions introduces significant complexity. Healthcare organizations, often lacking the necessary mathematical expertise, may struggle to implement and maintain these integrated systems. This complexity poses a practical challenge to the widespread adoption of such tools in the healthcare sector. Finding qualified experts who understand both soft sets and fuzzy logic is crucial but may not always be feasible.
- Risk of Overfitting: In cases such as Neuro-Adaptive Learning and ANFIS techniques, there is a risk of overfitting when using soft set extensions. Overfitting occurs when models perform well on training data but fail to generalize to new, unseen data. In healthcare, where diagnostic accuracy is paramount, overfitting can lead to misdiagnosis or inappropriate treatment recommendations, compromising patient safety.
- Handling Indeterminacy: While IndetermSoft Sets and IndetermHyperSoft Sets are designed to handle indeterminate and uncertain data, measuring and interpreting this uncertainty is complex. The subjectivity involved in quantifying indeterminacy can lead to inconsistent outcomes across different healthcare settings, making it difficult to standardize and validate results. The lack of standardized frameworks for uncertainty quantification remains a significant challenge.
- Interpretability and Transparency: The abstract nature of soft set-based models can make them difficult to interpret, particularly for healthcare practitioners who may not be familiar with these mathematical constructs. This lack of transparency can hinder trust and adoption among healthcare stakeholders, who need to understand the basis for diagnostic and treatment recommendations. Ensuring that soft set models are interpretable and transparent is crucial for their acceptance in clinical practice.

These challenges underscore the need for further research and development in soft set methodologies to ensure their successful integration into real-world healthcare applications. Addressing issues such as implementation complexity, computational intensity, risk of overfitting, handling indeterminacy, and enhancing interpretability will be critical for the future adoption of soft set-based tools in healthcare.

6. Conclusions

The evolution and adoption of soft sets, along with their extensions—such as HyperSoft Sets, IndetermSoft Sets, IndetermHyperSoft Sets, and TreeSoft Sets—represent a significant advancement in computational methodologies, especially in healthcare claims data analysis. These extensions offer innovative ways to model and analyze complex datasets characterized by uncertainty, imprecision, and indeterminacy, which are prevalent in healthcare data.

In the context of bioinformatics, where data is diverse and frequently noisy or incomplete [28,29], the adaptability of soft sets proves invaluable. They offer researchers a structured way to manage inherent uncertainties in biological data, such as those arising from gene expression profiles, protein interactions, and metabolic pathways [30,31]. By embracing fuzziness and imprecision, soft sets empower researchers to perform more accurate and robust analyses, revealing deeper insights into biological systems.

In healthcare, soft sets enable a nuanced representation of relationships within datasets, capturing complexities that traditional statistical methods may overlook. Given the often incomplete and ambiguous nature of healthcare claims data, soft sets provide a flexible framework for handling such uncertainty, improving the accuracy of data interpretation and decision-making processes.

Additionally, soft sets integrate seamlessly with other computational techniques, such as fuzzy logic, further enhancing their utility in data analysis across various fields. This flexibility makes them essential tools not only in healthcare but also in broader domains where managing uncertainty is critical.

In conclusion, soft sets and their extensions present a powerful framework for addressing the intricacies of healthcare claims data. Their ability to manage uncertainty, imprecision, and complexity holds great promise for improving diagnostics, personalized treatments, and overall decision-making in healthcare. As future research continues to explore the integration of soft sets with emerging technologies, these methodologies will play an increasingly pivotal role in healthcare, bioinformatics, and beyond.

Funding: This research received no external funding.

Institutional Review Board Statement: Not applicable.

Informed Consent Statement: Not applicable.

Data Availability Statement: As open sources, the following data collections are released (Browse by Research Unit, Center, or Department | UNM Digital Repository, https://digitalrepository.unm.edu/communities.html, accessed on 2 August 2024) along with the demonstrations of soft sets and their multifarious extensions (available at http://fs.unm.edu/NSS/ExtensionOfSoftSetToHypersoftSet.pdf; http://fs.unm.edu/NSS/IndetermSoftIndetermHyperSoft38.pdf, accessed on 2 August 2024). Additional information is available on request from the corresponding author.

Acknowledgments: The author is grateful to Florentin Smarandache from the Division of Mathematics, Physics, and Natural Sciences at the University of New Mexico, Gallup, SA, for his valuable assistance in the form of advice, evaluation, and review throughout the study period. Also, the author is grateful to the editors and reviewers who offered assistance in the form of advice, assessment, and checking during the study period.

Conflicts of Interest: The author declares no conflicts of interest.

References

1. Gîfu, D.; Trandabăț, D.; Cohen, K.; Xia, J. Special Issue on the Curative Power of Medical Data. *Data* **2019**, *4*, 85. [CrossRef]

2. Volosincu, M.; Lupu, C.; Gifu, D.; Trandabat, D. FII SMART at SemEval 2023 Task7: Multi-evidence Natural Language Inference for Clinical Trial Data. In Proceedings of the 17th International Workshop on Semantic Evaluation, SemEval-2023, Toronto, ON, Canada, 13–14 July 2023; Association for Computational Linguistics: Toronto, ON, Canada, 2023; pp. 212–220.
3. Thesmar, D.; Sraer, D.; Pinheiro, L.; Dadson, N.; Veliche, R.; Greenberg, P. Combining the Power of Artificial Intelligence with the Richness of Healthcare Claims Data: Opportunities and Challenges. *Pharm. Econ.* **2019**, *37*, 745–752. [CrossRef] [PubMed]
4. Molodtsov, D. Soft Set Theory First Results. *Comput. Math. Applic.* **1999**, *37*, 19–31. [CrossRef]
5. Smarandache, F.; Gîfu, D.; Teodorescu, M. Neutrosophic Elements in Discourse. *Soc. Sci. Educ. Res. Rev.* **2015**, *2*, 25–32.
6. Gifu, D. AI-backed OCR in Healthcare. *Procedia Comput. Sci.* **2022**, *207*, 1134–1143. [CrossRef]
7. Smarandache, F. Extension of Soft Set to Hypersoft Set, and then to Plithogenic Hypersoft Set. *Neutrosophic Sets Syst.* **2018**, *22*, 168–170. [CrossRef]
8. Smarandache, F. Introduction to the IndetermSoft Set and IndetermHyperSoft Set. *Neutrosophic Sets Syst.* **2022**, *50*, 629–650. [CrossRef]
9. Smarandache, F. Neutrosophic Function. In *Neutrosophic Precalculus and Neutrosophic Calculus*; Europa Nova: Brussels, Belgium, 2015; pp. 14–15.
10. Smarandache, F. *Neutrosophic Function, in Introduction to Neutrosophic Statistics*; Sitech & Education Publishing: Craiova, Romania, 2014; pp. 74–75.
11. Smarandache, F. Soft Set Product extended to HyperSoft Set and IndetermSoft Set Product extended to IndetermHyperSoft Set. *J. Fuzzy Ext. Appl.* **2022**, *3*, 313–316. [CrossRef]
12. Alkhazaleh, S.; Salleh, A.R.; Razak, S.; Hassan, N.; Ahmad, A.G. Multisoft Sets. In Proceedings of the 2nd International Conference on Mathematical Sciences, Kuala Lumpur, Malaysia, 30 November–2 December 2010; pp. 910–917.
13. Alqazzaz, A.; Sallam, K.M. Evaluation of Sustainable Waste Valorization using TreeSoft Set with Neutrosophic Sets. *Neutrosophic Sets Syst.* **2024**, *65*, 1.
14. Dhanalakshmi, G.; Sundarr, S.; Smarandache, F. Selection of the Best Process for Desalination Under a Treesoft Set Environment Using the Multi-criteria Decision-making Method. *Int. J. Neutrosophic Sci.* **2024**, *23*, 140–147. [CrossRef]
15. Smarandache, F. Foundation of the SuperHyperSoft Set and the Fuzzy Extension SuperHyperSoft Set: A New Vision. *Neutrosophic Syst. Appl.* **2023**, *11*, 48–51. [CrossRef]
16. Maji, P.; Biswas, R.; Roy, A.R. Intuitionistic Fuzzy Soft Sets. *J. Fuzzy Math.* **2001**, *9*, 589–602.
17. Zadeh, L.A. Fuzzy Sets and Their Application to Pattern Classification and Clustering Analysis. In *Classification and Clustering*; Van Ryzin, J., Ed.; Academic Press: Cambridge, MA, USA, 1997; pp. 251–299. [CrossRef]
18. Zimmermann, H.-J.; Zadeh, L.A.; Gaines, B.R. *Fuzzy Sets and Decision Analysis*; Elsevier: Amsterdam, The Netherlands, 1984.
19. Majumdar, P.; Samanta, S.K. Similarity Measure of Soft Sets. *New Math. Nat. Comput.* **2008**, *4*, 1–12. [CrossRef]
20. Majumdar, P.; Samanta, S.K. On Similarity and Entropy of Neutrosophic Sets. *J. Intell Fuzzy Syst.* **2014**, *26*, 1245–1252. [CrossRef]
21. Smarandache, F.; Abdel-Basset, M. (Eds.) *Neutrosofic Sets and Systems*; University of New Mexico, Educational Publisher Inc.: Ave Columbus, OH, USA, 2020; Volume 32.
22. Atanassov, K. Intuitionistic fuzzy sets. *Fuzzy Sets Syst.* **1986**, *20*, 87–96. [CrossRef]
23. Zou, Y.; Xiao, Z. Data Analysis Approaches of Soft Sets Under Incomplete Information. *Knowl. Based Syst.* **2008**, *21*, 941–945. [CrossRef]
24. Naz, M.; Shabir, M. On Fuzzy Bipolar Soft Sets, Their Algebraic Structures and Applications. *J. Intell. Fuzzy Syst.* **2014**, *26*, 1645–1656. [CrossRef]
25. Dhanalakshmi, V.; Bhaskaran, S. Applications of Soft Set Theory in Medical Image Analysis. *J. Med. Imaging Health Inform.* **2023**, *11*, 145–156.
26. Yang, X.; Zhao, Y. Insights into the Advantages and Specific Methods Used in Employing Soft Set Theory for Similar Purposes. *J. Med. Image Anal.* **2020**, *35*, 123–135.
27. Khan, A.; Gupta, R. Examination of Soft Set-Based Approaches in Medical Image Analysis: Evaluating Evidence in Medical Recommendations and Analyzing Factors Influencing Preventive Practices. *J. Med. Image Anal.* **2021**, *37*, 189–204.
28. Gîfu, D. Malaria Detection System. In Proceedings of the International Conference on Mathematical Foundations of Informatics (MFOI-2017), Chișinău, Moldova, 9–11 November 2017; Cojocaru, S., Gaindric, C., Drugus, I., Eds.; Institute of Mathematics and Computer Science, Academy of Sciences of Moldova: Chișinău, Moldova, 2017; pp. 74–78.
29. Gîfu, D. The Use of Decision Trees for Analysis of the Epilepsy. *Procedia Comput. Sci.* **2021**, *192*, 2844–2853. [CrossRef]
30. Gifu, D.; Trandabat, D.; Cohen, K.B.; Xia, J. The Curative Power of Medical Data. In Proceedings of the JCDL'18—18th ACM/IEEE on Joint Conference on Digital Libraries, Fort Worth, TX, USA, 3–6 June 2018; ACM: New York, NY, USA, 2018; pp. 431–433, ISBN 978-1-4503-5178-2. [CrossRef]
31. Curea, E.; Gîfu, D. A Framework for Medical Data Retrieval. In Proceedings of the Curative Power of Medical Data-MEDA 2017-, Selected Papers of the First International Workshop MEDA 2017, Constanța, Romania, 10–17 September 2017; Gîfu, D., Trandabăț, D., Eds.; "Alexandru Ioan Cuza" University Publishing House: Iași, Romania, 2018; pp. 41–51.

applied sciences

MDPI

Article

Quasi-Experimental Design for Medical Studies with the Method of the Fuzzy Pseudo-Control Group

Kiril Tenekedjiev [1,2,*], Daniela Panayotova [3,4], Mohamed Daboos [1], Snejana Ivanova [5], Mark Symes [2], Plamen Panayotov [3] and Natalia Nikolova [5,6]

1 Department of Computer Sciences, Varna Free University, 9007 Varna, Bulgaria; daboes2004@gmail.com
2 Australian Maritime College, University of Tasmania, Newnham, TAS 7248, Australia; mark.symes@utas.edu.au
3 Department of Cardiovascular Surgery and Angiology, Faculty of Medicine, Medical University—Varna "Prof. Dr. Paraskev Stoyanov", 9002 Varna, Bulgaria; dpanayotova7@gmail.com (D.P.); pl.panayotov@gmail.com (P.P.)
4 Department of Cardiac Surgery, St. Marina University Hospital, 9010 Varna, Bulgaria
5 Department of Information Technology, Nikola Vaptsarov Naval Academy, 9002 Varna, Bulgaria; s.ivanova13@abv.bg (S.I.); natalianik@gmail.com (N.N.)
6 Defence Science and Technology Group, Adelaide, SA 5111, Australia
* Correspondence: kiril.tenekedjiev@fulbrightmail.org

Featured Application: Any statistical analysis where a control group is absent, yet the study still needs to explore the effect of some sort of intervention over a population of objects. Medical data analysis naturally falls under this category of cases.

Abstract: (1) Background: Let the continuous parameter X be a proxy variable for the outcome of an intervention R. Quasi-experimental studies are designed to evaluate the effect of R over X when forming a randomized control group (without the intervention) is impractical or/and unethical. The most popular quasi-experimental design, the difference-in-differences (DID) method, uses four samples of X values (pre- and post-intervention experimental and pseudo-control groups). DID always quantitatively evaluates the effect of R over X. However, its practical significance is restricted by several (often unprovable) assumptions and by the monotonic preference requirement over X. We propose a novel fuzzy quasi-experimental computational approach that addresses those limitations. (2) Methods: A novel method of the fuzzy pseudo-control group (MFPCG) is introduced and formalized. It uses four fuzzy samples as input, exactly the same as DID. We practically determine and statistically compare the favorability of the differences in X before and after the intervention for the experimental and the pseudo-control groups in case of the more general hill preferences over X. MFPCG applies four modifications of fuzzy Bootstrap procedures to perform each of the nine statistical tests used. The new method does not use the assumptions of DID, but it does not always produce a positive or a negative answer, as MFPCG results are qualitative. It is not a competing methodology; as such, it should be used alongside DID. (3) Results: We assess the effect of annuloplasty that acts in conjunction with revascularization over two continuous parameters that characterize the condition of patients with ischemic heart disease complicated by moderate and moderate-to-severe ischemic mitral regurgitation. (4) Conclusions: The statistical results proved the favorable effect of annuloplasty on two parameters, both for patients with a relatively preserved medical state and patients with a relatively deteriorated medical state. We validate the MFPCG solution of the case study by comparing them with those from the fuzzy DID. We discuss the limitations and adaptability of MFPCG, which should warrant its use in other case studies and domains.

https://doi.org/10.3390/app15031370

Keywords: fuzzy samples; fuzzy Bootstrap procedures for statistical tests; medical data analysis; cluster of tests

1. Definition and Necessity of Pseudo-Control Groups

We explore the effect of a given intervention R over a continuous parameter X, which describes the status of objects in a population P, called a *target population*. Parameter X should be selected to be a proxy variable for the outcome of the intervention. To solve such a task, we would usually conduct an experiment to measure the values of X before and after intervention R for a set of objects from P, called an *experimental group* [1]. If we are only interested in the change in the parameter in the experimental group following the intervention, then we are at risk of reaching misleading conclusions. Some of the main reasons for this could be:

- If we observed a favorable change in X that is due to the cumulative effect of factors unaccounted for in the study rather than to intervention R (that only weakly contributed to the situation, did not contribute, or even contributed unfavorably), then our conclusion that the effect of R over X for objects from P was favorable would be incorrect.
- If we observed an unfavorable change in X that is due to the cumulative effect of factors unaccounted for in the study and not due to intervention R (that only weakly worsened the situation, did not contribute, or even contributed favorably), then our conclusion that the effect of R over X for objects from P was unfavorable would be incorrect.
- If we observed a negligible change in X that combined the favorable effect of R over X and the cumulative unfavorable effect of the factors unaccounted for in the study, then our conclusion that there was no effect of R over X for objects from P would be incorrect.
- If we observed a negligible change in X that combined the unfavorable effect of R over X and the cumulative favorable effect of the factors unaccounted for in the study, then our conclusion that there was no effect of R over X for objects from P would be incorrect.

Therefore, experiments use a *control* group comprising objects from P that are not subjected to the investigated intervention R [2]. Several methodologies generate adequate conclusions from experiments that use control and experimental groups. Often, if intervention R acts in conjunction with another base intervention, V, whose effect cannot be paused during the experiment (e.g., time), then parameter X is measured before and after the intervention. As a result, we can form four samples as follows:

1. E_b is the sample that contains the values of parameter X for the experimental group at the beginning of the experiment.
2. K_b is the sample that contains the values of parameter X for the control group at the beginning of the experiment.
3. E_e is the sample that contains the values of parameter X for the experimental group at the end of the experiment, after the group has been subjected to the base intervention V and the investigated intervention R.
4. K_e is the sample that contains the values of parameter X for the experimental group at the end of the experiment, after the group has been subjected to the base intervention V.

Since E_b and K_b are two samples drawn from the same population, we would not expect to find a statistically significant difference between them due to the very definition of control groups [3]. We can define the effect of the investigated intervention R over the selected parameter X as follows:

1. We test the samples E_e and K_e for equality:
   - If the values X in E_e are statistically significantly more favorable than in K_e, then intervention R over parameter X is proven to be statistically favorable.
   - If the values X in E_e are statistically significantly less favorable than in K_e, then intervention R over parameter X is proven to be statistically unfavorable.
   - If E_e and K_e have statistically indistinguishable values of X, then the effect of intervention R over parameter X is considered statistically unproven.
2. We test, for nullity, the change in X in the paired samples E_b and E_e and the change in X in the paired samples K_b and K_e:
   - If the temporal change (TC) in the experimental group is statistically significantly favorable, whereas the TC in the control group is statistically significantly unfavorable, then the effect of intervention R over parameter X is proven to be statistically favorable.
   - If the TC in the experimental group is not statistically significant, whereas the TC in the control group is statistically significantly unfavorable, then the effect of intervention R over parameter X is proven to be statistically favorable.
   - If the TC in the experimental group is statistically significantly unfavorable, whereas the TC in the control group is statistically significantly favorable, then the effect of intervention R over parameter X is proven to be statistically unfavorable.
   - If the TC in the experimental group is not statistically significant, whereas the TC in the control group is statistically significantly favorable, then the effect of intervention R over parameter X is proven to be statistically unfavorable.
   - If the TC in both groups are either simultaneously statistically significantly favorable, simultaneously statistically insignificant, or simultaneously statistically significantly unfavorable, then the effect of intervention R over parameter X is considered statistically unproven.

The procedures described above are forms of scientific experiments called *randomized control trials* (RCTs) [4]. Although there are different study designs for RCTs (e.g., single-blinded, double-blinded, parallel-group, cluster, pragmatic, noninferiority, etc.), the defining characteristic of the described scientific experiments is the (theoretical) possibility to allocate the participating items into treatment and control groups randomly.

In some experiments, the control group may be non-existent for various reasons. This is very typical in medical research that tests the effect of a medication or a medical procedure on humans. We shall describe three situations where using a classical control group is theoretically problematic and highly controversial from a practical point of view.

Sometimes, leaving patients without care is unethical (and even illegal). Therefore, some patients are assigned standard treatment (medication or procedure), whereas the remaining patients are assigned a new experimental treatment (medication or procedure) [?]. Ethical approvals for such studies are rarely granted, and only for treatments with years of preliminary lab testing. In that case, we have a special type of control group, because the experiment does not deal with the absolute effect of the innovative treatment but with the effect relative to the standard treatment.

At the same time, modern concepts favor evidence-based medicine [5]. The contemporary practice questions well-established procedures applied with a base treatment whose impact has not been thoroughly studied. It is practically impossible to experiment with a control group to prove the favorable effect of an established procedure. This is because one would struggle to explain to the individual patient, to their medical treatment team, to their insurance company, or to authorities why they did not receive treatment as per the best medical practice and instead were included in the control group, where the established procedure in question was omitted. At the very least, such an experiment would not receive approval from ethics committees, and the results would be inadmissible in reputable journals. An ethically admissible and legal way to overcome this situation is to choose the patients in the experiment to be as similar as possible regarding medical characteristics. Yet, their medical history should be different enough so that some of them (the experimental group) are assigned the investigated procedure and base treatment. In contrast, the rest are only assigned the base treatment based on the best judgment of their medical team. We assume that such patients form what we will call the *pseudo-control group*.

A similar situation arises when all required experimentation is conducted for a relatively new medication, which proves its favorable effect. However, the company that produces the medication took part (in one way or the other) in those experiments. The new medication, as a rule, is more expensive than its previous version(s), yet due to its favorable effect, it soon becomes the treatment norm, while at the same time, the higher price does not directly affect the patients as the medical insurance covers it. Modern research assumes that independent labs can replicate results from every published experiment. If discrepancies with the original study are identified, then they are immediately shared with the research community. This assumption is not valid for this new medication, though. Anyone with doubts about the new medication's favorable effect has no opportunity to experiment with a control group, as each patient should be given the best possible treatment. Again, the only possibility is to compare the effect of the medication in patients from the experimental group with that in patients with counterindications for that medication. The latter form a pseudo-control group because their medical condition differs from that of the patients in the experimental group.

Let us reformulate the problem at hand. We explore the effect of a given intervention (impact, influence) R in conjunction with another base intervention, V, over a given parameter X, which describes the outcome of objects in a target population, P. Assume that before and after interventions V and R, we have measured the values of X for a given group of objects from P, called the *experimental group*. We can identify the effect in question compared to the effect of the base intervention V over parameter X, which characterizes the status of objects from a population Q, similar to P, called a *pseudo-control population*. We assume that before and after intervention V, we have measured the values of X for a given group of objects from Q, called the *pseudo-control group*.

As a result, we can form four samples as follows:

1. E_b is the sample that contains the values of parameter X for the experimental group at the beginning of the experiment.
2. PC_b is the sample that contains the values of parameter X for the pseudo-control group at the beginning of the experiment.
3. E_e is the sample that contains the values of parameter X for the experimental group at the end of the experiment after the group has been subjected to the base intervention V and the investigated intervention R.
4. PC_e is the sample that contains the values of parameter X for the pseudo-control group at the end of the experiment after the group has been subjected to the base intervention V.

Scientific experiments that require the assessment of an intervention effect over a target population, without a control group that can be allocated initially by the random assignment of the study units, are called quasi-experiments [6]. Most published studies using that approach never even mention that they have performed quasi-experiments [7]. The fact that pseudo-control groups are traditionally called control groups does not help in that regard. There are numerous quasi-experimental designs (panel data analysis, nonequivalent control group designs, case–control design, etc.), but the most well-known and widely used pretest–posttest approaches are the difference-in-differences design (DID) and the regression discontinuity design (RDD).

DID, in its basic form, is equivalent to regression analysis over two dummy variables—one for the time period and one for the group membership. It is an easy-to-estimate quantitative method with understandable ideas [8]. It will always assess (correctly or incorrectly) the effect of intervention R over parameter X. However, the DID requires that all the assumptions of the least-squares model (the ordinary or the weighted one) hold [9]. One of the additional assumptions of DID is "the parallel trends assumption". The latter claims that the expected outcome for the treated and untreated populations would have been parallel if, counterfactually, no treatment was applied to both populations. This is a demanding assumption and rarely can be tested properly [10]. The same is true for the other assumptions of the DID [11]. Another major drawback of DID is that it can work only when the preferences over X are monotonic, which is rarely the case in medical studies. Last, but not least, DID is incapable of assessing the practical significance of the observed changes regardless of their statistical significance.

RDD is a nonequivalent control group design suitable for problems where a cutoff surface of some vector or scalar discriminant variable is defined. Each participating item in the experiment is allocated either to the experimental or pseudo-control groups, depending on which side of the cutoff surface the participant's discriminant variable is. If we select only those participants that are near the cutoff surface, we will form two almost randomly assigned reduced groups, with objects from one and the subpopulation (lying near the cutoff surface). The average treatment effect is easily estimated by comparing those new groups [12]. The idea of RDD is very understandable, but the main drawback is the requirement for huge sample sizes. This is very useful in big-data setups.

Experimental and pseudo-control groups occasionally contain objects whose membership to P and Q is unquestionable. In that case, the four samples above are crisp sets. On other occasions, however, there is ambiguity and uncertainty in the membership of an arbitrary object from the samples to the respective populations. In that more general case, we can model ambiguity by associating the values of X for a given object with a positive integer, μ, that takes values between 0 and 1, which is the degree of membership of the object to the respective group (where 1 indicates undoubted membership, whereas 0 indicates undoubted lack of membership). Therefore, the four samples can be considered fuzzy in line with the discussions in [13,14].

We shall explore the effect of intervention R over a selected parameter X by testing the equality of the populations P and Q before the intervention by comparing the samples E_b and PC_b, and after the intervention by comparing the samples E_e and PC_e. Comparing the statistical differences before and after the intervention will show one aspect of the effect of R over X.

Testing the equality of X in two populations using two fuzzy samples is a non-trivial task. Here are some reasons for that:

- The task depends on whether parameter X is discrete or continuous.
- We should conduct the task using several statistical tests whose results should match.
- The results from the tests should have high sensitivity and specificity, as judging the effect of intervention R over parameter X is based on the differences in the equality tests before and after the intervention.

A typical situation that creates pseudo-control groups is the experimental testing of medical procedures over patients. In such cases, we can use a pseudo-control group to assess the relative effect of the medical procedure compared to another procedure [15,16].

Let us assume that all participants in the experiment have similar medical characteristics, yet there are sufficient differences to stratify them into two groups. The pseudo-control group contains the other patients with indications only for the base intervention V according to the best judgment of their treatment physician or medical team. The experimental group contains patients with indications that make them suitable for intervention R in addition to the base intervention V.

In our work, we explore the case when the proxy variables for the outcome of the intervention are continuous parameters (e.g., X). In the next section, we review Bootstrap statistical tests for differences in two fuzzy samples, with X values drawn from two populations. The third problem, mentioned above, is the core of our paper. We shall solve this problem using a newly proposed quasi-experimental design called the method of the fuzzy pseudo-control group (MFPCG). Some ideas of MFPCG can be traced back to [15] (in the case of crisp samples) and to [16] (in the case of fuzzy samples).

2. State of the Art in Bootstrap Statistical Testing with Fuzzy Samples

Assume we have two one-dimensional (1D) samples of a continuous parameter Z, with a total of n_1 and n_2 number of observations each, respectively. The observations z_k^1 and z_k^2 of the first and second samples, respectively, belong to Population 1 and Population 2 with degrees of membership μ_k^1 and μ_k^2, respectively. We can then form Fuzzy sample 1 (denoted Z^1) and Fuzzy sample 2 (denoted Z^2):

$$Z^1 = \left\{ \left(z_1^1 - \mu_1^1\right), \left(z_2^1 - \mu_2^1\right), \ldots, \left(z_{n_1}^1 - \mu_{n_1}^1\right) \right\}, \tag{1}$$

$$Z^2 = \left\{ \left(z_1^2 - \mu_1^2\right), \left(z_2^2 - \mu_2^2\right), \ldots, \left(z_{n_2}^2 - \mu_{n_2}^2\right) \right\}. \tag{2}$$

We wish to explore how the different conditions to form the fuzzy samples influence the continuous 1D parameter Z values. In our setting, fuzzy samples are formed from two different populations, and we need to test whether Z from Population 1 has the same distribution as Z from Population 2.

We can use every non-fuzzy sample that describes a given random variable (r.v.) to approximate the cumulative distribution function (CDF) of that r.v. using an *empirical cumulative distribution function* (ECDF) [17]. The only condition to build ECDF is that the measurements in the sample should be independent and identically distributed (i.i.d.):

$$CDF_j(z) \approx ECDF_j(z) = \frac{1}{n_j} \sum_{\substack{k=1 \\ z_k^j \le z}}^{n_j} 1, \text{ for } z \in (-\infty; +\infty) \text{ and } j = 1, 2. \tag{3}$$

ECDF interprets the observations in Z^1 and Z^2 as non-fuzzy and neglects the information in the degrees of membership of the observations. Equation (3) assumes that we construct a discrete probability mass function (PMF), which approximates the density of the continuous r.v. Z. In this PMF, the probability that the r.v. takes an arbitrary value equals the relative frequency of that value in the sample.

We can use other CDF approximations under different assumptions for the observations in the sample (e.g., continuous linear, functional continuous linear, and granular continuous linear) [18].

Using the information in the degrees of membership from Fuzzy sample Z^1 and Fuzzy sample Z^2, we can derive a fuzzy empirical sample approximation of the CDF or an r.v. as a *fuzzy empirical distribution function* (FECDF). This is a generalization of the ECDF [19]:

$$CDF_j(z) \approx FECDF_j(z) = \sum_{\substack{k=1 \\ z_k^j \leq z}}^{n_j} \mu_k^i \Big/ \sum_{k=1}^{n_j} \mu_k^j, \text{ for } z \in (-\infty; +\infty) \text{ and } j = 1, 2. \quad (4)$$

In an implicit form [20], FECDF uses the probability mass function, yet here, the probability for an arbitrary value of the r.v. is the relative weight of the degrees of membership of that value in the fuzzy sample.

There are no analytical generalizations to calculate the p-value of most statistical tests over fuzzy samples (unlike crisp samples). An alternative approach is to use fuzzy Bootstrap simulation to calculate the conditional distributions of a given statistic if the null hypothesis, H_0 (that the populations have the same statistics or distributions), is true [21]. Bootstrap simulation is a computer-intensive technique that uses N pseudo-realities [22], where N is a large natural. It has proven effective for hypothesis testing over fuzzy data [23,24]. A fuzzy Bootstrap procedure only requires that the observations are i.i.d.

The fuzzy Bootstrap procedures we discuss below have four modifications each (denoted BM1 through BM4). Depending on how we form the synthetic samples, we have quasi-equal information generation (i.e., the synthetic samples have almost the same quantity of information as the original sample) and equal-size generation (i.e., the synthetic samples have the same number of fuzzy observations as the original sample). Regarding the type of CDF approximation, we can use either ECDF or FECDF. As a result, we can define the four Bootstrap Modifications:

- BM1: Fuzzy Bootstrap with quasi-equal-information generation using an ECDF. In each pseudo-reality, any synthetic sample is generated from the ECDF (constructed using (3) from the original sample) so that the degree of membership sum is almost identical to the same sum for the original sample. It is unlikely that the synthetic and original samples will have the same cardinality.
- BM2: Fuzzy Bootstrap with quasi-equal-information generation using a FECDF. In each pseudo-reality, any synthetic sample is generated from the FECDF (constructed using (4) from the original sample) so that the degree of membership sum is almost identical to the same sum at the original sample. It is unlikely that the synthetic and original samples will have the same cardinality.
- BM3: Fuzzy Bootstrap with equal-size generation using an ECDF. In each pseudo-reality, any synthetic sample is generated from the ECDF (constructed using (3) from the original sample) with cardinality equal to the cardinality of the original sample. It is unlikely that the synthetic and original samples will have the same degree of membership sums.
- BM4: Fuzzy Bootstrap with equal-size generation using a FECDF. In each pseudo-reality, any synthetic sample is generated from the FECDF (constructed using (4) from the original sample) with cardinality equal to the cardinality of the original sample. It is unlikely that the synthetic and original samples will have the same degree of membership sums.

We reiterate that these modifications are valid for all Bootstrap tests we present below.

The test statistic measures the difference between two sample CDFs when testing the equality of two population distributions. This assumes that the two populations have identical underlying continuous distributions.

There are three statistics classes when testing the equality of two continuous distributions. A typical representative of the quadratic class is the quadratic Anderson–Darling statistic and the Kramer–von Mises statistic [25]. The rank class uses metrics such as the Mann–Whitney U statistic and the Wilcoxon T statistic [26]. The most frequently used ones from the supremum class are the Kolmogorov–Smirnov [27] and its improved version—the Kuiper statistic (Ku) [28]. Ku is the sum of the supremum of positive differences and the supremum of the negative differences between two approximations of CDF based on the available samples:

$$Ku = \sup_z(CDF_1(z) - CDF_2(z)) + \sup_z(CDF_2(z) - CDF_1(z)). \tag{5}$$

The statistic (5) has the same sensitivity to deviations for all values of Z.

For continuous CDF, the estimate of the supremum requires non-trivial optimization and takes considerable time. The supremum in (5) is often replaced with a maximum, as suggested in [29]. In the case of fuzzy samples with FECDF approximation of CDF_1 and CDF_2, we can represent (5) as

$$Ku = \max_{k=1,2,\ldots,n_1}\left(FECDF_1\left(z_k^1\right) - FECDF_2\left(z_k^1\right)\right) + \max_{k=1,2,\ldots,n_2}\left(FECDF_2\left(z_k^2\right) - FECDF_1\left(z_k^2\right)\right). \tag{6}$$

The work [30] proves that in the case of FECDF calculated using (4)–(6), we can calculate Ku directly from the sample observations without the need to construct the FECDF:

$$\begin{aligned} Ku_r = {} & \max_{i=1,2,\ldots,n_1}\left(\sum_{\substack{k=1\\ z_k^1 \le z_i^1}}^{n_1} \mu_k^1 \Big/ \sum_{k=1}^{n_1}\mu_k^1 - \sum_{\substack{k=1\\ z_k^2 \le z_i^1}}^{n_2} \mu_k^2 \Big/ \sum_{k=1}^{n_2}\mu_k^2\right) \\ & + \max_{i=1,2,\ldots,n_2}\left(\sum_{\substack{k=1\\ z_k^2 \le z_i^2}}^{n_2} \mu_k^2 \Big/ \sum_{\substack{k=1\\ z_k^2 \le z_i^2}}^{n_2} \mu_k^2 - \sum_{\substack{k=1\\ z_k^1 \le z_i^2}}^{n_1} \mu_k^1 \Big/ \sum_{k=1}^{n_1}\mu_k^1\right). \end{aligned} \tag{7}$$

Dependence (7) brings down the calculation of Ku to a finite number of calculations of FECDF for given data points. The observations in the samples Z^1 and Z^2 are random; hence, Ku is an r.v., and Ku_r is one possible realization. The work [30] also offered a theorem to calculate the Kuiper statistic for fuzzy samples. It showed that (a) the statistic always exists; (b) the criterion is in the interval [0; 1]; (c) the supremum in (6) is a maximum; and (d) the criterion can be calculated using (7) with no more than (n_1 + n_2) calculations of the FECDF.

The non-fuzzy Bootstrap procedure constructs the conditional distributions of the Kuiper statistic when each observation in the samples (1) and (2) belongs with certainty to their respective populations if H_0 is true [31] (i.e., all degrees of membership in the sample equal to 1). The work [32] expands these procedures. It offers a numerical simulation algorithm to find the p-value of the statistical test for equality of the 1D continuous distributions of two populations, represented by the fuzzy samples (1) and (2).

In addition to exploring the distributions, we are also interested in knowing how the different conditions of obtaining the fuzzy samples impact the numerical characteristics of the distribution of the continuous 1D parameter in Population 1 and Population 2. This resembles the situation when the two fuzzy samples originate from two different populations. We shall explore the equality of the numerical characteristic C of the distribution law of an r.v. in Population 1 and Population 2. We need to test if Population 1 has the same

C as Population 2. The statistical tests calculate the value s of a given estimator S of the resemblance between the numerical characteristic estimates $\hat{c}_1$ and $\hat{c}_2$, that originate from fuzzy samples (1) and (2).

Some works, like [33], that discuss the procedures to assess the equality of arbitrary numerical characteristics (as presented above), also expand according to the type of the test (one-tailed or two-tailed). Then, we have eight variants of each fuzzy Bootstrap procedure.

Assume that M_1 and M_2 are the mean values for Populations 1 and 2, respectively. We can calculate the weighted mean values of the fuzzy samples (1) and (2), $\widehat{M}_1$ and $\widehat{M}_2$, respectively, which we will call *fuzzy sample means*:

$$\widehat{M}_j = \sum_{k=1}^{n_j} \mu_k^j z_k^j \Big/ \sum_{k=1}^{n_j} \mu_k^j, \text{ for } j = 1,2. \tag{8}$$

We will use the same notation for fuzzy sample p-quantile, fuzzy sample median, fuzzy sample variance, fuzzy sample STD, fuzzy sample interquartile range, fuzzy tests, etc. This aligns well with Zadeh's understanding that fuzzy logic is not logic that is fuzzy but rather crisp-rule logic dealing with fuzzy sets [34]. However, we never use fuzzy numbers in the whole paper, yet the samples (1) and (2) are still fuzzy, since the degree of membership of each observation measures how much that observation belongs to the respective population. This is the main component of Zadeh's idea, trying to formalize the fuzziness of concepts as part of the general uncertainty of the data.

For the test statistic, the works [32,33] use the difference,

$$\Delta_{1-2,r}^{mean} = \widehat{M}_1 - \widehat{M}_2 \tag{9}$$

The difference (9) is a realization of the random variable Δ_{1-2}^{mean}.

The work [32] presents a Bootstrap statistical test in eight variants to explore the difference in the means of two populations using fuzzy samples. The null hypothesis H_0 for all tests is that the populations have equal means. The alternative hypothesis H_1 varies depending on the test. The tests calculate the p-value, i.e., the probability of observing a difference between the means of the fuzzy samples as least as great as the measured one, if H_0 is true. The algorithms to calculate the p-values of those Bootstrap variants are also presented.

Assume that the elements of the fuzzy samples Z^1 and Z^2 from (1) and (2) are sorted to derive the sorted fuzzy samples, $Z^{1,sort}$ and $Z^{2,sort}$:

$$Z^{1,sort} = \left\{ \left(z_1^{1,sort} - \mu_1^{1,sort} \right), \left(z_2^{1,sort} - \mu_2^{1,sort} \right), \ldots, \left(z_{n_1}^{1,sort} - \mu_{n_1}^{1,sort} \right) \right\} \tag{10}$$

where $z_1^{1,sort} \le z_2^{1,sort} \le \ldots \le z_{n_1}^{1,sort}$,

$$Z^{2,sort} = \left\{ \left(z_1^{2,sort} - \mu_1^{2,sort} \right), \left(z_2^{2,sort} - \mu_2^{2,sort} \right), \ldots, \left(z_{n_1}^{2,sort} - \mu_{n_1}^{2,sort} \right) \right\} \tag{11}$$

where $z_1^{2,sort} \le z_2^{2,sort} \le z_3^{2,sort} \le \ldots \le z_{n_2}^{2,sort}$.

The work [33] offers a generalized procedure to calculate a fuzzy p-quantile of a distribution using sorted data from a fuzzy sample. The procedure uses the real function $q^j(.)$ from (12) for $p \in [0;1]$, which is linearly approximated on the nodes $\left(p_i^j, q_i^j\right)$ given in (13) (where $j = 1, 2$ refers to the sorted samples (10) and (11)):

$$q^j(p) = \begin{cases} q_i^j & \text{for } p = p_i^j \\ q_i^j + \dfrac{\left(q_{i+1}^j - q_i^j\right)\left(p - p_i^j\right)}{\left(p_{i+1}^j - p_i^j\right)} & \text{for } p_i^j < p < p_{i+1}^j \end{cases}, \text{ for } j = 1,2, \tag{12}$$

$$\left(p_i^j, q_i^j\right) = \begin{cases} \left(0, z_1^{j,sort}\right) & \text{for } i = 0 \\ \left(\frac{\mu_1^{j,sort}}{2}, z_1^{j,sort}\right) & \text{for } i = 1 \\ \left(\sum_{k=1}^{i-1} \mu_k^{j,sort} + \frac{\mu_i^{j,sort}}{2}, z_i^{j,sort}\right) & \text{for } i = 2,3,\ldots,n_j \\ \left(1, z_{n_j}^{j,sort}\right) & \text{for } i = n_j + 1 \end{cases}, \text{ for } j = 1,2. \tag{13}$$

The functions (12) assess the fuzzy p-quantile of the continuous r.v. Z using the sorted fuzzy samples (10) and (11).

Assume that MED_1 and MED_2 are the medians for Populations 1 and 2, respectively. We can calculate the fuzzy sample medians, $\widehat{MED}_1$ and $\widehat{MED}_2$, using the function (12) as follows:

$$\widehat{MED}_j = q^j(0.5), \text{ for } j = 1,2 \tag{14}$$

The test statistic in [33,35,36] is the difference:

$$\Delta_{1-2,r}^{med} = \widehat{MED}_1 - \widehat{MED}_2. \tag{15}$$

The difference (15) is a realization of the random variable Δ_{1-2}^{med}. The Bootstrap algorithms to test the equality of medians over non-fuzzy samples are presented in [35,36].

Assume that VAR_1 and VAR_2 are the variances for Populations 1 and 2, respectively. We can calculate the fuzzy sample variances, $\widehat{VAR}_1$ and $\widehat{VAR}_2$, as

$$\widehat{VAR}_j = \frac{\sum_{k=1}^{n_j} \mu_k^j \left(z_k^j - \widehat{M}_j\right)^2}{\sum_{k=1}^{n_j} \mu_k^j - max\left\{\mu_1^j, \mu_2^j, \ldots, \mu_{n_j}^j\right\}}, \text{ for } j = 1,2. \tag{16}$$

In (16), $\widehat{M}_j$ are the sample fuzzy means calculated using (8). For the test statistic, we can use the ratio

$$R_{1/2,r}^{var} = \widehat{VAR}_1 / \widehat{VAR}_2. \tag{17}$$

The ratio (17) is a realization of the random variable $R_{1/2}^{var}$. The work [37] presents algorithms for Bootstrap tests for the equality of variances over non-fuzzy samples.

Assume that IQR_1 and IQR_2 are the interquartile ranges of Populations 1 and 2, respectively. We can calculate the fuzzy sample interquartile ranges, $\widehat{IQR}_1$ and $\widehat{IQR}_2$, using the function (12):

$$\widehat{IQR}_j = q^j(0.75) - q^j(0.25), \text{ for } j = 1,2. \tag{18}$$

For the test statistic, we use the ratio

$$R_{1/2,r}^{iqr} = \widehat{IQR}_1 / \widehat{IQR}_2. \tag{19}$$

The ratio (19) is a realization of the random variable $R_{1/2}^{iqr}$. The work [38] presents algorithms for Bootstrap tests for the equality of interquartile ranges over non-fuzzy samples.

When the degrees of membership in (8), (13), (14), (16), and (18) equal 1, the formulae simplify to the well-known non-fuzzy sample estimates using the maximum likelihood estimates for the numerical characteristics of the random variable Z.

The work [39] constructs and uses algorithms for testing the equality of population medians, variances, and interquartile ranges over fuzzy samples by combining the fuzzy algorithms for the equality of population means from [32] with the non-fuzzy algorithms for the equality of population medians, variances, and interquartile intervals from [35–38].

Our paper does not claim any contributions to the Bootstrap statistical tests described in the current review section. Please refer to the references for details regarding those tests and their justification. In this study, we only implement those Bootstrap statistical tests to solve a challenging new problem.

Modern tendencies in statistical tests use a cluster of tests instead of single tests to explore the differences between two populations. Similar ideas are proposed in [39], where two populations are compared using a cluster of Bootstrap tests for means, medians, and lower/upper quartiles based on data from fuzzy samples.

3. The Method of the Fuzzy Pseudo-Control Group

For practical reasons, we sometimes need to use pseudo-control groups to explore a given effect. As we showed in Section 1, the standard approach is to define four fuzzy samples and compare the population characteristics pre- and post intervention. Section 2 shows that a sufficient number of Bootstrap tests can estimate the differences between the samples well. In this section, we shall introduce the MFPCG as one possible way to assess the effect using pseudo-control groups. This method may use several continuous parameters. We shall define the method for only a single parameter, but the application for the case of several parameters is trivial.

Sections 3.1–3.5 present the essence of each of the key stages of MFPCG as follows:

1. An expert-based definition of the optimal values of parameter X.
2. A favorability assessment of the differences between the populations.
3. The identification of the statistical significance of differences between populations.
4. The categorization of differences between populations.
5. The classification of the MFPCG result.

The realization of the method is not as straightforward as simply going through the five steps. After we choose the continuous parameter X, we can perform stage 1. We will quantify the prior (before the effect) differences between the target and the pseudo-control populations by performing stages 2, 3, and 4 over samples E_b and PC_b. Then, we will quantify the posterior (after the effect) differences between the target and the pseudo-control populations by performing stages 2, 3, and 4 over samples E_e and PC_e. Finally, we can perform stage 5 and quantify the effect over X. If the investigated effect can be demonstrated with other continuous parameters, we will repeat the same procedure for each one of them.

3.1. *An Expert-Based Definition of the Optimal Values of Parameter X*

Let Fuzzy sample 1 contain the values of the continuous parameter X and their degrees of membership for patients in the experimental group. In contrast, let Fuzzy sample 2 contain the values of X and their degrees of membership for patients in the pseudo-control group. We assume that the preferences over the values of parameter X are either monotonic or unimodal with a "flat" maximum within the range of X. Such preferences were referred to as hill preferences in [40]. In both cases, we can use expert input to define the optimal values of parameter X to be between $X_{d,opt}$ to $X_{u,opt}$. The outcome becomes less favorable as X decreases from $X_{d,opt}$, and as X increases from $X_{u,opt}$. All values between $X_{u,opt}$ to $X_{u,opt}$ are equally preferred by the expert.

When the expert preferences over X are monotonically increasing, we shall set that $X_{d,opt} = X_{u,opt} = +\infty$. Similarly, when the expert preferences over X are monotonically decreasing, then we shall set $X_{d,opt} = X_{u,opt} = -\infty$. Here, we use the fact that monotonic preferences are a special case of hill preferences.

Let ΔX be an expert-defined value of parameter X, such that any change in the parameter below this value is practically insignificant.

Preferences of this sort are widespread in the medical domain, where we very often encounter hill preferences and, at times, monotonic preferences. Valley preferences, as per [40], and multimodal preferences, as a rule, do not occur in medical practice.

3.2. A Favorability Assessment of the Difference Between Populations

For the experimental group, we can calculate the sample fuzzy numerical characteristics of the distribution of X from Fuzzy sample 1, denoted as follows: M_E—sample fuzzy mean value in the experimental group; MED_E—sample fuzzy median in the experimental group; VAR_E—sample fuzzy variance in the experimental group; IQR_E—sample fuzzy interquartile range in the experimental group.

Similarly, for the pseudo-control group, we can calculate the sample fuzzy numerical characteristics of the distribution of X from Fuzzy sample 2, denoted as follows: M_{PC}—sample fuzzy mean in the pseudo-control group; MED_{PC}—sample fuzzy median in the pseudo-control group; VAR_{PC}—sample fuzzy variance in the pseudo-control group; IQR_{PC}—sample fuzzy interquartile range in the pseudo-control group.

Each distribution has multiple measures of location and multiple measures of dispersion. For the sake of simplicity, from this point forward in the paper, the term "measures of location" will refer only to the mean and/or the median. Similarly, "measures of dispersion" will refer only to the variance (the squared standard deviation) and/or the interquartile range.

We will assume hill or monotonic preferences over the X values, as discussed in Section 3.1. Below, we present an algorithm to assess the favorability of differences between the fuzzy measures of location in the two populations.

Stage 2 Algorithm: A Favorability Assessment of the Difference Between the Fuzzy Central Tendencies of Two Populations

For fuzzy means:

If $|M_E - M_{PC}| < \Delta X$, or $\left(X_{d,opt} - \Delta X\right) < M_E < M_{PC} < (X_{u,opt} + \Delta X)$, or $\left(X_{d,opt} - \Delta X\right) < M_{PC} < M_E < (X_{u,opt} + \Delta X)$, then M_E is assumed to be neutral to M_{PC}.

If $M_{PC} \leq min\left\{X_{d,opt} - \Delta X, M_E - \Delta X\right\} \leq X_{d,opt} - \Delta X < M_E < X_{u,opt} + \Delta X$, or $\left(X_{d,opt} - \Delta X\right) < M_E < X_{u,opt} + dX \leq max\{X_{u,opt} + dX, M_E + dX\} \leq M_{PC}$, or $(X_{u,opt} + \Delta X) \leq M_E \leq (M_{PC} - \Delta X)$, or $(M_{PC} + \Delta X) \leq M_E \leq \left(X_{d,opt} - \Delta X\right)$, then M_E is assumed to be more favorable than M_{PC}.

If $M_E \leq min\left\{X_{d,opt} - \Delta X, M_{PC} - \Delta X\right\} \leq X_{d,opt} - \Delta X < M_{PC} < X_{u,opt} + \Delta X$, or $\left(X_{d,opt} - \Delta X\right) < M_{PC} < X_{u,opt} + dX \leq max\{X_{u,opt} + dX, M_{PC} + dX\} \leq M_E$, or $(X_{u,opt} + \Delta X) \leq M_{PC} \leq (M_E - \Delta X)$, or $(M_E + \Delta X) \leq M_{PC} \leq \left(X_{d,opt} - \Delta X\right)$, then M_E is assumed to be less favorable than M_{PC}.

If $M_E \leq \left(X_{d,opt} - \Delta X\right) < (X_{u,opt} + \Delta X) \leq M_{PC}$, or $M_{PC} \leq \left(X_{d,opt} - \Delta X\right) < (X_{u,opt} + \Delta X) \leq M_E$, then the favorability of M_E compared to M_{PC} is problem-specific and should be defined by an expert in the respective field. Such cases only rarely occur, as they indicate excessive medical intervention.

For fuzzy medians:

If either $|MED_E - MED_{PC}| < \Delta X$, or $\left(X_{d,opt} - \Delta X\right) < MED_E < MED_{PC} < (X_{u,opt} + \Delta X)$, or $\left(X_{d,opt} - \Delta X\right) < MED_{PC} < MED_E < (X_{u,opt} + \Delta X)$, then MED_E is assumed to be neutral to MED_{PC}.

If $MED_{PC} \leq min\left\{X_{d,opt} - \Delta X, MED_E - \Delta X\right\} \leq X_{d,opt} - \Delta X < MED_E < X_{u,opt} + \Delta X$, or $\left(X_{d,opt} - \Delta X\right) < MED_E < X_{u,opt} + dX \leq max\{X_{u,opt} + dX, MED_E + dX\} \leq$

MED_{PC}, or $(X_{u,opt} + \Delta X) \leq MED_E \leq (MED_{PC} - \Delta X)$, or $(MED_{PC} + \Delta X) \leq MED_E \leq \left(X_{d,opt} - \Delta X\right)$, then MED_E is assumed to be more favorable than MED_{PC}.

If $MED_E \leq min\left\{X_{d,opt} - \Delta X, MED_{PC} - \Delta X\right\} \leq X_{d,opt} - \Delta X < MED_{PC} < X_{u,opt} + \Delta X$, or $\left(X_{d,opt} - \Delta X\right) < MED_{PC} < X_{u,opt} + dX \leq max\{X_{u,opt} + dX, MED_{PC} + dX\} \leq MED_E$, or $(X_{u,opt} + \Delta X) \leq MED_{PC} \leq (MED_E - \Delta X)$, or $(MED_E + \Delta X) \leq MED_{PC} \leq \left(X_{d,opt} - \Delta X\right)$, then MED_E is assumed to be less favorable than MED_{PC}.

If $MED_E \leq \left(X_{d,opt} - \Delta X\right) < (X_{u,opt} + \Delta X) \leq MED_{PC}$, or $MED_{PC} \leq \left(X_{d,opt} - \Delta X\right) < (X_{u,opt} + \Delta X) \leq MED_E$, then the favorability of MED_E compared to MED_{PC} is problem-specific and should be defined by an expert in the respective field. Such cases only rarely occur, as they are an indication of excessive medical intervention.

If MFPCG is applied outside the medical domain, then valley preferences over X may be present, and we will need to adapt the Stage 2 Algorithm. However, if multimodal preferences are present, then the Stage 2 Algorithm is inapplicable and unadaptable.

3.3. The Identification of the Statistical Significance of Differences Between Populations

We shall use nine fuzzy statistical Bootstrap tests to explore the statistical significance of differences between the populations of X:

Test 1: Fuzzy Bootstrap Kuiper test for equality of population distributions (FBT1).
Test 2. Fuzzy two-tail Bootstrap test for equality of population means (FBT2).
Test 3. Fuzzy one-tail Bootstrap test for equality of population means (FBT3).
Test 4. Fuzzy two-tail Bootstrap test for equality of population medians (FBT4).
Test 5. Fuzzy one-tail Bootstrap test for equality of population medians (FBT5).
Test 6. Fuzzy two-tail Bootstrap test for equality of population variances (FBT6).
Test 7. Fuzzy one-tail Bootstrap test for equality of population variances (FBT7).
Test 8. Fuzzy two-tail Bootstrap test for equality of population interquartile ranges (FBT8).
Test 9. Fuzzy one-tail Bootstrap test for equality of population interquartile ranges (FBT9).

Let $Pvalue_i$ be the probability of incorrectly rejecting the null hypothesis in test i, where $i = 1, 2, \ldots, 9$. Let also α be the significance level of all tests with a value determined by the expert.

We present an algorithm to identify the statistical significance of differences between two populations using measures of location and dispersion.

Stage 3 Algorithm: Defining the Statistical Significance of Differences Between Two Populations

For distributions:

If $Pvalue_1 \leq \alpha$, then the population distributions are assumed to be statistically significantly different.

If $\alpha < Pvalue_1 < 2\alpha$, then the population distributions are assumed to be borderline statistically significantly different.

If $Pvalue_1 \geq 2\alpha$, then the population distributions are assumed statistically indistinguishable.

For means:

If $Pvalue_3 \leq Pvalue_2 \leq \alpha$ and $M_E > M_{PC}$, then the mean of the target population P is assumed to be statistically significantly greater than that of the pseudo-control population Q.

If $Pvalue_3 \leq Pvalue_2 \leq \alpha$ and $M_E < M_{PC}$, then the mean of the target population P is assumed to be statistically significantly smaller than that of the pseudo-control population Q.

If $Pvalue_3 \leq \alpha < Pvalue_2$ and $M_E > M_{PC}$, then the mean of the target population P is assumed to be borderline statistically significantly greater than that of the pseudo-control population Q.

If $Pvalue_3 \leq \alpha < Pvalue_2$ and $M_E < M_{PC}$, then the mean of the target population P is assumed to be borderline statistically significantly smaller than that of the pseudo-control population Q.

If $\alpha < Pvalue_3 \leq Pvalue_2$, then the mean of the target population P is assumed to be statistically indistinguishable from that of the pseudo-control population Q.

For medians:

If $Pvalue_5 \leq Pvalue_4 \leq \alpha$ and $MED_E > MED_{PC}$, then the median of the target population P is assumed to be statistically significantly greater than that of the pseudo-control population Q.

If $Pvalue_5 \leq Pvalue_4 \leq \alpha$ and $MED_E < MED_{PC}$, then the median of the target population p is assumed to be statistically significantly smaller than that of the pseudo-control population Q.

If $Pvalue_5 \leq \alpha < Pvalue_4$ and $MED_E > MED_{PC}$, then the median of the target population P is assumed to be borderline statistically significantly greater than that of the pseudo-control population Q.

If $Pvalue_5 \leq \alpha < Pvalue_4$ and $MED_E < MED_{PC}$, then the median of the target population P is assumed to be borderline statistically significantly smaller than that of the pseudo-control population Q.

If $\alpha < Pvalue_5 \leq Pvalue_4$, then the median of the target population P is assumed to be statistically indistinguishable from that of the pseudo-control population Q.

For variances:

If $Pvalue_7 \leq Pvalue_6 \leq \alpha$ and $VAR_E > VAR_{PC}$, then the variance of the target population P is assumed to be statistically significantly greater than that of the pseudo-control population Q.

If $Pvalue_7 \leq Pvalue_6 \leq \alpha$ and $VAR_E < VAR_{PC}$, then the variance of the target population P is assumed to be statistically significantly smaller than that of the pseudo-control population Q.

If $Pvalue_7 \leq \alpha < Pvalue_6$ and $VAR_E > VAR_{PC}$, then the variance of the target population P is assumed to be borderline statistically significantly greater than that of the pseudo-control population Q.

If $Pvalue_7 \leq \alpha < Pvalue_6$ and $VAR_E < VAR_{PC}$, then the variance of the target population P is assumed to be borderline statistically significantly smaller than that of the pseudo-control population Q.

If $\alpha < Pvalue_7 \leq Pvalue_6$, then the variance of the target population P is assumed to be statistically indistinguishable from that of the pseudo-control population Q.

For interquartile ranges:

If $Pvalue_9 \leq Pvalue_8 \leq \alpha$ and $IQR_E > IQR_{PC}$, then the interquartile range of the target population P is assumed to be statistically significantly greater than that of the pseudo-control population Q.

If $Pvalue_9 \leq Pvalue_8 \leq \alpha$ and $IQR_E < IQR_{PC}$, then the interquartile range of the target population P is assumed to be statistically significantly smaller than that of the pseudo-control population Q.

If $Pvalue_9 \leq \alpha < Pvalue_8$ and $IQR_E > IQR_{PC}$, then the interquartile range of the target population P is assumed to be borderline statistically significantly greater than that of the pseudo-control population Q.

If $Pvalue_9 \leq \alpha < Pvalue_8$ and $IQR_E < IQR_{PC}$, then the interquartile range of the target population P is assumed to be borderline statistically significantly smaller than that of the pseudo-control population Q.

If $\alpha < Pvalue_9 \leq Pvalue_8$, then the interquartile range of the target population p is assumed to be statistically indistinguishable from that of the pseudo-control population Q.

In the Stage 3 Algorithm, we are not ordering p-values of different statistical tests. Instead, what we aim to do is to calculate whether the one-tail and the two-tail tests are in compliance. In this sense, we explore four pairs of (one-tail—two-tail) tests—FBT2 and FBT3, FBT4 and FBT5, FBT6 and FBT7, and FBT8 and FBT9. If both tests in a pair reject the null hypothesis or if both tests in a pair fail to reject it, the result is clear. However, if the test results in a pair contradict, then there is no consensus in the statistical community as to which test should take precedence. In that case, we assume borderline statistical significance. The proposed Stage 3 Algorithm is a heuristic one that tries to encode common sense for application of statistical tests.

3.4. The Categorization of Differences Between Populations

Since we have defined the statistical significance and favorability of differences in parameter X between the target and the pseudo-control populations, we can now define the category C_t of the established differences in X in the two populations. C_t takes five different values, as follows:

Category 'C_{+1}'—the continuous parameter X indicates a statistically significant, more favorable condition in the target population than in the pseudo-control population.

Category '$C_{+1/2}$'—the continuous parameter X indicates borderline statistically significant, more favorable conditions in the target population than in the pseudo-control population.

Category 'C_0'—the continuous parameter X indicates a statistically insignificant difference in condition for the target and pseudo-control populations.

Category '$C_{-1/2}$'—the continuous parameter X indicates borderline statistically significant, less favorable conditions in the target population than in the pseudo-control population.

Category 'C_{-1}'—the continuous parameter X indicates statistically significant, less favorable conditions in the target population than in the pseudo-control population.

To improve the clarity and compactness of the presentation, we have introduced three conditions. The First Condition holds if the distributions of X in populations P and Q are statistically significantly different, and both characteristics of dispersion in the populations P and Q are not statistically different. The Second Condition holds if the distributions of X in populations P and Q are statistically significantly different, and both characteristics of dispersion in the populations P and Q are statistically indistinguishable. The Third Condition holds if the distributions of X in populations P and Q are borderline statistically significantly different and both characteristics of dispersion in populations P and Q are statistically indistinguishable.

We categorize the differences in the continuous parameter X between the two populations by consecutively testing the following 15 rules:

1. If one of the measures of the location of X in the target population P is statistically significantly more favorable than that in the pseudo-control population Q, whereas the other measure of location in the target population P is neither statistically significantly nor borderline statistically significantly less favorable than that of the pseudo-control population Q, then categorize in C_{+1}.
2. If one of the measures of location of X in the target population P is statistically significantly more favorable than that in the pseudo-control population Q, whereas the other measure of location in the target population P is borderline statistically significantly less favorable than that of the pseudo-control population Q, and the First Condition holds, then categorize in C_{+1}.
3. If one of the measures of location of X in the target population P is borderline statistically significantly more favorable than that in the pseudo-control population Q, whereas the other measure of location in the target population P is either borderline statistically significantly more favorable, or statistically indistinguishable, or neu-

tral to that in the pseudo-control population *Q*, and the First Condition holds, then categorize in C_{+1}.

4. If one of the measures of location of *X* in the target population *P* is statistically insignificantly more favorable than that in the pseudo-control population *Q*, whereas the other measure of location in the target population *P* is either statistically insignificantly more favorable or neutral compared to that in the pseudo-control population *Q*, and the Second Condition holds, then categorize in C_{+1}.
5. If one of the measures of location of *X* in the target population *P* is statistically significantly less favorable than that in the pseudo-control population *Q*, whereas the other measure of location in the target population *P* is neither statistically significantly nor borderline statistically significantly more favorable than that in the pseudo-control population *Q*, then categorize in C_{-1}.
6. If one of the measures of location of *X* in the target population *P* is statistically significantly less favorable than that in the pseudo-control population *Q*, whereas the other measure of location in the target population *P* is borderline statistically significantly more favorable than that in the pseudo-control population *Q*, and the First Condition holds, then categorize in C_{-1}.
7. If one of the measures of location of *X* in the target population *P* is borderline statistically significantly less favorable than that in the pseudo-control population *Q*, whereas the other measure of location in the target population *P* is either borderline statistically significantly less favorable, or statistically indistinguishable, or neutral compared to that in the pseudo-control population *Q*, and the First Condition holds, then categorize in C_{-1}.
8. If one of the measures of location of *X* in the target population *P* is statistically insignificantly less favorable than that in the pseudo-control population *Q*, whereas the other measure of location in the target population *P* is either statistically insignificantly less favorable or neutral compared to that in the pseudo-control population *Q*, and the Second Condition holds, then categorize in C_{-1}.
9. If one of the measures of location of *X* in the target population *P* is statistically significantly more favorable than that in the pseudo-control population *Q*, whereas the other measure of location in the target population *P* is borderline statistically significantly less favorable than that in the pseudo-control population *Q*, then categorize in $C_{+1/2}$.
10. If one of the measures of location of *X* in the target population *P* is borderline statistically significantly more favorable than that in the pseudo-control population *Q*, whereas the other measure of location in the target population *P* is either borderline statistically significantly more favorable, or statistically indistinguishable, or neutral with that in the pseudo-control population *Q*, then categorize in $C_{+1/2}$.
11. If one of the measures of location of *X* in the target population *P* is statistically insignificantly more favorable than that in the pseudo-control population *Q*, whereas the other measure of location in the target population *P* is either statistically insignificantly more favorable or neutral with that in the pseudo-control population *Q*, and the Third Condition holds, then categorize in $C_{+1/2}$.
12. If one of the measures of location of *X* in the target population *P* is statistically significantly less favorable than that in the pseudo-control population *Q*, whereas the other measure of location in the target population *P* is borderline statistically significantly more favorable than that in the pseudo-control population *Q*, then categorize in $C_{-1/2}$.
13. If one of the measures of location of *X* in the target population *P* is borderline statistically significantly less favorable than that in the pseudo-control population *Q*, whereas the other measure of location in the target population *P* is either borderline

statistically significantly less favorable, or statistically indistinguishable, or neutral with that in the pseudo-control population Q, then categorize in $C_{-1/2}$.

14. If one of the measures of location of X in the target population P is statistically insignificantly less favorable than that in the pseudo-control population Q, whereas the other measure of location in the target population P is either statistically insignificantly less favorable or neutral with that in the pseudo-control population Q, and the Third Condition holds, then categorize in $C_{-1/2}$.
15. If none of Rules 1 to 14 apply, then categorize in C_0.

Categorizing the differences between populations consecutively, applying the formulated fifteen rules, can be called the *rule-based approach*.

Alternatively, we can solve the same problem by constructing a discrete function that depends on two discrete variables and three logical variables.

The first input variable is the category C_M of the differences in the means of X in both populations. C_M has seven different discretes, as follows:

M_{00}—when the mean of X in the target population P is neutral compared to that in the pseudo-control population Q.

M_{+1}, $M_{+1/2}$, M_{+0}—when the mean of X in the target population P is, respectively, statistically significant, borderline statistically significant, or statistically insignificant and more favorable than that in the pseudo-control population Q.

M_{-1}, $M_{-1/2}$, M_{-0}—when the mean of X in the target population P is, respectively, statistically significant, borderline statistically significant, or statistically insignificant and less favorable than that in the pseudo-control population Q.

The second input variable is the category C_{MED} of the differences in the medians of X in both populations. C_{MED} has seven different discretes as follows:

MED_{00}—when the median of X in the target population P is neutral compared to that in the pseudo-control population Q.

MED_{+1}, $MED_{+1/2}$, MED_{+0}—when the median of X in the target population P is, respectively, statistically significant, borderline statistically significant, or statistically insignificant and more favorable than that in the pseudo-control population Q.

MED_{-1}, $MED_{-1/2}$, MED_{-0}—when the median of X in the target population P is, respectively, statistically significant, borderline statistically significant, or statistically insignificant and less favorable than that in the pseudo-control population Q.

The third input variable is the validity $Cond_1$ of the First Condition. $Cond_1$ takes the logical values 'T' and 'F' depending on whether the First Condition is true or false.

The fourth input variable is the validity $Cond_2$ of the Second Condition. $Cond_2$ takes the logical values 'T' and 'F' depending on whether the Second Condition is true or false.

The fifth input variable is the validity $Cond_3$ of the Third Condition. $Cond_3$ takes the logical values 'T' and 'F' depending on whether the Third Condition is true or false.

Now, we can define the function of categorization C_t as:

$$C_t = C_t(C_M, C_{MED}, Cond_1, Cond_2, Cond_3) \tag{20}$$

Table 1 presents the values of the discrete function C_t depending on the values of the input variables. The third column of the table depends on the logical variables $Cond_1$, $Cond_2$, and $Cond_3$ and is different in each case. If a line in that column is empty, then the categorization does not depend on the three logical variables.

Performing stage 4 of MFPCG using Table 1 can be called the *function-based approach*.

Table 1. The discrete categorization function C_t values depending on the C_M, C_{MED}, $Cond_1$, $Cond_2$, and $Cond_3$ input variables. The last column shows the rule that defines C_t.

C_M	C_{MED}	Generalized Condition	C_t	Rule
M_{+1}	MED_{+1}		C_{+1}	1
M_{+1}	$MED_{+1/2}$		C_{+1}	1
M_{+1}	MED_{+0}		C_{+1}	1
M_{+1}	MED_{00}		C_{+1}	1
M_{+1}	MED_{-0}		C_{+1}	1
M_{+1}	$MED_{-1/2}$	$Cond_1$ = T	C_{+1}	2
M_{+1}	$MED_{-1/2}$	$Cond_1$ = F	$C_{+1/2}$	9
M_{+1}	MED_{-1}		C_0	15
$M_{+1/2}$	MED_{+1}		C_{+1}	1
$M_{+1/2}$	$MED_{+1/2}$	$Cond_1$ = T	C_{+1}	3
$M_{+1/2}$	$MED_{+1/2}$	$Cond_1$ = F	$C_{+1/2}$	10
$M_{+1/2}$	MED_{+0}	$Cond_1$ = T	C_{+1}	3
$M_{+1/2}$	MED_{+0}	$Cond_1$ = F	$C_{+1/2}$	10
$M_{+1/2}$	MED_{00}	$Cond_1$ = T	C_{+1}	3
$M_{+1/2}$	MED_{00}	$Cond_1$ = F	$C_{+1/2}$	10
$M_{+1/2}$	MED_{-0}	$Cond_1$ = T	C_{+1}	3
$M_{+1/2}$	MED_{-0}	$Cond_1$ = F	$C_{+1/2}$	10
$M_{+1/2}$	$MED_{-1/2}$		C_0	15
$M_{+1/2}$	MED_{-1}	$Cond_1$ = T	C_{-1}	6
$M_{+1/2}$	MED_{-1}	$Cond_1$ = F	$C_{-1/2}$	12
M_{+0}	MED_{+1}		C_{+1}	1
M_{+0}	$MED_{+1/2}$	$Cond_1$ = T	C_{+1}	3
M_{+0}	$MED_{+1/2}$	$Cond_1$ = F	$C_{+1/2}$	10
M_{+0}	MED_{+0}	$Cond_2$ = T	C_{+1}	4
M_{+0}	MED_{+0}	$Cond_2$ = F and $Cond_3$ = T	$C_{+1/2}$	11
M_{+0}	MED_{+0}	$Cond_2$ = F and $Cond_3$ = F	C_0	15
M_{+0}	MED_{00}	$Cond_2$ = T	C_{+1}	4
M_{+0}	MED_{00}	$Cond_2$ = F and $Cond_3$ = T	$C_{+1/2}$	11
M_{+0}	MED_{00}	$Cond_2$ = F and $Cond_3$ = F	C_0	15
M_{+0}	MED_{-0}		C_0	15
M_{+0}	$MED_{-1/2}$	$Cond_1$ = T	C_{-1}	7
M_{+0}	$MED_{-1/2}$	$Cond_1$ = F	$C_{-1/2}$	13
M_{+0}	MED_{-1}		C_{-1}	5
M_{00}	MED_{+1}		C_{+1}	1
M_{00}	$MED_{+1/2}$	$Cond_1$ = T	C_{+1}	3
M_{00}	$MED_{+1/2}$	$Cond_1$ = F	$C_{+1/2}$	10
M_{00}	MED_{+0}	$Cond_2$ = T	C_{+1}	4
M_{00}	MED_{+0}	$Cond_2$ = F and $Cond_3$ = T	$C_{+1/2}$	11
M_{00}	MED_{+0}	$Cond_2$ = F and $Cond_3$ = F	C_0	15

Table 1. *Cont.*

C_M	C_{MED}	Generalized Condition	C_t	Rule
M_{00}	MED_{00}		C_0	15
M_{00}	MED_{-0}	$Cond_2$ = T	C_{-1}	8
M_{00}	MED_{-0}	$Cond_2$ = F and $Cond_3$ = T	$C_{-1/2}$	14
M_{00}	MED_{-0}	$Cond_2$ = F and $Cond_3$ = F	C_0	15
M_{00}	$MED_{-1/2}$	$Cond_1$ = T	C_{-1}	7
M_{00}	$MED_{-1/2}$	$Cond_1$ = F	$C_{-1/2}$	13
M_{00}	MED_{-1}		C_{-1}	5
M_{-0}	MED_{+1}		C_{+1}	1
M_{-0}	$MED_{+1/2}$	$Cond_1$ = T	C_{+1}	3
M_{-0}	$MED_{+1/2}$	$Cond_1$ = F	$C_{+1/2}$	10
M_{-0}	MED_{+0}		C_0	15
M_{-0}	MED_{00}	$Cond_2$ = T	C_{-1}	8
M_{-0}	MED_{00}	$Cond_2$ = F and $Cond_3$ = T	$C_{-1/2}$	14
M_{-0}	MED_{00}	$Cond_2$ = F and $Cond_3$ = F	C_0	15
M_{-0}	MED_{-0}	$Cond_2$ = T	C_{-1}	8
M_{-0}	MED_{-0}	$Cond_2$ = F and $Cond_3$ = T	$C_{-1/2}$	14
M_{-0}	MED_{-0}	$Cond_2$ = F and $Cond_3$ = F	C_0	15
M_{-0}	$MED_{-1/2}$	$Cond_1$ = T	C_{-1}	7
M_{-0}	$MED_{-1/2}$	$Cond_1$ = F	$C_{-1/2}$	13
M_{-0}	MED_{-1}		C_{-1}	5
$M_{-1/2}$	MED_{+1}	$Cond_1$ = T	C_{+1}	2
$M_{-1/2}$	MED_{+1}	$Cond_1$ = F	$C_{+1/2}$	9
$M_{-1/2}$	$MED_{+1/2}$		C_0	15
$M_{-1/2}$	MED_{+0}	$Cond_1$ = T	C_{-1}	7
$M_{-1/2}$	MED_{+0}	$Cond_1$ = F	$C_{-1/2}$	13
$M_{-1/2}$	MED_{00}	$Cond_1$ = T	C_{-1}	7
$M_{-1/2}$	MED_{00}	$Cond_1$ = F	$C_{-1/2}$	13
$M_{-1/2}$	MED_{-0}	$Cond_1$ = T	C_{-1}	7
$M_{-1/2}$	MED_{-0}	$Cond_1$ = F	$C_{-1/2}$	13
$M_{-1/2}$	$MED_{-1/2}$	$Cond_1$ = T	C_{-1}	7
$M_{-1/2}$	$MED_{-1/2}$	$Cond_1$ = F	$C_{-1/2}$	13
$M_{-1/2}$	MED_{-1}		C_{-1}	5
M_{-1}	MED_{+1}		C_0	15
M_{-1}	$MED_{+1/2}$	$Cond_1$ = T	C_{-1}	6
M_{-1}	$MED_{+1/2}$	$Cond_1$ = F	$C_{-1/2}$	12
M_{-1}	MED_{+0}		C_{-1}	5
M_{-1}	MED_{00}		C_{-1}	5
M_{-1}	MED_{-0}		C_{-1}	5

Table 1. *Cont.*

C_M	C_{MED}	Generalized Condition	C_t	Rule
M_{-1}	$MED_{-1/2}$		C_{-1}	5
M_{-1}	MED_{-1}		C_{-1}	5

3.5. The Classification of the MFPCG Result

Let b be an integer from the set $\{+1, +1/2, 0, -1/2, -1\}$ that coincides with the index of the category C_b, where the differences in the values of parameter X in the target population P and the pseudo-control population Q were categorized. Let e be an integer from the set $\{+1, +1/2, 0, -1/2, -1\}$ that coincides with the index of the category C_e, where the differences between the values of parameter X in the target population P and the pseudo-control population Q were categorized. The ordered pair (C_b, C_e) is the MFPCG result and depends on the data in the four samples: E_b, PC_b, E_e, and PC_e.

Using the MFPCG result, we can categorize the favorability and significance of the influence of the explored effect R over the selected parameter X into five classes, as follows:

Class 'YES+'—the effect R has a statistically significantly favorable influence over parameter X.

Class 'GR+'—the effect R has a borderline statistically significantly favorable influence over parameter X.

Class 'NO'—the effect R has neither statistically nor borderline statistically significant influence over parameter X.

Class 'GR−'—the effect R has a borderline statistically significantly unfavorable influence over parameter X.

Class 'YES−'—the effect R has a statistically significantly unfavorable influence over parameter X.

We perform the classification using an empirical rule that determines the influence of the effect over parameter X, using the MFPCG result:

$$\text{Classify the MFPCG result } (C_b,\ C_e) \text{ in } \begin{cases} \text{'YES+'} & \text{, if} \quad b - e < -1/2 \\ \text{'GR+'} & \text{, if} \quad b - e = -1/2 \\ \text{'NO'} & \text{, if} \quad b - e = 0 \\ \text{'GR}-\text{'} & \text{, if} \quad b - e = +1/2 \\ \text{'YES}-\text{'} & \text{, if} \quad b - e > +1/2 \end{cases} . \tag{21}$$

3.6. MFPCG Algorithm and Flowchat of the Method

Let the continuous parameters, X_1, X_2, …, and X_n, be proxies for the outcome of intervention R over the target population P compared with the pseudo-control population Q where R was not applied.

We shall integrate the five key stages shown in the previous subsections into a general algorithm of MFPCG for identifying the influence of R over X_1, X_2, …, and X_n using samples from the two populations.

MFPCG Algorithm

1. Select the significance level, α, and the number of pseudo-realities, N, of the Bootstrap statistical tests.
2. Set $i = 1$.
3. Choose $X = X_i$.
4. Extract from the database the fuzzy samples E_b, PC_b, E_e, and PC_e for this X.

5. Perform stage 1 of MFPCG and expertly determine for X the optimal value margins $X_{d,opt}$, $X_{u,opt}$, and the insignificant change threshold ΔX.
6. Perform stage 2 of MFPCG for E_b and PC_b.
7. Perform stage 2 of MFPCG for E_e and PC_e.
8. Repeat for Bootstrap Modification BMk (k = 1, 2, 3, 4):
    8.1. Perform stage 3 of MFPCG for E_b and PC_b using Bootstrap Modification BMk with N pseudo-realities for each Bootstrap test using significance level α.
    8.2. Perform stage 4 of MFPCG for E_b and PC_b using Bootstrap Modification BMk.
    8.3. Perform stage 3 of MFPCG for E_e and PC_e using Bootstrap Modification BMk with N pseudo-realities for each Bootstrap test using significance level α.
    8.4. Perform stage 4 of MFPCG for E_e and PC_e using Bootstrap Modification BMk.
    8.5. Perform stage 5 of MFPCG for Bootstrap Modification BMk and find the BMk class.
9. Set $i = i + 1$.
10. If $i < n$, then go to step 3. Otherwise, end the algorithm.

Apart from the method's main stages, the steps of the above algorithm are self-explanatory and trivial. In their entirety, the results answer the question of how R influences the continuous proxies X_1, X_2, …, and X_n. To determine R's overall influence, all $4n$ influences (for each Bootstrap Modification and each variable) need to be accumulated.

The flowchart of the method is given in Figure 1.

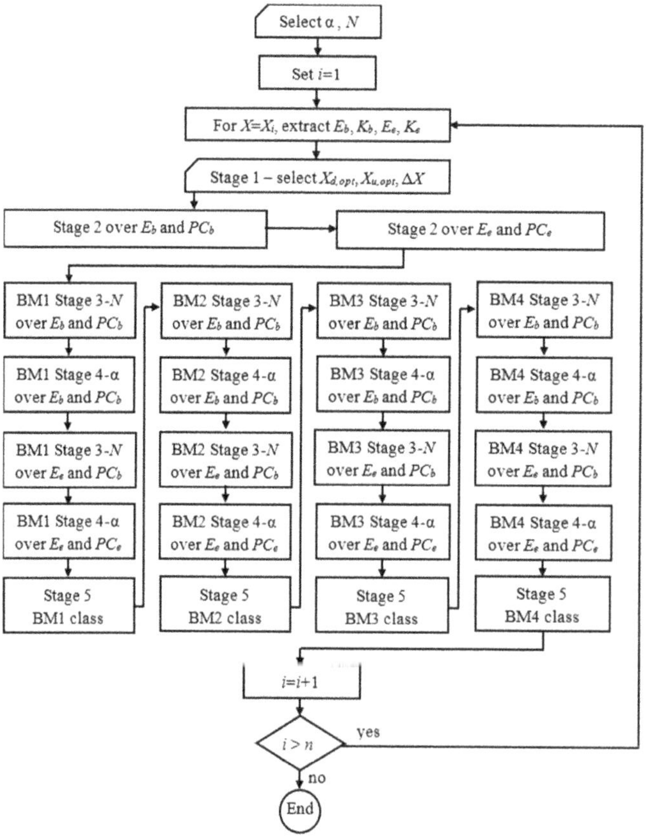

Figure 1. Flowchart of the MFPCG.

The MFPCG Algorithm and flowchart show the MFPCG results in four qualitative assessments for the favorability of intervention R over the target population for each of the proxies, X_i, of the intervention outcome. MFPCG does not need numerous assumptions to justify its conclusion, if any. The only notable exception is the hill preference assumption that, on the one hand, is easily proven if present and, on the other hand, is a significant relaxation of the monotonic preference assumption required in DID.

4. Annuloplasty Favorability Case Study

We shall illustrate our proposed method with a case study from medical practice.

Ischemic heart disease (IHD) (also known as coronary heart disease or coronary artery disease) is among the most common heart diseases worldwide. When IHD is additionally complicated with a secondary mitral regurgitation (*MR*), the mitral valve (MV) between the left heart chambers (the left atrium, LA, and the left ventricle, LV) does not fully close. Blood leaks backward across the valve and into the LA to form the regurgitation volume (RV). The prognosis for patients with ischemic *MR* (IMR) is worse than when the *MR* is caused by other conditions (e.g., primary *MR*, which is caused by a primary abnormality of one or more components of the valve apparatus—leaflets, chordae tendineae, papillary muscles, annulus, etc.). Such patients suffer an abnormality of the myocardium of the LV of the heart that leads to the remodeling of the LV and dislocation of the papillary muscles. This complex mechanism is the leading cause of IMR, which deteriorates over time and can cause various levels of heart failure [41–43]. Patients with mild IMR (also called grade I) usually undergo an isolated coronary artery bypass graft (CABG). Patients with severe IMR traditionally undergo a combined operation that includes mitral valve repair (MVRepair) through annuloplasty or valve replacement, combined with a coronary artery bypass (MVRepair + CABG). These surgical recommendations are well-accepted in medical practice [44].

When patients have moderate or moderate-to-severe IMR, the optimal treatment is rigorously debated due to factors such as recurring IMR several months to several years after surgery, long-term survival rates, etc. Research in favor of the combined intervention is proposed in [45–49]. Research that outlined the shortcomings of anuloplasty in such patients is provided in [50–52]. The available studies included comparatively small groups of patients, and the results are hard to compare, as the studies used different diagnostic criteria and operation techniques. Our analysis aims to demonstrate if annuloplasty positively influences patients with moderate and moderate-to-severe IMR.

Part of the patients with IMR in our study underwent MVRepair+CABG (group A), whereas the rest underwent only CABG (group B). The choice of surgical treatment in the case of IMR is not trivial, for the reasons outlined above. The choice of an approach faces the following difficulties:

(1) Traditionally, the classification of patients is based on subjective expertise. There is no specific measure of how typical a patient is to a given group.
(2) The groups are not homogenous. Therefore, comparing them is complicated.

Some patients are very suitable for a given procedure; others are clearly unsuitable for this procedure, but the decision is unclear and ambiguous for the remaining patients. A previous study offered two stratification algorithms to allocate the patients in each group into two comparatively more homogenous subgroups depending on the preoperative medical status of patients: comparatively preserved status (subgroups A_1 and B_1) and comparatively deteriorated status (subgroups A_2 and B_2) [53]. This allows us to avoid comparing the groups A and B. Instead, we will compare A_1 and B_1 on one hand and A_2 and B_2 on the other. As a result, we can adequately assess the effect of the annuloplasty.

We shall demonstrate the application of MFPCG to assess the effect of the annuloplasty (R) that acts in conjunction with the base intervention of revascularization (V) over two of the continuous parameters (X_1 and X_2), described in Section 4.1, that characterize the condition of the target population (P) of patients with moderate and moderate-to-severe IMR subjected to a combined procedure (MVRepair + CABG). The values of each parameter X for the patients in the experimental group A are measured before and after the combined procedure. We judge the effect of the annuloplasty in comparison with the effect of the isolated procedure over the same parameter X, which now characterizes the condition of the pseudo-control population (Q) of patients with severe IMR subjected to isolated revascularization (CABG). The values of parameter X are measured before and after the isolated CABG for the patients from the pseudo-control group B.

4.1. Database

The database for this case study contains the records of 169 patients with IHD (that required revascularization) and moderate and moderate-to-severe chronic IMR. The data are presented in [16]. The study was conducted among patients from the Clinic of Cardiovascular Surgery in UH "St. Marina", Varna (Bulgaria), who underwent surgery due to IHD complicated with *MR* in the period from 2007 to 2022. These patients were subjected to an MVRepair+CABG (group A) or to an isolated CABG (group B) [15]. In the study, each group was further divided into two comparatively homogenous subgroups:

- Those with a comparatively preserved medical state (A_1 and B_1)
- Those with a comparatively deteriorated medical state (A_2 and B_2).

The following parameters are measured and archived for each patient:

- 20 identifiers;
- 18 anamnesis and clinical preoperative parameters; and
- 13 three-dimensional (triple) echocardiographic parameters.

The parameters were collected as part of the patient's anamnesis or using echocardiographic equipment GE Vivid 7 PRO (till 2017) and GE Vivid 95 (afterward) (Minneapolis, MN, USA). All patients were subjected to transthoracic echocardiogram (TTE). The 13 three-dimensional parameters are measured in three different time intervals: (1) prior to surgery, (2) soon after surgery (from 5 to 30 days after surgery), and (3) late after surgery (from 6 to 54 months after surgery). So, each three-dimensional parameter contains three values at different time points. As a result, each patient is described with a 75-dimensional record that contains the above-listed parameters.

4.2. Division into Groups with Fuzzy Degrees of Membership

The work [54] presented three (one main and two auxiliary) fuzzy algorithms, which produce the degree of membership of each patient to a specific fuzzy subgroup based on the parameters available before the surgery (which are part of the 75-dimensional record for each patient). The procedures used the age of the patients, the 18 anamnesis and clinical preoperative parameters, and the preoperative values of the 13 three-dimensional echocardiographic parameters. The resulting degrees of membership coincide with the subjectively defined ones by the medical team, which are confirmed at the end of the measurement based on all parameters. Finding the degrees of membership of each patient is a form of classification that shows much better performance than other such classifiers. This is unsurprising given that the fuzzy algorithms form a specialized classifier that relies on object-specific knowledge, whereas the others are general classifiers. The fuzzy algorithms have substantially better performance measures than their crisp counterparts. That also is to be expected, since the former use more information than the latter, which incorrectly assumes that any patient is a typical representative of its group.

The main algorithm (MA) from [54] generates a fuzzy partition of the patients into two fuzzy sets (A and B) using their degrees of membership. Due to the lack of homogeneity in those two sets, the work proposed two auxiliary algorithms. They stratify each group into two homogenous subgroups according to medical state (comparatively preserved or comparatively deteriorated) using the conditional degrees of membership to the subgroups. This way, the approach is personalized and reduces the risk of incorrect decisions. It also allows for higher precision in allocating resources for the medical treatment of patients. The work compared the results of their approach with classical approaches, including Bayesian classifiers. The advantages of the classification achieved using the fuzzy algorithms were demonstrated using four criteria, including the ability of the algorithms to discern typical patients from outliers and generate a numerical estimate of the degree of typicality of patients to the subgroups.

In our paper, we use a slightly optimized version of those fuzzy algorithms. We also adapted the fuzzy algorithms to the new patient data obtained after [54] was published.

4.3. Assessing the Effect of Annuloplasty for Patients with Severe IMR Using Fuzzy Pseudo-Control Groups

We shall demonstrate the effect of annuloplasty according to two of the most significant integral diagnostic parameters that summarize the IMR status of the patient: *RF* (regurgitation fraction, in %) and *MR* (mitral regurgitation in an 8-level scale). Both parameters are measured three times: preoperatively (when the patient is admitted to the Clinic for cardiovascular surgery), early postoperatively (7–10 days after surgery), and late postoperatively (ambulatory check-ups from 6 to 54 months after surgery).

The *RF* (%) is interpreted through three separate parameters: preoperative regurgitation fraction (*Preop_RF*), early postoperative regurgitation fraction (*Early_Postop_RF*), and late postoperative regurgitation fraction (*Late_Postop_RF*). In each of its three forms, this parameter is a continuous variable measured in % and is calculated as the regurgitation volume divided by the total ejected volume (*LVEDV–LVESV*) [55]:

$$RF = 100 \times RV/(LVEDV - LVESV). \tag{22}$$

Here, *LVEDV* is the left ventricular end-systolic volume in mL, *LVESV* is the left ventricular end-diastolic volume in mL, and *RV* is the regurgitation volume through the MV in mL, which is the volume of blood that returns into the atrium through the mitral valve.

LVEDV and *LVESV* are calculated using a modified Simpson's rule with an apical 2nd and 4th chamber position, described in [56].

RV is measured from the 4th apical position using color and CW Doppler, and the radius of the proximal isovelocity surface area (*PISAr*) is manually measured using a magnified image and reduced Nyquist usually to 40–45, which allows us to outline the boundaries of *PISA* clearly. Each of the three parameters is measured three times, as a preoperative (*Preop_LVEDV*, *Preop_LVESV*, *Preop_RV*), early postoperative (*Early_Postop_LVEDV*, *Early_Postop_LVESV*, *Early_Postop_RVR*), and late postoperative (*Late_Postop_LVEDV*, *Late_Postop_LVESV*, *Late_Postop_RV*) parameter. In that sense, Equation (22) is three formulae, one per each period.

According to Section 3.1, expert estimates were obtained as follows: $X_{opt,d} = RF_{opt,d} = 0\%$, $X_{opt,up} = RF_{opt,up} = 1\%$, and $\Delta X = \Delta RF = 2\%$.

The grade of mitral regurgitation (*MR*) is measured by an 8-level scale: 0—lack of *MR*; 1—(grade 0–I) trivial *MR*; 2—(grade I) mild *MR*; 3—(grade I–II) mild-to-moderate *MR*; 4—(grade II) moderate *MR*; 5—(grade II–III) moderate-to-high *MR*; 6—(grade III) high *MR*; 7—(grade above III) severe *MR*. The grade of *MR* is presented through three parameters: preoperative grade of mitral regurgitation (*Preop_MR*), early postoperative grade of mitral regurgitation (*Early_Postop_MR*), and late postoperative grade of mitral regurgitation (*Late_Postop_MR*). Strictly speaking, *MR* is a discrete parameter, yet the large count of discretes (eight) allows for an approximation by a continuous parameter at a negligible discretization error. In this way, we illustrate the ability of MFPCG to assess the influence of the effect using a continuous parameter X, measured in an ordinal scale with five or more discretes.

According to Section 3.1, expert estimates were obtained as follows: $X_{opt,d} = MR_{opt,d} = 0$, $X_{opt,up} = MR_{opt,up} = 1$, and $\Delta X = \Delta MR = 0.5$.

On the one hand, we assess the effect of annuloplasty using MFPCG for patients with a relatively preserved medical state by comparing the values of both parameters for subgroups A_1 and B_1. We use four fuzzy samples for *RF* and four fuzzy samples for *MR*, as Sections 4.3.1 and 4.3.2 demonstrate. The fuzzy samples are formed using all patients with the necessary characteristics, regardless of whether those are typical or outliers.

On the other hand, we assess the same effect for patients with a relatively deteriorated medical state and compare the values of *MR* and *RF* for subgroups A_2 and B_2. We use four different fuzzy samples for *MR* and four different fuzzy samples for *RF*, as Sections 4.3.3 and 4.3.4 show. The fuzzy samples were also formed using all patients with the necessary characteristics, regardless of whether those are typical or outliers.

In essence, we should apply the MFPCG four times to solve the following tasks:

(Task 1) Assess the effect of annuloplasty over *RF* for patients with a relatively preserved medical state.

(Task 2) Assess the effect of annuloplasty over *MR* for patients with a relatively preserved medical state.

(Task 3) Assess the effect of annuloplasty over *RF* for patients with a relatively deteriorated medical state.

(Task 4) Assess the effect of annuloplasty over *MR* for patients with a relatively deteriorated medical state.

We solved the four tasks at a significance level of $\alpha = 0.05$. The Bootstrap simulation for each statistical test is performed with $N = 2000$ pseudo-realities.

We form four fuzzy samples for each of the four tasks, as described in Section 1:

- E_b is a fuzzy sample that contains the values of X and their degrees of membership to the experimental group A_i before the combined intervention.
- PC_b is a fuzzy sample that contains the values of X and their degrees of membership to the pseudo-control group B_i before the isolated intervention.
- E_e is a fuzzy sample that contains the values of X and their degrees of membership to the experimental group A_i late after the combined intervention.
- PC_e is a fuzzy sample that contains the values of X and their degrees of membership to the pseudo-control group B_i late after the isolated intervention.

4.3.1. Effect of Annuloplasty over RF for Patients with Relatively Preserved Medical State (Task 1)

In task 1, we use four fuzzy samples for *RF*, as described below.

E_b is a fuzzy sample that contains 34 values of *Preop_RF* and their degrees of membership to the experimental group A_1:

$E_b = \chi^{RF}_{A_1,preop}$ = {(57,0.630), (63,0.900), (42,0.630), (42,0.630), (57,0.360), (64,0.810), (39,0.810), (47,0.630), (55,0.900), (65,0.630), (37,0.630), (67,0.630), (65,0.490), (62,0.630), (65,0.700), (31,0.490), (53,0.630), (64,0.630), (44,0.630), (56,0.630), (68,0.700), (43,0.900), (55,0.630), (36,0.630), (55,0.490), (55,0.900), (68,0.630), (37,0.490), (64,0.630), (56,0.490), (49,0.630), (69,0.700), (45,0.900), (56,0.700)}.

PC_b is a fuzzy sample that contains 43 values of *Preop_RF* and their degrees of membership to the pseudo-control group B_1:

$PC_b = \chi^{RF}_{B_1,preop}$ = {(34,0.900), (62,0.810), (28,0.900), (38,0.900), (59,0.630), (51,0.810), (38,0.630), (39,0.900), (36,0.810), (28,0.900), (24,0.900), (59,0.630), (38,0.490), (49,0.810), (40,0.900), (59,0.630), (35,0.630), (47,0.630), (24,0.490), (48,0.810), (25,0.900), (38,0.490), (34,0.900), (32,0.900), (21,0.490), (37,0.810), (22,0.630), (26,0.900), (34,0.810), (29,0.630), (36,0.900), (36,0.630), (60,0.490), (20,0.630), (21,0.900), (32,0.900), (15,0.900), (19,0.900), (31,0.700), (41,0.700), (36,0.700), (39,0.700), (21,0.357)}.

E_e is a fuzzy sample that contains 32 values of *Late_Postop_RF* and their degrees of membership to the experimental group A_1:

$E_e = \chi^{RF}_{A_1,Lpostop}$ = {(0,0.630), (37,0.900), (27,0.630), (43,0.630), (0,0.360), (24,0.810), (18,0.810), (12,0.630), (0,0.900), (0,0.630), (0,0.630), (0,0.630), (0,0.630), (13,0.700), (0,0.630), (0,0.630), (0,0.630), (0,0.630), (0,0.700), (0,0.900), (17,0.630), (12,0.630), (0,0.490), (0,0.900), (0,0.630), (0,0.490), (0,0.630), (18,0.490), (0,0.630), (8,0.700), (7,0.900), (0,0.700)}.

PC_e is a fuzzy sample that contains 41 values of *Late_Postop_RF* and their degrees of membership to the pseudo-control group B_1:

$PC_e = \chi^{RF}_{B_1,Lpostop}$ = {(0,0.900), (43,0.810), (6,0.900), (13,0.900), (88,0.630), (39,0.810), (48,0.630), (12,0.900), (65,0.810), (14,0.900), (0,0.900), (48,0.490), (41,0.810), (11,0.900), (38,0.630), (12,0.630), (14,0.630), (36,0.490), (58,0.810), (27,0.900), (0,0.490), (19,0.900), (24,0.900), (65,0.490), (23,0.630), (12,0.900), (43,0.810), (10,0.630), (18,0.900), (30,0.630), (41,0.490), (23,0.630), (0,0.900), (21,0.900), (33,0.900), (12,0.900), (0,0.700), (22,0.700), (0,0.700), (24,0.700), (0,0.357)}.

Table 2 presents the numerical characteristics of the four fuzzy samples.

Table 2. The numerical characteristics and change favorability for the *RF* fuzzy samples for groups A_1 and B_1.

Sample	E_b	PC_b	R Favorability	E_e	PC_e	R Favorability
No. of observations	34	43	N/A	32	41	N/A
Fuzzy mean, %	54	35.5	unfavorable	7.79	24.2	favorable
Fuzzy median, %	55.1	35.2	unfavorable	0	20.7	favorable
Fuzzy STD, %	10.8	11.8	N/A	12.1	20.1	N/A
Fuzzy IQR, %	19.9	12.3	N/A	12.8	26.6	N/A

First, let us assess the influence of annuloplasty on the preoperative *RF* values.

According to Section 3.2, from $RF_{u,opt} + \Delta RF = 1 + 2 = 3\% \leq M_{PC} = 35.5\% \leq (M_E - \Delta RF) = 54 - 2 = 52\%$, it follows that M_E is less favorable than M_{PC}. This is indicated in column four of Table 2. From $RF_{u,opt} + \Delta RF = 1 + 2 = 3\% \leq MED_{PC} = 35.2\% \leq (MED_E - \Delta RF) = 55.1 - 2 = 53.1\%$, it follows that MED_E is less favorable than MED_{PC}. This is indicated in column four of Table 2.

Line two of Table 3 presents the *p*-values for the nine Bootstrap statistical tests for the BM1 Bootstrap. According to the Stage 3 Algorithm, since $Pvalue_1 = 0 \leq \alpha = 0.05$, then the preoperative population distributions of *RF* are assumed to be statistically significantly different. Since $Pvalue_3 = 0 \leq Pvalue_2 = 0 \leq \alpha = 0.05$ and $M_E = 54\% > M_{PC} = 35.5\%$, then the preoperative mean in the target population A_1 is assumed to be statistically significantly greater than that in the pseudo-control population B_1. Since $Pvalue_5 = 0 \leq Pvalue_4 = 0 \leq \alpha = 0.05$ and $MED_E = 55.1\% > MED_{PC} = 35.2\%$, then the preoperative median of the target population A_1 is assumed to be statistically significantly greater than that in the pseudo-control population B_1. Since $\alpha = 0.05 < Pvalue_7 = 0.248 \leq Pvalue_6 = 0.4995$, then the preoperative variance of the target population A_1 is assumed statistically indistinguishable from that in the pseudo-control population B_1. Since $\alpha = 0.05 < Pvalue_9 = 0.0975 \leq Pvalue_8 = 0.169$, then the preoperative interquartile interval of the target population A_1 is assumed statistically indistinguishable from that in the pseudo-control population B_1.

Table 3. The p-values of the fuzzy Bootstrap statistical tests in MFPCG for parameter RF, comparing subgroups A_1 and B_1.

Modification	Time	FBT1	FBT2	FBT3	FBT4	FBT5	FBT6	FBT7	FBT8	FBT9
BM1	Preop	0.0000	0.0000	0.0000	0.0000	0.0000	0.4995	0.2480	0.1690	0.0975
BM1	Late_Postop	0.0010	0.0000	0.0000	0.0000	0.0000	0.0335	0.0270	0.1870	0.1800
BM2	Preop	0.0000	0.0000	0.0000	0.0000	0.0000	0.5360	0.2565	0.1785	0.1170
BM2	Late_Postop	0.0010	0.0000	0.0000	0.0005	0.0000	0.0285	0.0160	0.1745	0.1495
BM3	Preop	0.0000	0.0000	0.0000	0.0000	0.0000	0.5310	0.2670	0.2075	0.1155
BM3	Late_Postop	0.0010	0.0000	0.0000	0.0010	0.0000	0.0340	0.0320	0.1735	0.1670
BM4	Preop	0.0000	0.0000	0.0000	0.0000	0.0000	0.5410	0.2420	0.1720	0.1135
BM4	Late_Postop	0.0000	0.0000	0.0000	0.0005	0.0000	0.0320	0.0195	0.1500	0.1300

We obtained detailed results for the other three Bootstrap Modifications. Their p-values are given in lines 4, 6, and 8 of Table 3.

Let us categorize the differences between A_1 and B_1 using the BM1 Bootstrap. Section 3.4 defines the values of the five input variables of the discrete categorization function (20). The preoperative differences in the means of RF in the populations A_1 and B_1 are $C_M = M_{-1}$ (the preoperative mean of RF in the target population A_1 is statistically significantly less favorable than that in the pseudo-control population B_1). The preoperative differences in the medians of RF in the populations A_1 and B_1 are $C_{MED} = MED_1$ (the preoperative median of RF in the target population A_1 is statistically significantly less favorable than that in the pseudo-control population B_1). $Cond_1$ = T, since the distributions of RF in populations A_1 and B_1 are statistically significantly different, and the two characteristics of dispersion in populations A_1 and B_1 are not statistically different. $Cond_2$ = T, since the distributions of RF in populations A_1 and B_1 are statistically significantly different, and both characteristics of dispersion in populations A_1 and B_1 are statistically indistinguishable. $Cond_3$ = F, since the distributions of RF in the populations A_1 and B_1 are not borderline statistically significantly different.

According to the last line of Table 1, the preoperative differences in the continuous parameter RF between the two populations A_1 and B_1 are categorized as $C_t = C_{-1}$. We can see from the same line of Table 1 that we have applied Rule 5: if one of the measures of location of RF in the target population A_1 is statistically significantly less favorable than that in the pseudo-control population B_1, whereas the other measure of location in the target population A_1 is neither statistically significantly nor borderline statistically significantly more favorable than that in the pseudo-control population B_1, then categorize in C_{-1}.

Columns 3 to 9 on line two of Table 4 show the input variables' values and the categorization function's values. We obtained similar results for the remaining three Bootstrap Modifications shown in lines 4, 6, and 8 of Table 4.

Let us now assess the influence of annuloplasty on the late postoperative RF values.

According to Section 3.2, from $RF_{u,opt} + \Delta RF = 1 + 2 = 3\% \leq M_E = 7.79\% \leq (M_{PC} - \Delta RF) = 24.2\% - 2\% = 22.2\%$, it follows that M_E is more favorable than M_{PC}. This is indicated in column seven of Table 2. From $RF_{d,opt} - \Delta RF = 0 - 2 = -2\% < MED_E = 0\% < RF_{u,opt} + \Delta RF = 1 + 2 = 3\% \leq max\{RF_{u,opt} - \Delta RF, MED_E + \Delta RF\} =$

$max\{0-2, 0+2\} = 2\% \leq MED_{PC} = 20.7\%$, it follows that MED_E is more favorable than MED_{PC}. This is indicated in column seven of Table 2.

Table 4. The MFPCG diagnostics of the influence of R on a continuous parameter RF, comparing subgroups A_1 and B_1.

Modification	Time	C_M	C_{MED}	$Cond_1$	$Cond_2$	$Cond_3$	C_t	Rule	Result of MFPCG	Class
BM1	Preop	M_{-1}	MED_{-1}	T	T	F	C_{-1}	5	$(C_b, C_e) = (C_{-1}, C_{+1})$	YES+
BM1	Late_Postop	M_{+1}	MED_{+1}	F	F	F	C_{+1}	1		
BM2	Preop	M_{-1}	MED_{-1}	T	T	F	C_{-1}	5	$(C_b, C_e) = (C_{-1}, C_{+1})$	YES+
BM2	Late_Postop	M_{+1}	MED_{+1}	F	F	F	C_{+1}	1		
BM3	Preop	M_{-1}	MED_{-1}	T	T	F	C_{-1}	5	$(C_b, C_e) = (C_{-1}, C_{+1})$	YES+
BM3	Late_Postop	M_{+1}	MED_{+1}	F	F	F	C_{+1}	1		
BM4	Preop	M_{-1}	MED_{-1}	T	T	F	C_{-1}	5	$(C_b, C_e) = (C_{-1}, C_{+1})$	YES+
BM4	Late_Postop	M_{+1}	MED_{+1}	F	F	F	C_{+1}	1		

Line three of Table 3 presents the p-values for the nine Bootstrap statistical tests for the first Bootstrap Modification.

The p-values of the nine Bootstrap statistical tests for BM1 Bootstrap are given on line three of Table 3. According to Section 3.3, since $Pvalue_1 = 0.01 \leq \alpha = 0.05$, then the late postoperative population distributions of RF are assumed to be statistically significantly different. Since $Pvalue_3 = 0 \leq Pvalue_2 = 0 \leq \alpha = 0.05$ and $M_E = 7.79\% < M_{PC} = 24.2\%$, then the late postoperative mean of the target population A_1 is assumed to be statistically significantly smaller than that in the pseudo-control population B_1. Since $Pvalue_5 = 0 \leq Pvalue_4 = 0 \leq \alpha = 0.05$ and $MED_E = 0\% < MED_{PC} = 20.7\%$, then the late postoperative median of the target population A_1 is assumed to be statistically significantly smaller than that in the pseudo-control population B_1. Since $Pvalue_7 = 0.027 \leq Pvalue_6 = 0.0335 \leq \alpha = 0.05$ and $VAR_E = 12.1^2 < VAR_{PC} = 20.1^2$, then the late postoperative variance of the target population A_1 is assumed to be statistically significantly smaller than that in the pseudo-control population B_1. Since $\alpha = 0.05 < Pvalue_9 = 0.18 \leq Pvalue_8 = 0.187$, the late postoperative interquartile range of the target population A_1 is assumed statistically indistinguishable from that in the pseudo-control population B_1.

Detailed results can be obtained for the other three Bootstrap Modifications. Their p-values are in lines 5, 7, and 9 of Table 3.

Let us categorize the difference between A_1 and B_1 using BM1 Bootstrap. According to Section 3.4, we can define the values of the five input variables of the discrete function of categorization (20). The late postoperative differences in the means of RF in the populations A_1 and B_1 are $C_M = M_{+1}$ (the late postoperative mean of RF in the target population A_1 is statistically significantly more favorable than that in the pseudo-control population B_1). The late postoperative differences in the medians of RF in the populations A_1 and B_1 are $C_{MED} = MED_{+1}$ (the late postoperative median of RF in the target population A_1 is statistically significantly more favorable than that in the pseudo-control population B_1). $Cond_1$ = F, since the variances in the populations A_1 and B_1 are statistically different. $Cond_2$ = F, since the variances in the populations A_1 and B_1 are statistically distinguishable. $Cond_3$ = F, since the distributions of RF in the populations A_1 and B_1 are not borderline statistically significantly discernible.

According to the first line of Table 1, the late postoperative differences in the continuous parameter RF between the populations A_1 and B_1 are categorized as $C_t = C_{+1}$. The same line in Table 1 shows that we have applied Rule 1: if one of the measures of location of RF in the target population A_1 is statistically significantly more favorable than that in the pseudo-control population B_1, whereas the other measure of location in the target population A_1 is neither statistically significantly nor borderline statistically significantly less favorable than that in the pseudo-control population B_1, then categorize in C_{+1}.

Columns 3 to 9 on line three of Table 4 show the input variables' values and the categorization function's values. We obtained similar results for the remaining three Bootstrap Modifications, shown in lines 5, 7, and 9 of Table 4.

According to Section 3.5, the result from MFPCG for BM1 Bootstrap is $(C_b, C_e) = (C_{-1}, C_{+1})$. That result is in line two of column 10 of Table 4. Hence, $b = -1$, and $e = 1$. According to Equation (21), the result (C_b, C_e) is classified in class 'YES+' since $b - e = (-1) - 1 = -2 < -1/2$. The resulting class shows that according to BM1 Bootstrap, the influence of annuloplasty has a statistically significantly favorable influence over parameter RF in populations A_1 and B_1. This is indicated in line two of the last column of Table 4.

Similar results can be obtained for the other three Bootstrap Modifications. The results are in lines 4, 6, and 8 of Table 4.

4.3.2. Effect of Annuloplasty over MR for Patients with Relatively Preserved Medical State (Task 2)

In task 2, we use four fuzzy samples for MR, as described below.

E_b is a fuzzy sample that contains 34 values of *Preop_MR* and their degrees of membership to the experimental group A_1:

$E_b = \chi^{MR}_{A_1,preop}$ = {(5,0.630), (6,0.900), (4,0.630), (6,0.630), (4,0.360), (6,0.810), (5,0.810), (4,0.630), (6,0.900), (6,0.630), (4,0.630), (5,0.630), (5,0.490), (5,0.630), (6,0.700), (4,0.490), (4,0.630), (6,0.630), (5,0.630), (5,0.630), (6,0.700), (6,0.900), (6,0.630), (4,0.630), (4,0.490), (6,0.900), (4,0.630), (5,0.490), (5,0.630), (5,0.490), (5,0.630), (7,0.700), (6,0.900), (6,0.700)}.

PC_b is a fuzzy sample that contains 43 values of *Preop_MR* and their degrees of membership to the pseudo-control group B_1:

$PC_b = \chi^{MR}_{B_1,preop}$ = {(3,0.900), (3,0.810), (3,0.900), (3,0.900), (4,0.630), (4,0.810), (4,0.630), (3,0.900), (4,0.810), (3,0.900), (3,0.900), (4,0.630), (4,0.490), (4,0.810), (3,0.900), (4,0.630), (4,0.630), (4,0.630), (4,0.490), (4,0.810), (3,0.900), (4,0.490), (3,0.900), (3,0.900), (4,0.490), (4,0.810), (4,0.630), (3,0.900), (4,0.810), (4,0.630), (3,0.900), (4,0.630), (4,0.490), (4,0.630), (3,0.900), (3,0.900), (3,0.900), (3,0.900), (3,0.700), (3,0.700), (4,0.700), (4,0.700), (4,0.357)}.

E_e is a fuzzy sample that contains 32 values of *Late_Postop_MR* and their degrees of membership to the experimental group A_1:

$E_e = \chi^{MR}_{A_1,Lpostop}$ = {(0,0.630), (2,0.900), (2,0.630), (4,0.630), (2,0.360), (4,0.810), (2,0.810), (2,0.630), (0,0.900), (0,0.630), (1,0.630), (0,0.630), (0,0.630), (1,0.700), (0,0.630), (0,0.630), (0,0.630), (0,0.630), (0,0.700), (0,0.900), (2,0.630), (2,0.630), (0,0.490), (0,0.900), (0,0.630), (0,0.490), (0,0.630), (2,0.490), (0,0.630), (1,0.700), (1,0.900), (0,0.700)}.

PC_e is a fuzzy sample that contains 41 values of *Late_Postop_MR* and their degrees of membership to the pseudo-control group B_1:

$PC_e = \chi^{MR}_{B_1,Lpostop}$ = {(2,0.900), (2,0.810), (2,0.900), (2,0.900), (5,0.630), (4,0.810), (4,0.630), (2,0.900), (6,0.810), (1,0.900), (1,0.900), (3,0.490), (2,0.810), (2,0.900), (4,0.630), (1,0.630), (2,0.630), (4,0.490), (4,0.810), (4,0.900), (1,0.490), (1,0.900), (2,0.900), (5,0.490), (4,0.630), (2,0.900), (4,0.810), (2,0.630), (2,0.900), (2,0.630), (4,0.490), (3,0.630), (0,0.900), (2,0.900), (4,0.900), (2,0.900), (0,0.700), (1,0.700), (0,0.700), (2,0.700), (0,0.357)}.

The numerical realization of MFPCG for task 2 is given in Tables 5–7, which have a similar structure to Tables 2–4 described in Section 4.3.1.

Table 5. The numerical characteristics and change favorability for the *MR* fuzzy samples for groups A_1 and B_1.

Sample	E_b	PC_b	*R* Favorability	E_e	PC_e	*R* Favorability
No. of observations	34	43	N/A	32	41	N/A
Fuzzy mean	5.28	3.48	unfavorable	0.878	2.4	favorable
Fuzzy median	5	3	unfavorable	0	2	favorable
Fuzzy STD	0.865	0.507	N/A	1.2	1.46	N/A
Fuzzy IQR	1	1	N/A	2	2	N/A

Table 6. The *p*-values of the fuzzy Bootstrap statistical tests in MFPCG for parameter *MR*, comparing subgroups A_1 and B_1.

Modification	Time	FBT1	FBT2	FBT3	FBT4	FBT5	FBT6	FBT7	FBT8	FBT9
BM1	Preop	0.0000	0.0000	0.0000	0.0000	0.0000	0.0000	0.0000	1.0000	0.9985
BM1	Late_Postop	0.0000	0.0000	0.0000	0.0115	0.0010	0.3015	0.1735	1.0000	0.5240
BM2	Preop	0.0000	0.0000	0.0000	0.0000	0.0000	0.0005	0.0000	1.0000	0.9875
BM2	Late_Postop	0.0010	0.0000	0.0000	0.0080	0.0010	0.3480	0.1570	1.0000	0.5735
BM3	Preop	0.0000	0.0000	0.0000	0.0005	0.0000	0.0000	0.0000	1.0000	0.9980
BM3	Late_Postop	0.0010	0.0000	0.0000	0.0080	0.0020	0.3000	0.1715	1.0000	0.4940
BM4	Preop	0.0000	0.0000	0.0000	0.0000	0.0000	0.0000	0.0000	1.0000	0.9945
BM4	Late_Postop	0.0000	0.0000	0.0000	0.0080	0.0005	0.3165	0.1450	1.0000	0.5945

Table 7. The MFPCG diagnostics of the influence of *R* on a continuous parameter *MR*, comparing subgroups A_1 and B_1.

Modification	Time	C_M	C_{MED}	$Cond_1$	$Cond_2$	$Cond_3$	C_t	Rule	Result of MFPCG	Class
BM1	Preop	M_{-1}	MED_{-1}	F	F	F	C_{-1}	5	$(C_b, C_e) = (C_{-1}, C_{+1})$	YES+
BM1	Late_Postop	M_{+1}	MED_{+1}	T	T	F	C_{+1}	1		
BM2	Preop	M_{-1}	MED_{-1}	F	F	F	C_{-1}	5	$(C_b, C_e) = (C_{-1}, C_{+1})$	YES+
BM2	Late_Postop	M_{+1}	MED_{+1}	T	T	F	C_{+1}	1		
BM3	Preop	M_{-1}	MED_{-1}	F	F	F	C_{-1}	5	$(C_b, C_e) = (C_{-1}, C_{+1})$	YES+
BM3	Late_Postop	M_{+1}	MED_{+1}	T	T	F	C_{+1}	1		
BM4	Preop	M_{-1}	MED_{-1}	F	F	F	C_{-1}	5	$(C_b, C_e) = (C_{-1}, C_{+1})$	YES+
BM4	Late_Postop	M_{+1}	MED_{+1}	T	T	F	C_{+1}	1		

4.3.3. Effect of Annuloplasty over RF for Patients with Relatively Deteriorated Medical State (Task 3)

In task 3, we use four fuzzy samples for *RF*, as described below.

E_b is a fuzzy sample that contains 53 values of *Preop_RF* and their degrees of membership to the experimental group A_2:

$E_b = \chi^{RF}_{A_2,preop}$ = {(66,0.306), (46,0.630), (68,0.700), (65,0.900), (71,0.490), (61,0.700), (58,0.810), (50,0.810), (64,0.490), (50,0.306), (47,0.900), (53,0.900), (41,0.630), (51,0.306), (70,0.900), (65,0.700), (54,0.700), (33,0.810), (66,0.810), (71,0.490), (60,0.630), (54,0.810), (61,0.490), (50,0.490), (34,0.630), (63,0.700), (69,0.700), (63,0.900), (38,0.900), (64,0.700), (71,0.630), (60,0.700), (63,0.490), (73,0.700), (68,0.700), (43,0.700), (43,0.810), (59,0.700),

(59,0.900), (65,0.490), (74,0.900), (50,0.700), (73,0.700), (82,0.700), (70,0.900), (50,0.900), (76,0.700), (51,0.630), (77,0.900), (43,0.900), (63,0.700), (68,0.630), (48,0.630)}.

PC_b is a fuzzy sample that contains 39 values of *Preop_RF* and their degrees of membership to the pseudo-control group B_2:

$PC_b = \chi^{RF}_{B_2,preop}$ = {(50,0.490), (49,0.490), (46,0.357), (38,0.260), (31,0.630), (35,0.490), (26,0.700), (21,0.700), (31,1.000), (48,0.490), (28,0.630), (24,1.000), (43,0.510), (39,0.630), (24,0.490), (46,0.630), (50,0.357), (55,0.630), (39,0.700), (54,1.000), (47,1.000), (50,0.700), (56,0.810), (30,0.490), (47,1.000), (30,0.700), (41,0.700), (57,1.000), (60,1.000), (48,0.490), (45,0.357), (35,0.260), (44,0.630), (30,0.510), (43,0.260), (40,0.357), (53,1.000), (23,1.000), (74,1.000)}.

E_e is a fuzzy sample that contains 44 values of *Late_Postop_RF* and their degrees of membership to the experimental group A_2:

$E_e = \chi^{RF}_{A_2,Lpostop}$ = {(0,0.700), (42,0.900), (0,0.490), (0,0.700), (0,0.810), (0,0.810), (14,0.490), (31,0.306), (20,0.900), (11,0.700), (0,0.810), (10,0.490), (0,0.630), (21,0.810), (10,0.490), (0,0.490), (0,0.630), (0,0.700), (20,0.700), (7,0.900), (13,0.900), (0,0.700), (12,0.700), (18,0.490), (24,0.700), (0,0.700), (0,0.700), (19,0.810), (0,0.700), (29,0.900), (0,0.490), (0,0.900), (0,0.700), (25,0.700), (0,0.700), (0,0.900), (0,0.900), (6,0.700), (0,0.630), (0,0.900), (11,0.900), (0,0.700), (0,0.630), (0,0.630)}.

PC_e is a fuzzy sample that contains 32 values of *Late_Postop_RF* and their degrees of membership to the pseudo-control group B_2:

$PC_e = \chi^{RF}_{B_2,Lpostop}$ = {(43,0.490), (35,0.490), (53,0.630), (0,0.700), (0,0.700), (7,1.000), (21,0.490), (15,1.000), (11,0.510), (44,0.630), (25,0.490), (78,0.630), (0,0.357), (77,0.630), (70,1.000), (57,1.000), (11,0.700), (66,0.490), (28,1.000), (0,0.700), (48,0.700), (76,1.000), (45,0.490), (19,0.357), (23,0.260), (10,0.630), (13,0.510), (32,0.260), (29,0.357), (16,1.000), (15,1.000), (47,1.000)}.

Tables 8–10 provide the numerical realization of MFPCG for task 3. These tables have a similar structure to Tables 2–4 described in Section 4.3.1.

Table 8. The numerical characteristics and change favorability for the *RF* fuzzy samples for groups A_2 and B_2.

Sample	E_b	PC_b	R Favorability	E_e	PC_e	R Favorability
No. of observations	53	39	N/A	44	32	N/A
Fuzzy mean, %	59	42.6	unfavorable	7.89	32.8	favorable
Fuzzy median, %	61	44.7	unfavorable	0	27.1	favorable
Fuzzy STD, %	11.9	13.2	N/A	11.1	25.6	N/A
Fuzzy IQR, %	18	21	N/A	13.4	39.1	N/A

Table 9. The *p*-values of the fuzzy Bootstrap statistical tests in MFPCG for parameter *RF*, comparing subgroups A_2 and B_2.

Modification	Time	FBT1	FBT2	FBT3	FBT4	FBT5	FBT6	FBT7	FBT8	FBT9
BM1	Preop	0.0000	0.0000	0.0000	0.0000	0.0000	0.4730	0.2180	0.5005	0.3030
BM1	Late_Postop	0.0000	0.0000	0.0000	0.0020	0.0020	0.0000	0.0000	0.0460	0.0460
BM2	Preop	0.0000	0.0000	0.0000	0.0010	0.0010	0.4715	0.3350	0.6020	0.4405
BM2	Late_Postop	0.0005	0.0000	0.0000	0.0025	0.0025	0.0000	0.0000	0.0475	0.0475
BM3	Preop	0.0000	0.0000	0.0000	0.0035	0.0030	0.4670	0.1880	0.5025	0.2865
BM3	Late_Postop	0.0005	0.0000	0.0000	0.0000	0.0000	0.0000	0.0000	0.0570	0.0570
BM4	Preop	0.0000	0.0000	0.0000	0.0020	0.0020	0.4475	0.3070	0.5635	0.4270
BM4	Late_Postop	0.0000	0.0000	0.0000	0.0015	0.0015	0.0000	0.0000	0.0475	0.0475

Table 10. The MFPCG diagnostics of the influence of R on a continuous parameter RF, comparing subgroups A_2 and B_2.

Modification	Time	C_M	C_{MED}	$Cond_1$	$Cond_2$	$Cond_3$	C_t	Rule	Result of MFPCG	Class
BM1	Preop	M_{-1}	MED_{-1}	T	T	F	C_{-1}	5	$(C_b, C_e) = (C_{-1}, C_{+1})$	YES+
BM1	Late_Postop	M_{+1}	MED_{+1}	F	F	F	C_{+1}	1		
BM2	Preop	M_{-1}	MED_{-1}	T	T	F	C_{-1}	5	$(C_b, C_e) = (C_{-1}, C_{+1})$	YES+
BM2	Late_Postop	M_{+1}	MED_{+1}	F	F	F	C_{+1}	1		
BM3	Preop	M_{-1}	MED_{-1}	T	T	F	C_{-1}	5	$(C_b, C_e) = (C_{-1}, C_{+1})$	YES+
BM3	Late_Postop	M_{+1}	MED_{+1}	F	F	F	C_{+1}	1		
BM4	Preop	M_{-1}	MED_{-1}	T	T	F	C_{-1}	5	$(C_b, C_e) = (C_{-1}, C_{+1})$	YES+
BM4	Late_Postop	M_{+1}	MED_{+1}	F	F	F	C_{+1}	1		

4.3.4. Effect of Annuloplasty over MR for Patients with Relatively Deteriorated Medical State (Task 4)

In task 4, we use four fuzzy samples for MR, as described below.

E_b is a fuzzy sample that contains 53 values of *Preop_MR* and their degrees of membership to the experimental group A_2:

$E_b = \chi^{MR}_{A_2,preop}$ = {(5,0.306), (5,0.630), (6,0.700), (6,0.900), (4,0.490), (6,0.700), (6,0.810), (6,0.810), (6,0.490), (4,0.306), (5,0.900), (6,0.900), (4,0.630), (4,0.306), (6,0.900), (6,0.700), (5,0.700), (4,0.810), (5,0.810), (5,0.490), (4,0.630), (6,0.810), (5,0.490), (5,0.490), (4,0.630), (6,0.700), (6,0.700), (6,0.900), (6,0.900), (6,0.700), (5,0.630), (6,0.700), (6,0.490), (6,0.700), (6,0.700), (6,0.700), (5,0.810), (5,0.700), (6,0.900), (5,0.490), (7,0.900), (7,0.700), (7,0.700), (7,0.700), (6,0.900), (6,0.900), (6,0.700), (6,0.630), (7,0.900), (6,0.900), (6,0.700), (6,0.630), (6,0.630)}

PC_b is a fuzzy sample that contains 38 values of *Preop_MR* and their degrees of membership to the pseudo-control group B_2:

$PC_b = \chi^{MR}_{B_2,preop}$ = {(4,0.490), (4,0.490), (3,0.260), (4,0.630), (4,0.490), (3,0.700), (3,0.700), (4,1.000), (4,0.490), (4,0.630), (4,1.000), (4,0.510), (4,0.630), (4,0.490), (4,0.630), (4,0.357), (4,0.630), (3,0.700), (4,1.000), (4,1.000), (3,0.700), (4,0.810), (4,0.490), (4,1.000), (3,0.700), (3,0.700), (4,1.000), (3,1.000), (4,0.490), (3,0.357), (3,0.260), (4,0.630), (4,0.510), (4,0.260), (4,0.357), (5,1.000), (4,1.000), (7,1.000)}.

E_e is a fuzzy sample that contains 44 values of *Late_Postop_MR* and their degrees of membership to the experimental group A_2:

$E_e = \chi^{MR}_{A_2,Lpostop}$ = {(0,0.700), (5,0.900), (0,0.490), (2,0.700), (0,0.810), (0,0.810), (2,0.490), (2,0.306), (2,0.900), (1,0.700), (0,0.810), (2,0.490), (0,0.630), (1,0.810), (1,0.490), (0,0.490), (0,0.630), (0,0.700), (2,0.700), (2,0.900), (1,0.900), (0,0.700), (2,0.700), (2,0.490), (2,0.700), (0,0.700), (0,0.700), (1,0.810), (0,0.700), (2,0.900), (0,0.490), (0,0.900), (0,0.700), (2,0.700), (0,0.700), (0,0.900), (0,0.900), (1,0.700), (0,0.630), (0,0.900), (1,0.900), (0,0.700), (0,0.630), (0,0.630)}.

PC_e is a fuzzy sample that contains 32 values of *Late_Postop_MR* and their degrees of membership to the pseudo-control group B_2:

$PC_e = \chi^{MR}_{B_2,Lpostop}$ = {(4,0.490), (4,0.490), (5,0.630), (1,0.700), (0,0.700), (2,1.000), (2,0.490), (2,1.000), (2,0.510), (4,0.630), (3,0.490), (4,0.630), (2,0.357), (5,0.630), (4,1.000), (4,1.000), (2,0.700), (5,0.490), (4,1.000), (0,0.700), (4,0.700), (4,1.000), (5,0.490), (2,0.357), (2,0.260), (1,0.630), (1,0.510), (2,0.260), (2,0.357), (2,1.000), (2,1.000), (5,1.000)}.

The numerical realization of MFPCG for task 4 is given in Tables 11–13, which have a similar structure to Tables 2–4 described in Section 4.3.1.

Table 11. The numerical characteristics and change favorability for the *MR* fuzzy samples for groups A_2 and B_2.

Sample	E_b	PC_b	*R* Favorability	E_e	PC_e	*R* Favorability
No. of observations	53	38	N/A	44	32	N/A
Fuzzy mean	5.7	3.92	unfavorable	0.827	2.92	favorable
Fuzzy median	6	4	unfavorable	0	2.64	favorable
Fuzzy STD	0.802	0.813	N/A	1.13	1.53	N/A
Fuzzy IQR	1	0.101	N/A	2	2	N/A

Table 12. The *p*-values of the fuzzy Bootstrap statistical tests in MFPCG for parameter *MR*, comparing subgroups A_2 and B_2.

Modification	Time	FBT1	FBT2	FBT3	FBT4	FBT5	FBT6	FBT7	FBT8	FBT9
BM1	Preop	0.0000	0.0000	0.0000	0.0000	0.0000	0.9650	0.4540	0.5010	0.4145
BM1	Late_Postop	0.0000	0.0000	0.0000	0.0005	0.0000	0.1550	0.0915	1.0000	0.5060
BM2	Preop	0.0000	0.0000	0.0000	0.0000	0.0000	0.9675	0.6010	0.5290	0.3650
BM2	Late_Postop	0.0000	0.0000	0.0000	0.0000	0.0000	0.1925	0.0775	1.0000	0.5125
BM3	Preop	0.0000	0.0000	0.0000	0.0000	0.0000	0.9690	0.4135	0.5175	0.4340
BM3	Late_Postop	0.0000	0.0000	0.0000	0.0005	0.0000	0.1795	0.1165	1.0000	0.4925
BM4	Preop	0.0000	0.0000	0.0000	0.0000	0.0000	0.9690	0.6085	0.5365	0.3895
BM4	Late_Postop	0.0000	0.0000	0.0000	0.0005	0.0000	0.1885	0.0860	1.0000	0.5335

Table 13. The MFPCG diagnostics of the influence of *R* on a continuous parameter *MR*, comparing subgroups A_2 and B_2.

Modification	Time	C_M	C_{MED}	$Cond_1$	$Cond_2$	$Cond_3$	C_t	Rule	Result of MFPCG	Class
BM1	Preop	M_{-1}	MED_{-1}	T	T	F	C_{-1}	5	$(C_b, C_e) = (C_{-1}, C_{+1})$	YES+
BM1	Late_Postop	M_{+1}	MED_{+1}	T	T	F	C_{+1}	1		
BM2	Preop	M_{-1}	MED_{-1}	T	T	F	C_{-1}	5	$(C_b, C_e) = (C_{-1}, C_{+1})$	YES+
BM2	Late_Postop	M_{+1}	MED_{+1}	T	T	F	C_{+1}	1		
BM3	Preop	M_{-1}	MED_{-1}	T	T	F	C_{-1}	5	$(C_b, C_e) = (C_{-1}, C_{+1})$	YES+
BM3	Late_Postop	M_{+1}	MED_{+1}	T	T	F	C_{+1}	1		
BM4	Preop	M_{-1}	MED_{-1}	T	T	F	C_{-1}	5	$(C_b, C_e) = (C_{-1}, C_{+1})$	YES+
BM4	Late_Postop	M_{+1}	MED_{+1}	T	T	F	C_{+1}	1		

4.4. Summary

In the annuloplasty favorability case study, the MFPCG Algorithm (Section 3.6) was applied two times. Let *U* be the super-population of patients diagnosed with IHD and moderate and moderate-to-severe IMR with indications for surgery. In both applications, $X_1 = RF$ and $X_2 = MR$. In the first application, *P* is the population from *U* consisting of patients with indications for combined surgery who have a relatively preserved medical state (subgroup A_1 comprises patients from *P*); *Q* is the population of *U* consisting of patients with indications for an isolated intervention who have a relatively preserved medical state (subgroup B_1 comprises patients from *Q*). In the second application, *P* is the population of *U* consisting of patients with indications for combined surgery who have a relatively deteriorated medical state (subgroup A_2 comprises patients from P); Q is the population of U consisting of patients with indications for an isolated intervention who have relatively deteriorated medical state (subgroup B_2 comprises patients from Q).

5. Validation of the Case Study Conclusions

5.1. External Validation

Each of the four tasks formulated in Section 3 is solved four times depending on the modification of the Bootstrap tests performed.

Tables 4, 7, 10 and 13 show that for each of the sixteen solutions, we obtain the following MFPCG result: $(C_b, C_e) = (-1, +1)$, with the MFPCG category: 'YES+', as described in Section 3.5. In their entirety, the results show a favorable effect of annuloplasty on the analyzed parameters, both for patients with a relatively preserved medical state and patients with a relatively deteriorated medical state.

These conclusions are in accordance with the conclusions in [15,57–59], which is an external validation of the MFPCG results for annuloplasty favorability. This affirmative result is an improvement over the aforementioned publications in the following ways:

- In this study, we used data for all available patients, whereas the cited sources analyzed the data after rejecting outliers (which comprised about 20% of the data).
- In our study, we prove every influence using four different Bootstrap Modifications, improving the conclusions' statistical credibility. Our approach uses a cluster of tests instead of individual p-values, which is in accordance with the modern trends in data analysis [33,39].
- Here, we discuss the typicality of patients to a respective subgroup for the first time, whereas in earlier works, the classification is considered absolute (crisp).
- The statistical support for a favorable effect of annuloplasty is efficiently completed using only two integral parameters. In contrast, the earlier works used a double-digit count of parameters to reach the same conclusions.

5.2. Fuzzy DID Method (FDID)

For the sake of internal validation, we will compare the acquired conclusions on the annuloplasty favorability with the results of the DID method. To improve the comparability of DID and MFFCG results, we developed a fuzzy DID that uses Bootstrap in the four discussed modifications to estimate the confidence interval (CI) of the average treatment effect (*ATE*):

FDID Algorithm

1. Select the significance level, α, and the number of pseudo-realities, N, to construct the Bootstrap CIs.
2. Set $i = 1$.
3. Choose $X = X_i$.
4. Extract from the database the fuzzy samples E_b, PC_b, E_e, and PC_e for this X.
5. Estimate the fuzzy mean values of the four samples $M_{E,b}$, $M_{PC,b}$, $M_{E,e}$, and $M_{PC,e}$ using (8).
6. Estimate the fuzzy DID estimator as the *ATE*:

$$ATE = (M_{E,e} - M_{PC,e}) - (M_{E,b} - M_{PC,b}) \tag{23}$$

7. Find the index of the empirical $\alpha/2$-quantile from the Bootstrap distribution of *ATE*, as $Nd = \text{round}(N \times \alpha/2)$.
8. Find the index of the empirical $(1-\alpha/2)$-quantile from the Bootstrap distribution of *ATE*, as $Nu = \text{round}(N - N \times \alpha/2)$.

9. Repeat for Bootstrap Modification BMk (k = 1, 2, 3, 4):
    9.1. Repeat for pseudo-reality r (r = 1, 2, ..., N):
        9.1.1. From sample E_b, generate $sE_{b,r}$, using Bootstrap Modification BMk.
        9.1.2. From sample PC_b, generate $sPC_{b,r}$, using Bootstrap Modification BMk.
        9.1.3. From sample E_e, generate $sE_{e,r}$, using Bootstrap Modification BMk.
        9.1.4. From sample PC_e, generate $sPC_{e,r}$, using Bootstrap Modification BMk.
        9.1.5. Estimate the fuzzy mean values of the four synthetic samples $sM_{E,b,r}$, $sM_{PC,b,r}$, $sM_{E,e,r}$, and $sM_{PC,e,r}$ using (8).
        9.1.6. Estimate the fuzzy DID estimator as $sATE_r$ in the r-th pseudo-reality:

$$sATE_r = (sM_{E,e,r} - sM_{PC,e,r}) - (sM_{E,b,r} - sM_{PC,b,r}) \quad (24)$$

    9.2. Sort the synthetic $sATE_r$ in ascending order and obtain $sATE_{sort,r}$ (r = 1, 2, ..., N).
    9.3. Estimate the Reverse Percentile 100 × (1 − α)%-CI for ATE using Bootstrap Modification BMk:

$$\Pr\{2 \times ATE - sATE_{sort,Nu} < ATE < 2 \times ATE - sATE_{sort,Nd}\} = 1 - \alpha \quad (25)$$

10. Set $i = i+1$.
11. If $i < n$, then go to step 3. Otherwise, end the algorithm.

5.3. Case Study Solved with FDID

In essence, we should apply the FDID four times to solve the four tasks formulated in Section 4.3. For the sake of comparability, we solved the four tasks at a significance level of $\alpha = 0.05$, and the Bootstrap CIs were calculated with $N = 2000$ pseudo-realities.

5.3.1. FDID Solution of Task 1 (Effect of Annuloplasty over RF for A_1 and B_1 Patients)

First, we will solve task 1, as described in Section 4.3, using the fuzzy DID method. We shall use the four samples given in Section 4.3.1. Table 14 shows the fuzzy mean values of the four samples. The ATE for task 1 is (−43.9%), given on line 4, column 4 of the table. Those results are illustrated in Figure 2, which shows the three temporal functions of the fuzzy means in A_1, B_1, and the counterfactual of A_1, along with ATE. After applying the algorithm of the fuzzy DID, we obtained four Reverse Percentile 95%-CIs for ATE in task 1:

- For BM1, $\Pr\{-43.7 < ATE < -26.1\} = 0.95$;
- For BM2, $\Pr\{-44.6 < ATE < -27.1\} = 0.95$;
- For BM3, $\Pr\{-44.1 < ATE < -26\} = 0.95$;
- For BM4, $\Pr\{-44.4 < ATE < -26.9\} = 0.95$.

Table 14. Fuzzy means of RF, % for subgroups A_1 and B_1.

	A_1 (E)	B_1 (PC)	Difference (D)
Preop (b)	$M_{E,b} = +54$, %	$M_{PC,b} = +35.5$, %	$D_b = +18.5$, %
Postop (e)	$M_{E,e} = +7.79$, %	$M_{PC,e} = +24.2$, %	$D_e = -16.4$, %
Temporal change (TC)	$TC_E = -46.2$, %	$TC_{PC} = -11.3$, %	$ATE = -34.9$, %

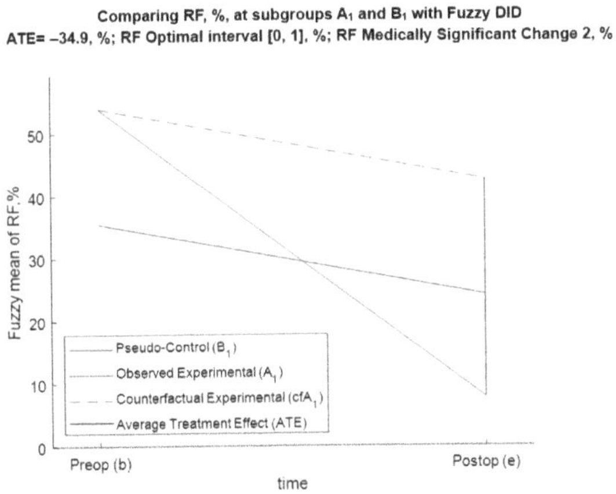

Figure 2. DID graphical illustration for task 1.

5.3.2. FDID Solution of Task 2 (Effect of Annuloplasty over MR for A_1 and B_1 Patients)

We shall use the four samples given in Section 4.3.2. Table 15 shows the fuzzy mean values of the four samples. The *ATE* for task 2 is (–3.31%), given on line 4, column 4 of the table. Those results are illustrated in Figure 3, which shows the three temporal functions of the fuzzy means in A_1, B_1, and the counterfactual of A_1, along with *ATE*. After applying the algorithm of the fuzzy DID, we obtained four Reverse Percentile 95%-CIs for *ATE* in task 2:

- For BM1, $\Pr\{-3.97 < ATE < -2.67\} = 0.95$;
- For BM2, $\Pr\{-3.91 < ATE < -2.54\} = 0.95$;
- For BM3, $\Pr\{-4 < ATE < -2.64\} = 0.95 = 0.95$;
- For BM4, $\Pr\{-3.9 < ATE < -2.54\} = 0.95 = 0.95$.

Table 15. Fuzzy means of *MR*, % for subgroups A_1 and B_1.

	A_1 *(E)*	B_1 *(PC)*	**Difference (*D*)**
Preop (*b*)	$M_{E,b} = +5.28$, %	$M_{PC,b} = +3.48$, %	$D_b = +1.8$, %
Postop (*e*)	$M_{E,e} = +0.878$, %	$M_{PC,e} = +2.4$, %	$D_e = -1.52$, %
Temporal change (TC)	$TC_E = -4.4$, %	$TC_{PC} = -1.08$, %	$ATE = -3.31$, %

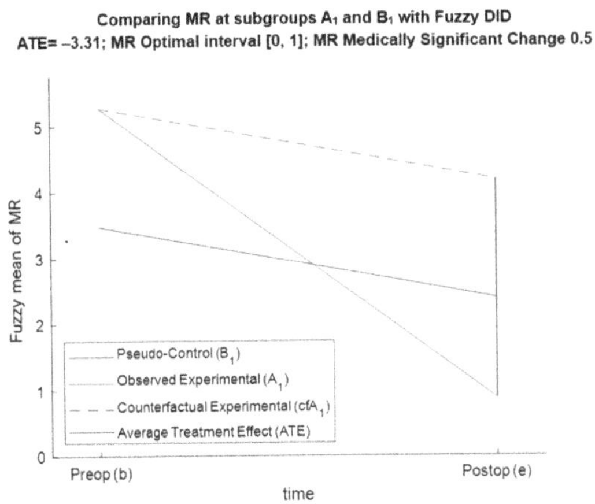

Figure 3. DID graphical illustration for task 2.

5.3.3. FDID Solution of Task 3 (Effect of Annuloplasty over RF for A_2 and B_2 Patients)

We shall use the four samples given in Section 4.3.3. Table 16 shows the fuzzy mean values of the four samples. The *ATE* for task 3 is (–41.4%), given on line 4, column 4 of the table. Those results are illustrated in Figure 4, which shows the three temporal functions of the fuzzy means in A_2, B_2, and the counterfactual of A_2, along with *ATE*. After applying the algorithm of the fuzzy DID, we obtained four Reverse Percentile 95%-CIs for *ATE* in task 3:

- For BM1, $\Pr\{-52.5 < ATE < -29.5\} = 0.95$;
- For BM2, $\Pr\{-54.5 < ATE < -29.7\} = 0.95$;
- For BM3, $\Pr\{-52.7 < ATE < -30.5\} = 0.95$;
- For BM4, $\Pr\{-54 < ATE < -29.9\} = 0.95$.

Table 16. Fuzzy means of *RF*, % for subgroups A_2 and B_2.

	A_2 (*E*)	B_2 (*PC*)	Difference (*D*)
Preop (*b*)	$M_{E,b} = +59$, %	$M_{PC,b} = +42.6$, %	$D_b = +16.4$, %
Postop (*e*)	$M_{E,e} = +7.89$, %	$M_{PC,e} = +32.8$, %	$D_e = -24.9$, %
Temporal change (TC)	$TC_E = -51.1$, %	$TC_{PC} = -9.78$, %	$ATE = -41.4$, %

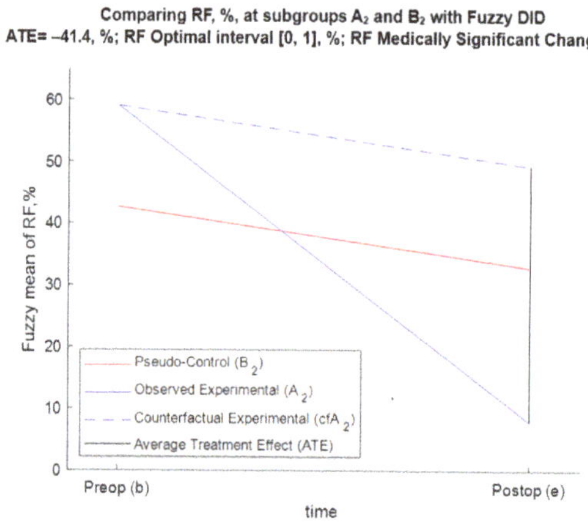

Figure 4. DID graphical illustration for task 3.

5.3.4. FDID Solution of Task 4 (Effect of Annuloplasty over MR for A_2 and B_2 Patients)

We shall use the four samples given in Section 4.3.4. Table 17 shows the fuzzy mean values of the four samples. The *ATE* for task 4 is (−3.87%), given on line 4, column 4 of the table. Those results are illustrated in Figure 5, which shows the three temporal functions of the fuzzy means in A_2, B_2, and the counterfactual of A_2, along with *ATE*. After applying the algorithm of the fuzzy DID, we obtained four Reverse Percentile 95%-CIs for *ATE* in task 4:

- For BM1, $\Pr\{-4.62 < ATE < -3.17\} = 0.95$;
- For BM2, $\Pr\{-4.56 < ATE < -3.1\} = 0.95$;
- For BM3, $\Pr\{-4.63 < ATE < -3.15\} = 0.95$;
- For BM4, $\Pr\{-4.62 < ATE < -3.09\} = 0.95$.

Table 17. Fuzzy means of MR, % for subgroups A_2 and B_2.

	A_2 (E)	B_2 (PC)	Difference (D)
Preop (b)	$M_{E,b} = +5.7$, %	$M_{PC,b} = +3.92$, %	$D_b = +1.78$, %
Postop (e)	$M_{E,e} = +0.827$, %	$M_{PC,e} = +2.92$, %	$D_e = -2.09$, %
Temporal change (TC)	$TC_E = -4.87$, %	$TC_{PC} = -1$, %	$ATE = -3.87$, %

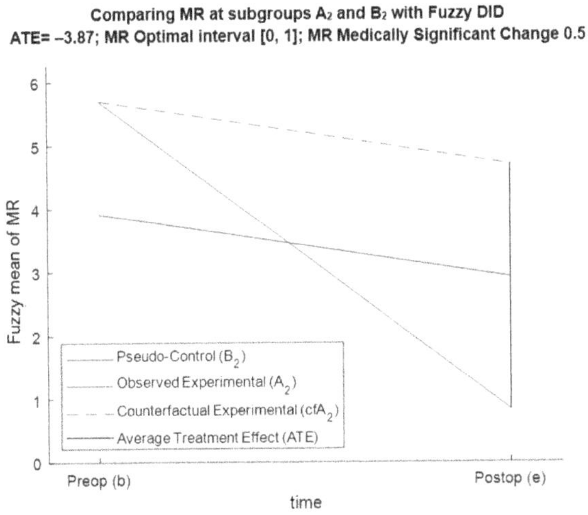

Figure 5. DID graphical illustration for task 4.

5.4. Internal Validation with FDID

According to Section 5.3, each of the four tasks was solved four times depending on the Bootstrap Modification used to construct the CIs of ATE. For each of the 16 solutions, we obtain an ATE that is statistically significant and practically favorable. This shows the favorable effect of annuloplasty on the analyzed parameters for both subgroups A_1 and B_1, and subgroups A_2 and B_2.

The conclusions from FDID are in accordance with the conclusions from MFPCG from Section 5.1, which internally validate the results of MFPCG. The affirmative result of MFPCG relates to the affirmative result of FDID in the following ways:

- The results from FDID are conditional upon the assumptions of the method. We do not have a way of proving the parallel trend assumption, as shown in Figures 2–5. We also cannot prove that, in this particular case, the classical normal linear regression model (CNLRM) assumptions [9,60] about nullity, homoskedasticity, normality, correlation, multicollinearity, and linearity hold.
- Both methods use data for all available patients without rejecting outliers.
- Both methods use a cluster of tests instead of individual p-values.
- Both methods consider the typicality of patients to a respective subgroup.
- MFPCG produces qualitative results that annuloplasty is favorable for patients with an average or average-to-severe IMR. At the same time, the FDID produced quantitative results as to how much the annuloplasty improved the outcome for those patients compared with patients with isolated CABG.

5.5. Internal Validation with Fuzzy RDD (FRDD)

For the sake of internal validation, we also compared the acquired conclusions on the annuloplasty favorability with the results of the RDD method. To improve the comparability of RDD and MFFCG results, we developed a fuzzy RDD (FRDD) that uses Bootstrap in the four discussed modifications, on the one hand, to estimate the CIs of ATE, and on the other hand, to identify whether the reduced E_b and PC_b have statistically indistinguishable X_i values. There is no obvious scalar discriminant variable that separates the experimental and the control groups. The main challenge was that, in our example, the assignment to the experimental or control groups was performed by the main algorithm from [54]. MA produces a degree of membership to the combined-operation group (μ_A) and to the isolated-procedure group ($\mu_B = 1 - \mu_A$) for each patient. The closer μ_A and μ_B are, the nearer the patient is to the hypothetical cutoff surface of the vector discriminant variable. So, we estimated that the reduced fuzzy samples rE_b, and rE_e are derived from E_b and E_e by purging all patients with $\mu_A > \mu_{cutoff}$ (for some pre-selected values of μ_{cutoff}). Similarly, the reduced fuzzy samples rPC_b and rPC_e are derived from PC_b and PC_e by purging all patients with $\mu_B > \mu_{cutoff}$. If at least one of the four reduced samples has a cardinality less than six, or its sum of degrees of membership is less than 3, then we consider that the restriction is too strict for any additional data processing, and the method does not produce a result. If not, then using the four Bootstrap Modifications, we can test whether rE_b and rPC_b are statistically different. If they are not, then the method does not produce a result. However, if E_b is statistically indistinguishable from PC_b, then we can unite the two samples into the fuzzy sample U_b and estimate its fuzzy mean value, $M_{U,b}$, using (8). In that case, we can safely assume that the fuzzy mean values of rE_b and rPC_b are equal and coincide with the fuzzy mean value of U_b:

$$M_{rE,b} = M_{rPC,e} = M_{U,b} \tag{26}$$

Then, the fuzzy RDD estimator of the outcome is the reduced ATE $(rATE)$:

$$rATE = (M_{rE,e} - M_{rPC,e}) \tag{27}$$

Here, FRDD acts almost the same as RCT, since the reduced pseudo-control group is indistinguishable from the experimental group, and we can at least mentally assume a random partition of the patients. Formula (27) is a special case of the (25) under the assumption (26). We will finish the FRDD Algorithm by calculating the four Reverse Percentile $100 \times (1 - \alpha)$%-CI for $rATE$ using Bootstrap Modification BMk with the method described in the FDID Algorithm.

We have not provided the FRDD Algorithm in this paper, since its application turned out to be unsuccessful. For $\mu_{cutoff} = 0.7$, the cardinality of the reduced samples was between 8 and 18 for all four tasks. That was enough to compare rE_b and rPC_b. However, for tasks 2, 3, and 4, the 20 most important tests (4 for identity of distributions, 8 for equality of fuzzy means, and 8 for equality of fuzzy medians) all have p-values of zero. For task 1, there was a mixed bag of results—the eight tests for equality of fuzzy means had p-values less than α, the eight tests for equality of fuzzy medians showed borderline statistical significance, and only one of the tests for identity of distributions showed statistical significance. Overall, there is sufficient evidence that, for task 1, rE_b and rPC_b are different. Thus, the entire algorithm failed.

For $\mu_{cutoff} = 0.69$, the cardinality of the reduced samples was between 1 and 4 for all four tasks. Since the cardinality was less than 6, the FRDD failed again.

The failure of FRDD to solve any of the four tasks in the annuloplasty favorability case study was expected due to the limitations of RDD, discussed in Section 1.

6. Discussion and Conclusions

6.1. Basic Idea and Adaptability of MFPCG

The MFPCG Algorithm may seem complicated to practitioners. Yet, it reflects a simple idea—in the absence of a control group, it is sometimes possible to prove a statistical influence of R with a pseudo-control group using a certain parameter X. For example, R has a favorable influence over X if there is a statistically significantly less favorable value in the experimental group before R, and more favorable values after R, in comparison to the pseudo-control group. Then, the differences between the control and pseudo-control groups are irrelevant to the statistical conclusions. The latter cannot be rejected by showing that the pseudo-control group is different from the experimental group. For that reason, the method has the potential to be of use.

However, such conclusions are not always possible, e.g., before and after intervention R, X is less favorable in the experimental group than in the pseudo-control group.

MFPCG has considerable adaptability (and even parametrization in future developments). The version we proposed in this paper should only be interpreted as general guidance. It is sufficient only to follow the key ideas and philosophy of the approach. Every time the method is applied, it is likely that some steps ought to be modified to adjust to that specific problem and its need for classification. Therefore, the method's applicability is broader than our discussion could allude to. The values proposed in Section 3 are robust, yet every practitioner can modify them to fit their specific task. Future researchers can even adapt the name of the method, since some fuzzy purists would have issues with our interpretation of fuzziness, in line with the discussion in Section 2 on that matter. We are perfectly happy if researchers call our novel approach the Method of the Weighted Pseudo-Control Group (MWPCG).

Stage 4 of MFPCG summarizes the results from stages 2 and 3. It has the highest potential to adapt to the specific problem by modifying the proposed rules and/or formulating new ones. This also refers to how stage 4 is formalized. In Section 3.4, we presented two approaches to suit people with different propensities to formalization. The rule-based approach is relatively compact. The function-based approach achieves the same categorization of the differences between populations with less effort and required attention from the practitioner. Both approaches are algorithmically equivalent. However, choosing one over the other is a prerogative of the practitioner applying the method. We can also develop a third approach, where the inputs are all possible combinations of the five input parameters from Section 3.4. We can develop a table similar to Table 2, with columns C_M, C_{MED}, $Cond_1$, $Cond_2$, $Cond_3$, C_t, and *Rule*. That table should have $7 \times 7 \times 2 \times 2 \times 2 = 319$ rows (note that Table 2 is a compact version of that 319-row table). Performing stage 4 of MFPCG with that extended table can be called the *explicit function-based approach*. The user's preference shall dictate which approach would be used. The descending order of the three approaches regarding compactness is: 1- the rule-based, 2- the function-based, and 3- the explicit function-based. However, that order coincides with the ascending order of logical simplicity. Therefore, the choice of approach depends on the user's trade-off between compact presentation and logical complexity.

From the flowchart in Figure 1 and the MFPCG Algorithm, we can see that our novel method can be adapted for parallel computing. The Stage 2 blocks can be calculated independently. The same applies to the four BMk meta-blocks (each including two Stage-3 blocks, two Stage-4 blocks, and one Stage-5 block). The whole section in the flowchart regarding X_i can be calculated as n independent parallel processes. The most time-consuming parts of the discussed algorithm are the eight Stage-3 blocks. In each of them, we calculate nine statistical tests. Each one of those blocks can be calculated as five independent parallel processes (it is not computationally efficient to separate a one-tailed statistical test from its two-tailed counterpart). Finally, each of those five independent parallel processes can be separated into N subprocesses estimating the individual independent pseudo-realities. It thus follows that the sky is the limit as far as parallel computing is concerned. As a result, we claim that the MFPCG can solve big-data problems.

6.2. Limitations of MFPCG

The first limitation of MFPCG is that, in its current form, it cannot deal with valley preferences as defined in [40]. The method would need to undergo significant restructuring to adapt to such preferences. However, if the preferences are multi-modal, no major adaptation would help. Luckily, such preferences are very rare in medical studies.

A second limitation is that sometimes MFPCG cannot assess the favourability of the intervention. MFPCG works by comparing the qualitative differences between the experimental and the control groups before and after the intervention. For example, if before and after intervention R, X is more favorable in the experimental group than in the pseudo-control group, then no conclusion can be reached regardless of the relative magnitude of this favourability.

Another major limitation of MFPCG transpires in the case where a significant factor changes in the experimental group differently from the way it changes in the pseudo-control group. For example, such a situation would arise if the medical team focused its efforts on patients with base intervention V and investigated intervention R more than on those with only V intervention. This can occur due to financial considerations or due to cognitive biases. Mathematically, this is a likely problem and causes concern. However, such cases are rare in medical research that is free from fraudulent or unethical activities. This limitation is an Achilles heel for any quasi-experiment designs and is not unique to MFPCG.

6.3. Synergies of MFPCG, FRDD, and FDID

It should be clear by now that MFPCG, FRDD, and FDID are all making causal inferences between the intervention R and the outcome. However, the three methods considerably differ:

- FDID always produces a quantitative assessment of the influence, and FRDD sometimes produces a quantitative assessment of the influence, whereas MFPCG sometimes produces a qualitative assessment of that influence.
- FRDD and FDID apply only to monotonic preferences over X, whereas MFPCG deals with hill preferences that are very applicable in medical studies, especially in the current age of overmedication in Western societies.
- FDID uses many assumptions that are hard to verify (the same is true to a smaller extent about FRDD), unlike MFPCG.
- FRDD and FDID only deal with mean values, whereas the more complex MFPCG operates on distributions, means, medians, standard deviations, and interquartile ranges.
- FRDD and FDID are incapable of assessing the practical significance of observed changes regardless of their statistical significance, whereas this aspect is incorporated in MFPCG.
- FRDD and FDID are easy to implement, whereas MFPCG is computationally challenging.
- There is considerable knowledge of how to implement and modify FRDD and FDID to deal with different problems since these are well known, whereas MFPCG is a new approach.

The above considerations show that MFPCG is not an alternative to FRDD or FDID but rather a complement. The three methods should be used in conjunction:

(1) We should always start by applying FRDD. It generally works when there are large experimental and pseudo-control groups. The quantitative result, if any, statistically proves that the pseudo-control sample is, in fact, the control one, since there is no statistically significant difference between the pre-intervention samples. If the values of X in the fuzzy samples are in the region of monotonic preferences, the results of FRDD would be useful.
(2) We then try MFPCG. If the method works, it will provide a very reliable qualitative assessment of the positive or negative influence of the intervention R.
(3) We can finish with FDID. The reliability of the quantitative result depends on the validity of the assumptions of the method. If the values of X in the fuzzy samples are in the region of monotonic preferences, the results of FDID would be useful.

6.4. Applications of MFPCG

Our expectations are that the fuzzy sample input of MFPCG would facilitate its application, since it allows for encoding the uncertainty and ambiguity in the data. The latter is a modern trend in statistical data analysis. Using fuzzy samples in medical research is a well-established practice. The works [13,14] describe their successful use in medical case studies. On the other hand, MFPCG follows the trend that statistical inference should be based on a cluster of tests as opposed to one test. This approach is proposed and motivated in medical case studies in [39,61,62]. The size of the cluster of tests is quadrupled by the fuzziness of the data. As the flowchart of MFPCG shows, the influence of R over X_i is determined by 72 fuzzy statistical tests. In most cases, we will use not one but n parameters X_i. Consequently, the influence of R over parameters X_i is determined using $72n$ statistical tests (in the special case of crisp samples, those two values decrease to 18 and $18n$, respectively). On the one hand, we can interpret the uncertainty of data in a way that enhances the comprehension of the studied effect. On the other hand, we respond to recent criticism of the single p-value concept [63].

The proposed MFPCG was invented to solve problems in medical studies. It can be applied in experimental quantitative research for solving problems from econometrics, education, statistics, public administration, social sciences, political science, sports management, etc. Of course, in those new areas, it is more likely to encounter multi-modal preferences, which could prevent us from using the method.

6.5. Future Research

Future research should focus on some MFPCG modifications while preserving its key philosophy. It is also worth testing the implementation of the method over other databases from other areas of knowledge, as the existence of control groups might be an issue in areas outside medical research.

Some of the members of the team of authors are currently developing a new method that unites FDID and FRDD, which can provide a different perspective on the problem of assessing the influence of an intervention over a target population.

Author Contributions: Conceptualization, K.T., N.N. and M.D.; methodology, K.T, S.I., N.N. and M.D.; software, K.T. and M.S.; validation, K.T., M.S., S.I. and M.D.; investigation, P.P., D.P., K.T., N.N., S.I. and M.D.; data curation, P.P. and D.P.; writing—original draft preparation, D.P., S.I., M.D. and M.S.; writing—review and editing, K.T., N.N. and D.P.; supervision, N.N. and P.P.; funding acquisition, K.T. All authors have read and agreed to the published version of the manuscript.

Funding: This research was funded by the University of Tasmania/Australian Maritime College (RT.112222).

Institutional Review Board Statement: The study was conducted in accordance with the Declaration of Helsinki, and approved by the Ethics in Research Committee of Medical University—Varna "Prof. Dr. Paraskev Stoyanov" (protocol 026-188/30 December 2021).

Informed Consent Statement: Informed consent was obtained from all subjects involved in the study.

Data Availability Statement: The original contributions presented in the study are included in the article, further inquiries can be directed to the corresponding author.

Acknowledgments: The authors would like to sincerely thank the anonymous reviewers and the academic editor who helped to substantially improve this paper.

Conflicts of Interest: The authors declare no conflicts of interest.

References

1. Hinkelmann, K.; Kempthorne, O. *Design and Analysis of Experiments, Volume I: Introduction to Experimental Design*, 2nd ed.; Wiley Series of Probability and Statistics: Washington, DC, USA, 2008.
2. Bailey, R.A. *Design of Comparative Experiments*; Cambridge University Press: Cambridge, UK, 2008; ISBN 978-0-521-68357-9.
3. Everitt, B.S. *The Cambridge Dictionary of Statistics*; Cambridge University Press: Cambridge, UK, 2002; ISBN 0-521-81099-X.
4. Chalmers, T.C.; Smith, H.; Blackburn, B.; Silverman, B.; Schroeder, B.; Reitman, D.; Ambroz, A. A method for assessing the quality of a randomized control trial. *Control. Clin. Trials* **1981**, *2*, 31–49. [CrossRef]
5. Eddy, D.M. Evidence-based medicine: A unified approach. *Health Aff.* **2005**, *24*, 9–17. [CrossRef]
6. Robson, L.S.; Shannon, H.S.; Goldenhar, L.M.; Hale, A.R. Quasi-experimental and experimental designs: More powerful evaluation designs. In *Guide to Evaluating the Effectiveness of Strategies for Preventing Work Injuries*; Department of Health and Human Services, National Institute for Occupational Safety and Health: Cincinnati, OH, USA, 2001; pp. 29–42.
7. Kampenes, V.B.; Dybå, T.; Hannay, J.E.; Sjøberg, D.I.K. A systematic review of quasi-experiments in software engineering. *Inf. Softw. Technol.* **2009**, *51*, 71–82. [CrossRef]
8. Roth, J.; Sant'Anna, P.H.C.; Bilinski, A.; Poe, J. What's trending in difference-in-differences? A synthesis of the recent econometrics literature. *J. Econom.* **2023**, *235*, 2218–2244. [CrossRef]
9. Poole, M.A.; O'Farrell, P.N. The assumptions of the linear regression model. *Trans. Inst. Br. Geogr.* **1971**, *52*, 145–158. [CrossRef]
10. Ryan, A.M.; Burgess, J.F., Jr.; Dimick, J.B. Why we should not be indifferent to specification choices for difference-in-differences. *Health Res. Educ. Trust.* **2015**, *50*, 1211–1235. [CrossRef]
11. Abadie, A. Semiparametric difference-in-differences estimators. *Rev. Econ. Stud.* **2005**, *72*, 1–19. [CrossRef]
12. Imbens, G.; Lemieux, T.H. Regression Discontinuity Designs: A Guide to Practice. National Bureau of Economic Research Technical Working Paper 337. 2007. Available online: http://www.nber.org/papers/t0337 (accessed on 10 January 2025).
13. Nikolova, N.; Rodríguez, R.M.; Symes, M.; Toneva, D.; Kolev, K.; Tenekedjiev, K. Outlier detection algorithms over fuzzy data with weighted least squares. *Int. J. Fuzzy Syst.* **2021**, *23*, 1234–1256. [CrossRef]
14. Farkas, Á.Z.; Farkas, V.J.; Gubucz, I.; Szabó, L.; Bálint, K.; Tenekedjiev, K.; Nagy, A.I.; Sótonyi, P.; Hidi, L.; Nagy, Z.; et al. Neutrophil extracellular traps in thrombi retrieved during interventional treatment of ischemic arterial diseases. *Thromb. Res.* **2019**, *175*, 46–52. [CrossRef]
15. Mihaylova, N. Bootstrap-Based Simulation Platform for Analysis of Medical Information. Ph.D. Thesis, Nikola Vaptsarov Naval Academy, Varna, Bulgaria, 2015.
16. Panayotova, D. Application of echocardiographic methods for fuzzy stratification determining the volume of surgery in patients with ischemic mitral regurgitation. In *Medical Academic Repository*; Medical University: Varna, Bulgaria, 2023. Available online: https://repository.mu-varna.bg/handle/nls/3461 (accessed on 23 December 2024).
17. Faugeras, O.P. Maximal coupling of empirical copulas for discrete vectors. *J. Multivar. Anal.* **2015**, *137*, 179–186. [CrossRef]
18. Tenekedjiev, K.; Dimitrakiev, D.; Nikolova, N. Building frequentist distributions of continuous random variables. *Mach. Mech.* **2002**, *47*, 164–168.
19. Gao, S.; Zhong, Y.; Gu, C. Random weighting estimation of confidence intervals for quantiles. *Aust. N. Z. J. Stat.* **2013**, *55*, 43–53. [CrossRef]
20. Poe, G.; Giraud, K.; Loomis, J. Computational methods for measuring the difference of empirical distributions. *Am. J. Agric. Econ.* **2005**, *87*, 353–365. [CrossRef]
21. Wasserman, L. The Bootstrap and the Jackknife. In *All of Nonparametric Statistics*; Springer Texts in Statistics; Springer: New York, NY, USA, 2006; pp. 27–41. [CrossRef]
22. Henderson, R. The Bootstrap: A technique for data-driven statistics. Using computer-intensive analyses to explore experimental data. *Clin. Chim. Acta* **2005**, *359*, 1–26. [CrossRef]

23. González-Rodríguez, G.; Montenegro, M.; Colubi, A.; Gil, M.-A. Bootstrap techniques and fuzzy random variables: Synergy in hypothesis testing with fuzzy data. *Fuzzy Sets Syst.* **2006**, *157*, 2608–2613. [CrossRef]
24. Politis, D. Computer-intensive methods in statistical analysis. *Signal Process. Mag.* **1998**, *15*, 39–55. [CrossRef]
25. Chernobai, A.; Rachev, S.T.; Fabozzi, F.J. Composite goodness-of-fit tests for left-truncated loss samples. In *Handbook of Financial Econometrics and Statistics*; Lee, C.F., Lee, J., Eds.; Springer: New York, NY, USA, 2015; pp. 575–596. [CrossRef]
26. Groebner, D.F.; Shannon, P.W.; Fry, P.C. *Business Statistics—A Decision-Making Approach*, 10th ed.; Pearson: London, UK, 2018; pp. 387–434.
27. Böhm, W.; Hornik, K. A Kolmogorov-Smirnov test for r samples. *Res. Rep. Ser. Dep. Stat. Math.* **2010**, *105*, 103–125. [CrossRef]
28. Lemeshko, B.; Gobrunova, A.A. Application and power of the nonparametric Kuiper, Watson, and Zhang tests of goodness-of-fit. *Meas. Tech.* **2013**, *56*, 465–475. [CrossRef]
29. Press, W.H.; Teukolsky, S.A.; Vetterling, W.T.; Flannery, B.P. *Numerical Recipes—The Art of Scientific Computing*, 3rd ed.; Cambridge University Press: New York, NY, USA, 2007; Volume 732, p. 737.
30. Nikolova, N.; Ivanova, S.; Chin, C.; Tenekedjiev, K. Calculation of the Kolmogorov-Smirnov and Kuiper statistics over fuzzy samples. *Proc. Jangjeon Math. Soc.* **2017**, *20*, 269–311.
31. Nikolova, N.; Chai, S.; Ivanova, S.; Kolev, K.; Tenekedjiev, K. Bootstrap Kuiper testing of the identity of 1D continuous distributions using fuzzy samples. *Int. J. Comput. Intell. Syst.* **2015**, *8*, 63–75. [CrossRef]
32. Nikolova, N.; Mihaylova, N.; Tenekedjiev, K. Bootstrap tests for mean value differences over fuzzy samples. *IFAC-PapersOnLine* **2015**, *48*, 7–14. [CrossRef]
33. Tenekedjiev, K.; Nikolova, N.; Rodriguez, R.M.; Hirota, K. Bootstrap testing of central tendency nullity over paired fuzzy samples. *Int. J. Fuzzy Syst.* **2021**, *23*, 1934–1954. [CrossRef]
34. Zadeh, L.A. Fuzzy logic. In *Granular, Fuzzy, and Soft Computing*; Lin, T.Y., Liau, C.J., Kacprzyk, J., Eds.; Encyclopedia of Complexity and Systems Science Series; Springer: New York, NY, USA, 2009; pp. 19–49. [CrossRef]
35. Bickel, P.J.; Ren, J.-J. The Bootstrap in hypothesis testing. *Lect. Notes-Monogr. Ser.* **2001**, *36*, 91–112. Available online: http://www.jstor.org/stable/4356107 (accessed on 5 January 2025).
36. Wehrens, R.; Putter, H.; Buydens, L.M.C. The Bootstrap: A tutorial. *Chemom. Intell. Lab. Syst.* **2000**, *54*, 35–52. [CrossRef]
37. Cahoy, D.O. A Bootstrap test for equality of variances. *Comput. Stat. Data Anal.* **2010**, *54*, 2306–2316. [CrossRef]
38. Greco, L.; Luta, G.; Wilcox, R. On testing the equality between interquartile ranges. *Comput. Stat.* **2024**, *39*, 2873–2898. [CrossRef]
39. Hidi, L.; Komorowicz, E.; Kovács, G.I.; Szeberin, Z.; Garbaisz, D.; Nikolova, N.; Tenekedjiev, K.; Szabó, L.; Kolev, K.; Sótonyi, P. Cryopreservation moderates the thrombogenicity of arterial allografts during storage. *PLoS ONE* **2021**, *16*, e0255114. [CrossRef] [PubMed] [PubMed Central]
40. Nikolova, N.; Hirota, K.; Kobashikawa, C.; Tenekedjiev, K. Elicitation of non-monotonic preferences of a fuzzy rational decision maker. *Inf. Technol. Control.* **2006**, *4*, 36–50.
41. Coats, A.J.S.; Anker, S.D.; Baumbach, A.; Alfieri, O.; von Bardeleben, R.S.; Bauersachs, J.; Bax, J.J.; Boveda, S.; Čelutkienė, J.; Cleland, J.G.; et al. The management of secondary mitral regurgitation in patients with heart failure: A joint position statement from the Heart Failure Association (HFA), European Association of Cardiovascular Imaging (EACVI), European Heart Rhythm Association (EHRA), and European Association of Percutaneous Cardiovascular Interventions (EAPCI) of the ESC. *Eur. Heart J.* **2021**, *42*, 1254–1269. [CrossRef] [PubMed] [PubMed Central]
42. Mazin, I.; Arad, M.; Freimark, D.; Goldenberg, I.; Kuperstein, R. The prognostic role of mitral valve regurgitation severity and left ventricle function in acute heart failure. *J. Clin. Med.* **2022**, *11*, 4267. [CrossRef] [PubMed] [PubMed Central]
43. Vajapey, R.; Kwon, D. Guide to functional mitral regurgitation: A contemporary review. *Cardiovasc. Diagn. Ther.* **2021**, *11*, 781–792. [CrossRef] [PubMed] [PubMed Central]
44. Chan, K.M.; Punjabi, P.P.; Flather, M.; Wage, R.; Symmonds, K.; Roussin, I.; Rahman-Haley, S.; Pennell, D.J.; Kilner, P.J.; Dreyfus, G.D.; et al. Coronary artery bypass surgery with or without mitral valve annuloplasty in moderate functional ischemic mitral regurgitation: Final results of the Randomized Ischemic Mitral Evaluation (RIME) trial. *Circulation* **2012**, *126*, 2502–2510. [CrossRef] [PubMed]
45. Cully, M. Mitral valve repair with CABG surgery. *Nat. Rev. Cardiol.* **2013**, *10*, 6. [CrossRef] [PubMed]
46. Acker, M.A.; Parides, M.K.; Perrault, L.P.; Moskowitz, A.J.; Gelijns, A.C.; Voisine, P.; Smith, P.K.; Hung, J.W.; Blackstone, E.H.; Puskas, J.D.; et al. Mitral-valve repair versus replacement for severe ischemic mitral regurgitation. *N. Engl. J. Med.* **2014**, *370*, 23–32. [CrossRef] [PubMed]
47. Goldstein, D.; Moskowitz, A.J.; Gelijns, A.C.; Ailawadi, G.; Parides, M.K.; Perrault, L.P.; Hung, J.W.; Voisine, P.; Dagenais, F.; Gillinov, A.M.; et al. Two-year outcomes of surgical treatment of severe ischemic mitral regurgitation. *N. Engl. J. Med.* **2016**, *374*, 344–353. [CrossRef]
48. Andalib, A.; Chetrit, M.; Eberg, M.; Filion, K.B.; Thériault-Lauzier, P.; Lange, R.; Buithieu, J.; Martucci, G.; Eisenberg, M.; Bolling, S.F.; et al. A systematic review and meta-analysis of outcomes following mitral valve surgery in patients with significant functional mitral regurgitation and left ventricular dysfunction. *J. Heart Valve Dis.* **2016**, *25*, 696–707.

49. Dayan, V.; Soca, G.; Cura, L.; Mestres, C.A. Similar survival after mitral valve replacement or repair for ischemic mitral regurgitation: A meta-analysis. *Ann. Thorac. Surg.* **2014**, *97*, 758–765. [CrossRef]
50. Lio, A.; Miceli, A.; Varone, E.; Canarutto, D.; Di Stefano, G.; Della Pina, F.; Gilmanov, D.; Murzi, M.; Solinas, M.; Glauber, M. Mitral valve repair versus replacement in patients with ischaemic mitral regurgitation and depressed ejection fraction: Risk factors for early and mid-term mortality dagger. *Interdiscip. Cardiovasc. Thorac. Surg.* **2014**, *19*, 64–69. [CrossRef]
51. LaPar, D.J.; Ailawadi, G.; Isbell, J.M.; Crosby, I.K.; Kern, J.A.; Rich, J.B.; Speir, A.M.; Kron, I.L. Mitral valve repair rates correlate with surgeon and institutional experience. *J. Thorac. Cardiovasc. Surg.* **2014**, *148*, 995–1003; Discussion 3–4. [CrossRef]
52. Maltais, S.; Schaff, H.V.; Daly, R.C.; Suri, R.M.; Dearani, J.A.; Sundt, T.M., 3rd; Enriquez-Sarano, M.; Topilsky, Y.; Park, S.J. Mitral regurgitation surgery in patients with ischemic cardiomyopathy and ischemic mitral regurgitation: Factors that influence survival. *J. Thorac. Cardiovasc. Surg.* **2011**, *142*, 995–1001. [CrossRef] [PubMed]
53. Panayotov, P.; Panayotova, D.; Nikolova, N.; Donchev, N.; Ivanova, S.; Mircheva, L.; Petrov, V.; Tenekedjiev, K. Algorithms for formal stratification of patients with ischemic mitral regurgitation. *Scr. Sci. Medica* **2018**, *50*, 33–38. [CrossRef]
54. Nikolova, N.; Panayotov, P.; Panayotova, D.; Ivanova, S.; Tenekedjiev, K. Using fuzzy sets in surgical treatment selection and homogenizing stratification of patients with significant chronic ischemic mitral regurgitation. *Int. J. Comput. Intell. Syst.* **2019**, *12*, 1075–1090. [CrossRef]
55. Oxorn, D.C.; Otto, C.M. *Atlas of Intraoperative Transesophageal Echocardiography*; W.B. Saunders Company: Philadelphia, PA, USA, 2006.
56. Armstrong, W.F.; Ryan, T.H. *Feigenbaum's Echocardiography*, 7th ed.; Lippincott Williams & Wilkins: Philadelphia, PA, USA, 2010.
57. Charles, E.J.; Kronn, I.L. Data, not dogma, for ischemic mitral regurgitation. *J. Thorac. Cardiovasc. Surg.* **2017**, *154*, 137–138. [CrossRef] [PubMed]
58. Doig, F.; Lu, Z.-Q.; Smith, S.; Naidoo, R. Long term survival after surgery for ischaemic mitral regurgitation: A single centre Australian experience. *Heart Lung Circ.* **2021**, *30*, 612–619. [CrossRef] [PubMed]
59. El-Hag-Aly, M.A.; El Swaf, Y.F.; Elkassas, M.H.; Hagag, M.G.; Allam, H.K. Moderate ischemic mitral incompetence: Does it worth more ischemic time? *Gen. Thorac. Cardiovasc. Surg.* **2020**, *68*, 492–498. [CrossRef]
60. Gujarati, D. *Basic Econometrics*, 4th ed.; Tata McGraw Hill: New York, NY, USA, 2004; pp. 148–149+378+947–948.
61. Raska, A.; Kálmán, K.; Egri, B.; Csikós, P.; Beinrohr, L.; Szabó, L.; Tenekedjiev, K.; Nikolova, N.; Longstaff, C.; Roberts, I.; et al. Synergism of red blood cells and tranexamic acid in the inhibition of fibrinolysis. *J. Thromb. Haemost.* **2024**, *22*, 794–804. [CrossRef]
62. Tóth, E.; Beinrohr, L.; Gubucz, I.; Szabó, L.; Tenekedjiev, K.; Nikolova, N.; Nagy, A.I.; Hidi, L.; Sótonyi, P.; Szikora, I.; et al. Fibrin to von Willebrand factor ratio in arterial thrombi is associated with plasma levels of inflammatory biomarkers and local abundance of extracellular DNA. *Thromb. Res.* **2022**, *209*, 8–15. [CrossRef]
63. Lytsy, P. P in the right place: Revisiting the evidential value of *p*-values. *J. Evid. Based Med.* **2018**, *11*, 288–291. [CrossRef] [PubMed] [PubMed Central]

applied sciences

MDPI

Perspective

The Critical Link in the Successful Application of Advanced Clinical Decision Making—Revisiting the Physician–Patient Relationship from a Practical and Pragmatic Perspective

Franco Musio

Department of Medicine, University of Virginia School of Medicine—Inova Fairfax Campus, Falls Church, VA 22033, USA; frmusio@gmail.com

Abstract: Advanced clinical decision making has been rapidly evolving, primarily due to the ever-expanding field of healthcare technologies. Moreover, the physician–patient relationship has taken on new complexions, particularly in the realm of shared decision making, which champions patient autonomy, leading to contemporary "personalized medicine". Models currently studied and employed in clinical decision making and the bonds between physician and patient will be explored to include their intricate interrelationships. Furthermore, both clinical decision making and the physician–patient relationship demonstrate dynamic reciprocal associations with each other in a synergistic fashion. Novel schematics will be highlighted for the elucidation of these labyrinthine processes, and real-life clinical examples will be shared. A strong bond between physicians and patients, particularly through the exercise of shared decision making, is inherent and necessary for the effectuation of clinical decisions and treatment plans. The vital ingredients of trust, empathy, and communication will be elaborated upon as underpinning the goals of thorough and meticulous patient care. Ultimately, the physician–patient relationship acts as a "filter" through which the processes of decision making must pass in order to be implemented. As such, the strength of this alliance is critical in today's complex era of advanced healthcare technologies.

Keywords: clinical decision making; physician–patient relationship; healthcare; communication; trust; problem solving

1. Introduction

Advanced clinical decision making is entering into a new ever-complex era due to rapidly developing health care technologies spearheaded by accelerating artificial intelligence. In 2023, 17.6% of the gross domestic product (GDP) of the United States was spent on healthcare (4.8 trillion dollars), with the greatest percentage based on clinical decisions by physicians [1]. The importance of this is also reflected in contentions that erroneous decision making is now one of the top three causes of death in the US and likely around the world [2]. Conversely, the above is greatly outweighed by the exercise of judicious medical science problem solving leading to the curing of diseases, longer life spans, and vastly improved quality of life for many patients globally. Notwithstanding the wonderous breakthroughs enabling up-to-date clinical decision making, in the majority of cases, these processes would not have been possible without a strong physician–patient relationship. This perspective is based on my interactions with thousands of patients and a similar number of colleagues over many years in my practice of medicine in the fields of nephrology/internal medicine. My interpretation and use of models of clinical decision making and the physician–patient relationship are in their representations as frameworks for problem solving and delivery of care, particularly in the treatment of multifaceted and intricate diseases.

Both clinical decision making and the physician–patient relationship are construed by models with the purpose of applying more concrete structures to formulations that are often nebulous and ill-defined. Four separate models of clinical decision-making "processes" will be explored, although it should be noted that there are intersections and overlapping aspects of each in day-to-day practice. Likewise, four separate models of the physician–patient relationship will be presented, which similarly demonstrate overlapping features in the realities of clinical practice. Rapidly advancing healthcare technologies and mass media are greatly influencing the physician–patient relationship and leveraging its dynamics to a more collaborative alliance of shared decision making. Emphasis is thus placed upon patient autonomy in contemporary "patient-centered care". Moreover, the elements of trust, empathy, and communication will be discussed as the true foundations for a solid association between physicians and patients.

Intricate schematic representations will be posited, and real-life clinical examples will be interspersed throughout the sections of this perspective. Briefly, three separate paradigms (with sub-paradigms) will be proposed, represented by two- and three-dimensional geometric figures: the four models of clinical decision making, the four models of the physician–patient relationship, and the multifaceted relationships and interconnections between the models of clinical decision making and the physician–patient relationship. The sequential order of these analyses in this perspective is based on the central importance of the physician–patient relationship as the "catalyst" for clinical decision making and, thus, the ultimate purpose of healthcare. These precepts will become more tangible as this perspective develops. Effectively, my strong leanings favor the model of shared decision making for both clinical decision making and the physician–patient relationship, which will be elaborated upon.

At a higher level, the physician–patient relationship acts as a "rate-limiting step" for the execution of clinical decisions. Furthermore, this alliance interacts with and develops its characteristics from the models of clinical decision making. Interestingly, the inverse will also become apparent—that is, the processes of clinical decision making also interact with and develop their characteristics from the models of the physician–patient relationship. The main thesis of this perspective, therefore, is the inductively derived precept that the execution and ultimate effectuation of clinical decision making is accomplished by its filtering and distillation through the medium of the physician–patient relationship. In this vein, the current vast literature concerning clinical decision making and the physician–patient relationship will be distinguished from my opinions and personal perspectives, gleaned and refined throughout my years of medical practice.

The intent of this perspective is to serve as a framework of critical thinking for the scientific and medical communities. The overriding objective is to shed insight into the constructs and components integral to modern-day patient care, particularly those of a complex nature. Ultimately, the aim is to assist scientists, clinicians, and all professionals directly or indirectly involved in the healthcare field in the advancement of their appreciation of the mechanics of the entities of clinical decision making and the physician–patient relationship. In point of fact, I wish to share my "epiphany", which will come to light through the unfolding of this perspective piece, that a synergism and reciprocal interrelationships exist between the two. In sum, a "bird's eye view" of this intricate topic will be presented to the scientific and medical communities in this Special Issue of Advanced Decision Making in Clinical Medicine.

This compendium will be partitioned into main segments (and their subsegments), with the intent of sequentially introducing descriptions, concepts, and precepts in a building block fashion, ultimately leading to conclusions and their synthesis:

1. The processes of clinical decision making: the four models, with clinical examples,
2. The integral role of the physician–patient relationship: historical notes of the four models, with clinical examples,
3. The variables of trust, empathy, and communication: hallmarks of shared decision making,
4. Neurobiological, psychosocial, and behavioral components of clinical practice,
5. The essential role of the physician–patient relationship for the effectuation of advanced clinical decision making.

2. Discussion

2.1. The Processes of Clinical Decision Making: The Four Models, with Clinical Examples

2.1.1. Overview

The skeletal framework of clinical decision making is predicated on the steps involved in hypotheco-deductive reasoning adapted from the scientific method: hypothesis generation, evaluation, refinement, and verification [3]. The more recent literature describes slight variations of the above, although the root of medical decision making is based on a stepwise process of validations in the initial and subsequent face-to-face encounters with patients [4]. More "ornate" frameworks exist based on the complexity of the individual cases, with advanced clinical decision making in clinical medicine now able to insert its "tentacles" within and between any number of steps of this elaborate paradigm (Figure 1). In fact, such a scaffold may be applied to various degrees to a universal approach in the applications of scientific inquiry and pursuits of many different disciplines. The preeminent processes in clinical decision making currently encompass four models:

- Rational Model,
- Evidence-Based Model,
- Intuitive Model,
- Participatory/Shared Decision-Making Model.

The Rational Model emanates from the study of cognitive science, which consists of critical thinking, metacognition (thinking about thinking), introspection, reflection, and communication [5,6]. This approach pre-supposes adequate data and information for well-defined and structured clinical scenarios coupled with the availability of the required time. This process can optimally be used in cases such as those of slow-growing (or even aggressive) malignancies or long-term conditions, including chronic kidney, pulmonary, and heart disease, in which a number of possible diagnostic studies, imaging techniques, and laboratory and genetic analyses are available for the evaluation and treatment of the specific malady.

The Evidence-Based Model parallels the Rational Model as it is predicated on high-quality research engendering empirical pathways, practice guidelines, and clinical decision rules, although it also includes the wishes of the patient [7,8]. Conversely, in my opinion, the many nuances, variables, and anecdotal elements so often present in clinical medicine and contributing to its "art form" are not wholly emphasized in this model. By way of illustration, this process of decision making is not optimal in all cases, such as with certain complex illnesses in which the infusion of packed red blood cells would likely benefit the patient. The above would occur only through the implementation of transfusion thresholds higher than those recommended by societal guidelines (as the guidance is currently based on a trigger of a low level of hemoglobin to administer transfusions). Another example would include the treatment of hypertension, in which adherence to current guidelines from a number of medical societies is not always applicable and appropriate for all patients. These would include those with cerebrovascular and renovascular diseases, which often require higher blood pressures for the adequate perfusion of blood to these tissue beds. As a result, although beneficial in many circumstances, this approach is not always tailored to the individual manifesting unique pathophysiological characteristics.

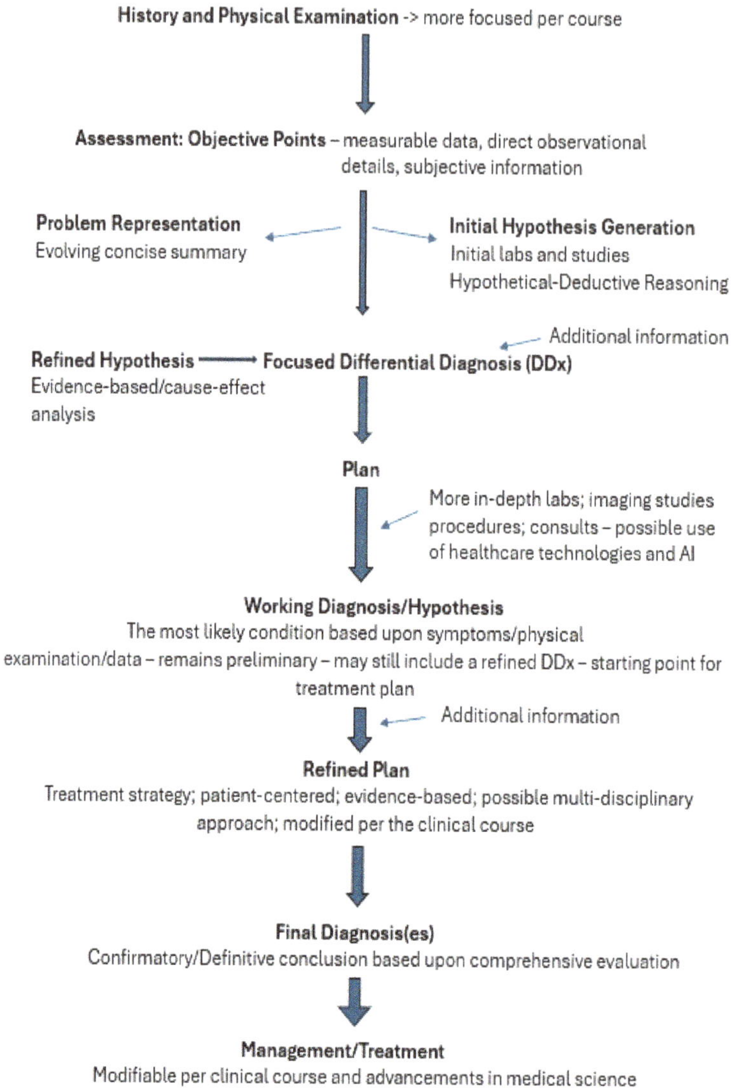

Figure 1. Diagnostic Paradigm of Clinical Decision Making.

The Intuitive Model employs spontaneous decisions based on the physician's combination of experience, wisdom, instincts, and, at times, emotions [9]. This unique approach is frequently utilized in acute and critical circumstances, such as those seen in the Emergency Departments with cardiac arrests or intraoperatively when unanticipated anatomical challenges or complications (such as hemorrhage) spontaneously occur. Under these conditions, the decision-making process must take place very rapidly, and, at times, immediately due to the emergent nature of the condition. Instinctual responses based on the experience of the physician are thus required at times. Also, it is rare that a decision using this model cannot be retraced and adjusted in the setting of the unpredictability of the challenges being addressed.

The Participatory/Shared Decision-Making Model is as much a process for decision making as the mainstream model for the physician–patient relationship itself, in which patient autonomy and patient-centered care are highlighted. The shared decision-making process appears to be abetted by the rapid growth of medical science and mass media, leading to multiple diagnostic approaches and treatments that were not available until the last decade or even more recently. As a result, the process of arriving at a decision is based on the contribution of both the physician and the patient in a climate of respect for each other's system of values and goals [10–13]. A prime example of this model of decision making occurs in the arena of hematology–oncology, in which the very rapid advancement of diagnostics and medications/treatments now leads to multiple potential options of care, which require significant input from the patient/family. In addition, my own field of nephrology has rapidly grown such that multiple treatment regimens for many different types of kidney diseases now appear to also oblige the involvement of the patient and their family.

These prodigious advancements in the medical sciences have also affected my practice as the greater part of my current decision-making processes is based on this model of Participatory/Shared Decision Making. Interestingly, studies over the last twenty years reflect improved outcomes with the application of this model of clinical decision making, particularly among patients with diabetes mellitus and systemic lupus erythematosus [14,15]. Anecdotal experiences also favor this "prototypical" model in my personal discerning and formation of decisions. Patients are typically keenly aware of the dynamics, distinctions, and subtleties of their own bodies; thus, they are well-positioned to contribute in a collaborative fashion to the determination of the plan of action for their specific disease process/processes. However, this model of decision making may not be preferred by all physicians (and patients) due to a number of potential circumstances, which will be explored later.

2.1.2. Geometric Paradigms for the Interrelationships of the Models for Clinical Decision Making

As a means of conceptualizing the intricacies of these four models of clinical decision making, a novel metaphorical geometric schematic paradigm will be proposed (never previously introduced in the literature): a 3-dimensional tetrahedral triangular pyramid composed of four triangular-plane figure faces, six straight edges, and four vertices (Figure 2).

This geometric figure represents the summation and integration of the four models of clinical decision making as a Principal paradigm. Each vertex represents one individual model of clinical decision making, with the entire geometric figure consisting of and broken down into four separate metaphorical plane figure "triangulations" with the following reciprocal relationships:

- Sub-paradigm a: Participatory/SDM Model—Evidence-Based Model—Rational Model (Figure 3a),
- Sub-paradigm b: Participatory/SDM Model—Evidence-Based Model—Intuitive Model (Figure 3b),
- Sub-paradigm c: Participatory/SDM Model—Rational Model—Intuitive Model (Figure 3c),
- Sub-paradigm d: Evidence-Based Model—Rational Model—Intuitive Model (Figure 3d).

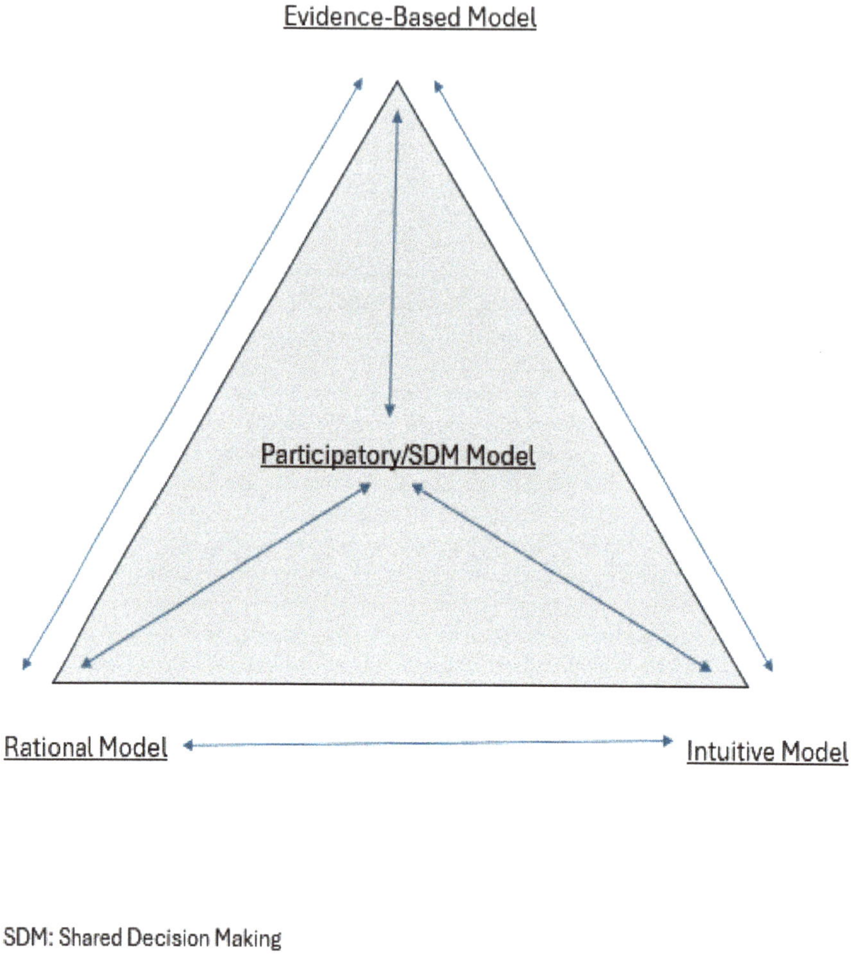

Figure 2. The Principal paradigm represented as a tetrahedral pyramid metaphorically demonstrating the summation and integration of the all the reciprocal relationships of the four models of clinical decision making.

The purpose of the principal paradigm and the sub-paradigms is to improve on the concept that "real-life" clinical decision making is based simply on individual models. Rather, this metaphorical tetrahedral triangular pyramid consisting of four triangles illustrates the confluence of the four models required for real-life clinical decision making. The double-sided arrows are placed between the vertices in a similar fashion to that of a symbol used in mathematics or logic: each vertex representing a single model is "true" only if each of the other three vertices is also "true". Each model is interconnected geometrically, although also in actuality; that is, each model of clinical decision making has a two-directional relationship with each of the other models. The translation to the real-life practice of medicine is that decision making cannot be based on just one model, but rather a composite with varying degrees of contribution by all four models.

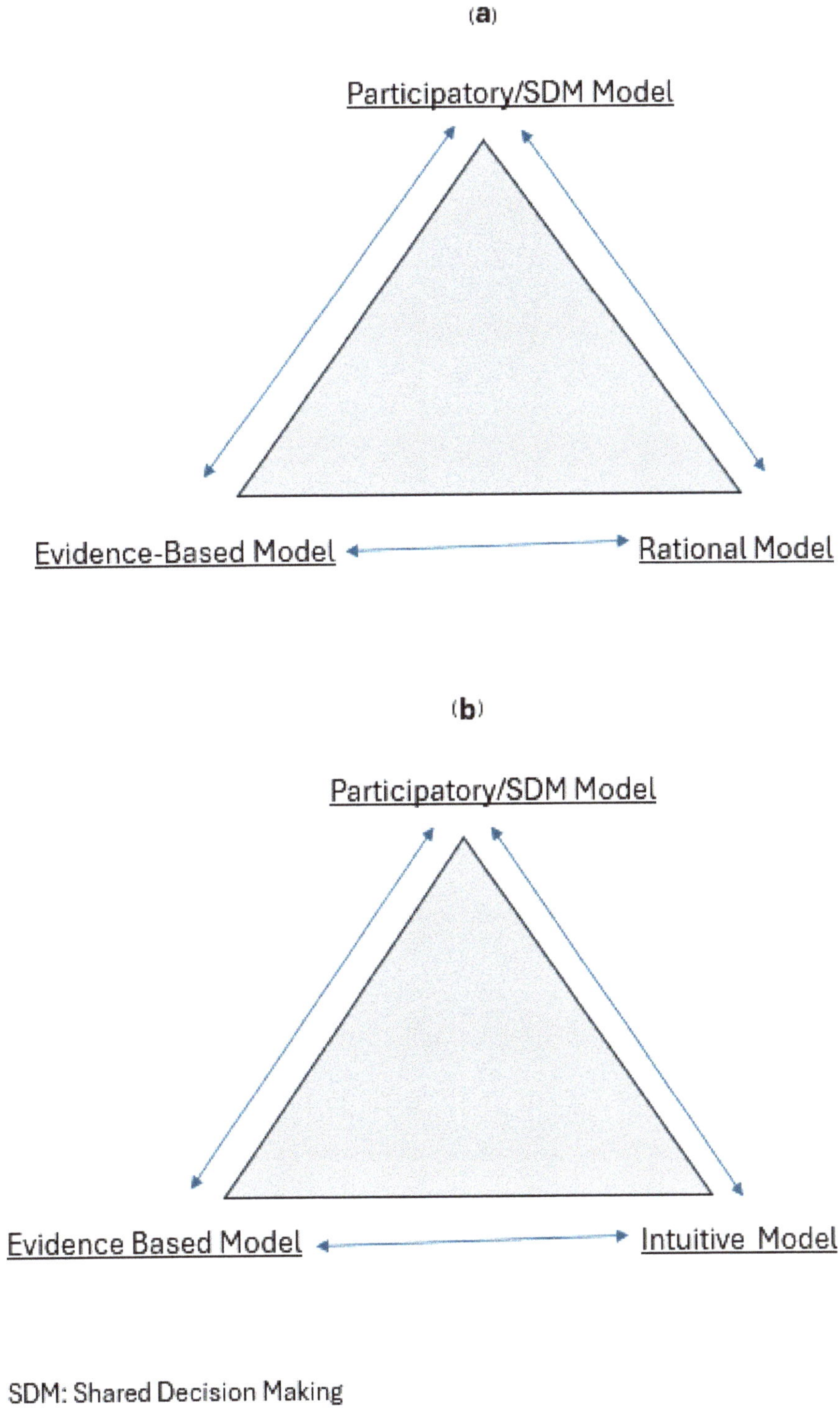

Figure 3. *Cont.*

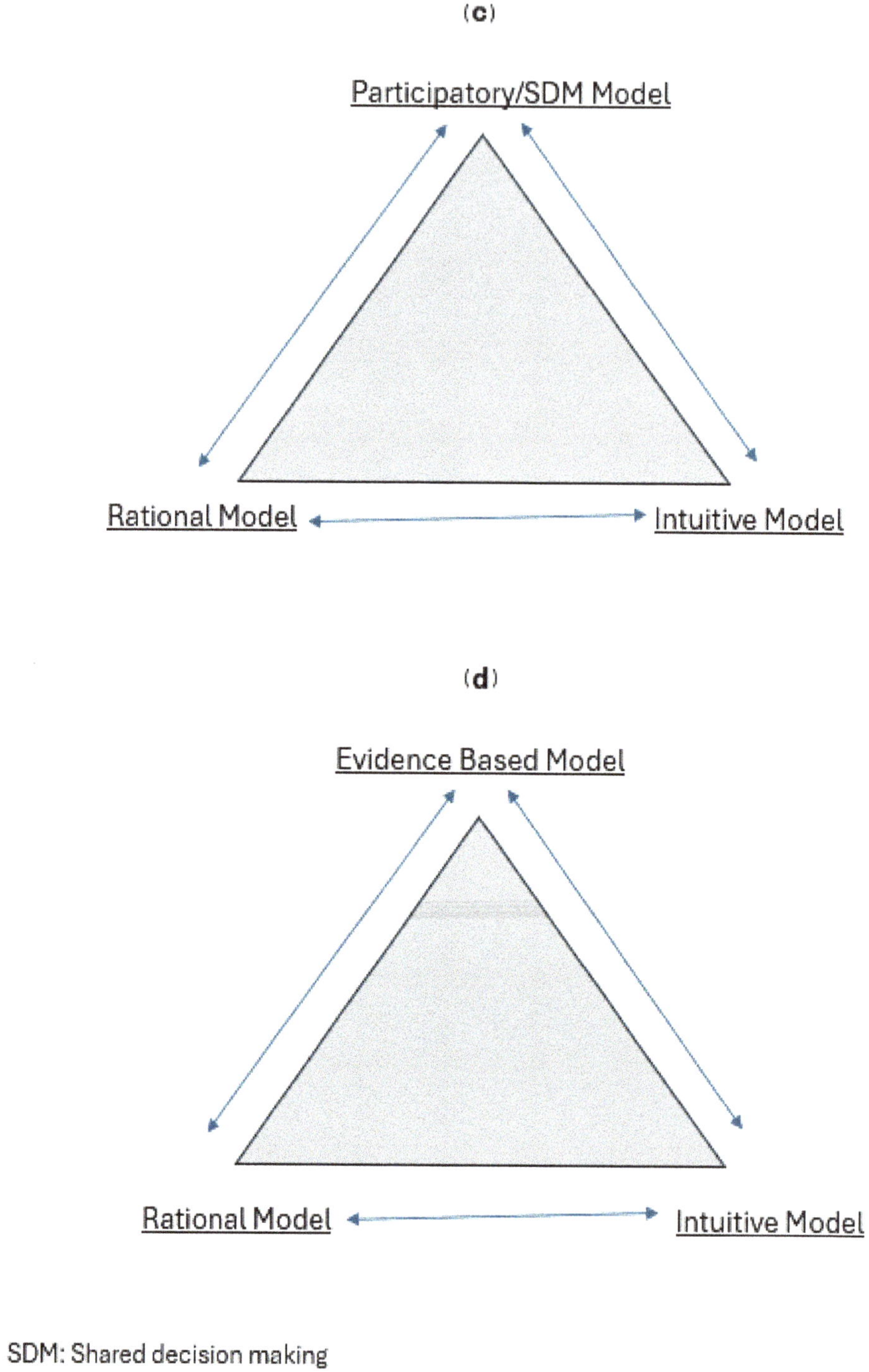

Figure 3. (**a**–**d**) The four separate triangular sub-paradigms which as a composite constitute the principal tetrahedral pyramid depicted in Figure 2. These plane figures metaphorically subtype all the interrelationships involved in clinical decision making.

For further elaboration, the essence of the four separate metaphorical "triangulations" is that the individual decision-making models in real-life medical practice cannot be utilized in isolation; rather realistic and tangible patient care is based on a synthesis of elements from multiple models. In order for the tetrahedral pyramid to take geometric form, each individual vertex must share a straight line with and thus be connected to each of the other three remaining individual vertices. The integration of the above, therefore, results in the confluence of all four models of clinical decision making in the care of patients. That is, one individual model (as represented by one individual vertex) does not exist in isolation, but rather in a fluid and dynamic interaction of various proportionate degrees with the other three individual models (likewise represented by individual vertices).

At a higher level, the four separate metaphorical triangulations, similarly, cannot exist in isolation, but rather as a convergence with each of the other individual triangles in order for the tetrahedral pyramid to take its geometric form. As with the individual vertices, a fluid and dynamic interaction exists in various proportionate degrees within and between each entire triangle (each representing three individual models of clinical decision making). As a result, an intermingling of all the models again occurs in the composition of the entire metaphorical tetrahedral pyramid. Moreover, certain models of clinical decision making also contribute to a greater or lesser extent in the overall decision-making process for each individual patient based on multiple factors: the availability of data, the complexity of the medical problem(s), the multiple nuances and exceptions seen in the particular disease process(es), the availability of resources and clinical expertise in addressing the medical problem(s), and the cooperation and wishes of the patient, in addition to other considerations.

2.1.3. Clinical Examples of the Convergence of the Models of Clinical Decision Making

Real-life examples of the intersection of the models of clinical decision making abound in the day-to-day practice of medicine. An example would be the care of a complex renal transplant patient with many comorbidities in the intensive care unit facing sepsis, hemolysis (breakdown of red blood cells), respiratory failure, and progressive renal failure from an overwhelming infection. The multiple models/processes essential in attaining the decisions required in the care of this patient may often change in regard to their relative contributions and consequences, although they may still interact with each other based on the undulating courses of the diseases and conditions themselves. The participation of the patient (to the extent possible) and the family is paramount, although a rational overview of the clinical course, at times using evidence-based strategies, as well as involving elements of clinical intuition by the physician are all important components of arriving at the advanced care decisions required in this and many other complicated cases requiring multiple specialists at tertiary and quaternary care institutions. Patients requiring a lower amount of involved care, for example, those with a single clinician caring for a less critically ill individual than the former, also require varying models (with various relative contributions) in the decision-making processes. Such an example would be represented by a hemodialysis patient in the outpatient setting experiencing fluid retention and hypertension, with complications during treatments, such as fluctuating hypotension and hypertension, cramping, and malaise, ultimately leading to suboptimal treatments. The attending nephrologist and patient must often use the process of shared decision making, particularly in this case as the patient will need to gainfully participate in and agree to the treatment plans. The clinician will also need to utilize rational and evidence-based decision-making processes (possibly with some intuition) in arriving at the solutions in the care of this particular patient. As the course continues, the models remain interrelated with each other, although their relative contributions to the overall treatment plan may change.

2.2. The Integral Role of the Physician–Patient Relationship: Historical Notes of the Four Models, with Clinical Examples

2.2.1. Overview

The objective of this segment is to diverge from the models of clinical decision making discussed in the previous segment and focus on the separate models of the physician–patient relationship. The interlocking and reciprocal relationship between the overall models of clinical decision making and those of the physician–patient relationship will be elaborated in Segment V.

The modern-day study of the physician–patient relationship commenced with the writings of Talcot Parsons, Professor of Sociology at Harvard University, who described and championed an asymmetric Paternalistic Model, in which the physician acts as a fatherly figure and as a trained and institutionally certified expert caring autonomously and knowing the best course of action, with no input by the patient [16]. In rare circumstances, elements of this model may still be applicable. This professionally dominant model was preeminent following World War Two until the mid-1960s, during a period coined as the Golden Age of Medicine. This period served as the springboard for the evolution of the physician–patient relationship due to the growing "commodification" of healthcare, in which the medical landscape was forced to change due to numerous external pressures to include insurance companies, the rapidly growing pharmaceutical industry, and federal governments around the world [17].

In 1972, Robert Veatch, Professor Emeritus of Medical Ethics and Philosophy at Georgetown University, was the first to accommodate to the new medical landscape by proposing four models of the physician–patient relationship, upon which all the subsequent literature and scholarly discussion has been based: Priestly Model, Engineering Model, Contractual Model, and Collegial Model [18]. Parenthetically, I am honored to have been a student of Professor Veatch in my early collegiate years. Similar to the Paternalistic Model, the Priestly Model assumes that the physician makes all the medical decisions without input from the patient or recognition of their system of values. The Engineering/Scientific Model can be construed as the antithesis of the above and as the foundation of a consumerism approach, in which the patient asymmetrically makes the medical decision after the data, technical information, and options are presented by the physician. Both the Contractual and Collegial Models are very similar, with slight variations, in which a collaboration exists between the physician and patient, thus presaging shared decision making in the current era of patient autonomy and patient-centered care.

Twenty years later, Ezekiel Emanuel and Linda Emanuel, from the Dana Farber Cancer Institute (Boston, MA, USA) and the Kennedy School of Government of Harvard University, respectively, elaborated upon four models of the physician–patient relationship (paralleling those of Veatch), which remain the basis for current-day scholarship and practice: Paternalistic Model, Informative Model, Interpretive Model, and the Deliberative/Shared Decision-Making Model [19]. The Paternalistic and Informative Models retain their age-old characteristics. The latter is based on Veatch's Engineering/Scientific Model, which portrays the physician as the provider of information and the patient as the consumer, thus representing a relationship presupposing the modern-day "commodification" of medicine. Examples of the above include the not-so-infrequent patient referred to as the "doctor shopper", who will often admit that they have not been satisfied with their previous physicians (or the advice given); therefore, multiple different clinicians are sought. In my experience, these patients typically do not seek partnerships or alliances in their interactions with physicians.

On the other hand, the Interpretive Model connotes a collaborative relationship between the physician and the patient, with the nuance that the physician acts as a counselor of sorts, assisting the patient in understanding their own value systems and goals in arriving at treatment plans. In this case, the physician does not inject his or her own system of values and thus uses those of the patient as the basis for recommendations in the treatment plan. This relationship is often close and highly productive, although without true involvement of the physician's own preferences. Occasionally, I utilize this Interpretive Model style of interaction and seek to highlight the patient's own set of principles and morals; thus, I will not elaborate on my personal recommendations and preferences. However, I certainly share my experiences and interpretations of the medical condition/s (as well as those of my colleagues and the medical community) with the patient in a collaborative fashion. An example would be that of an elderly, although "physiologically fit", patient with a certain kidney disease, in which the treatments are evolving and are not clear-cut. This patient has previously clarified their wishes of "allowing nature to take its course", which will be revisited by myself, and thus, the aggressivity of the medication and treatment regimen would require tailoring. Although my personal preference and recommendations in cases such as these, at times, would be to pursue a more aggressive plan of action, it would oppose the patient's value system and preferences; therefore, a milder regimen with fewer potential side effects would be chosen.

The Deliberative Model is synonymous with and the template for the current era of shared decision making between the physician and the patient. Spurred by the prodigious mass media in tandem with rapidly accelerating medical science, the patient is now approaching a more central role in clinical decision making and in their engagement in the physician–patient relationship. As such, the modern-day bond between the two involves the physician analyzing and presenting the scientific data in the context of the patient's case, giving recommendations for courses of action and treatment with mutual input from the patient regarding their preferences. Both the physician and the patient share each other's personal system of values, although the final decision is typically arrived at by the patient.

I principally prefer this latter relationship model, although I also appreciate the intersection of the other models of the physician–patient relationship in fostering unions with patients. This may be illustrated with nephrological diseases such as glomerulonephritides (inflammation of the microscopic filtering portion of the kidneys) and other renal diseases, in which many forms may exist as primary or secondary conditions. The treatment paradigms have become more numerous and diverse due to ongoing research such that "one size does not fit all". There are now multiple medications, immunosuppressive, biological, and non-biological agents, and procedures that are employed in the arsenal for the treatment of kidney diseases. As a result, treatment plans must consider variables such as age, sex, ongoing comorbid issues, and psychological/social/cultural issues, which require input and mutual discussion between the physician and the patient. I will make clear my recommendations and preferences to be followed by deliberation in a collaborative fashion, although ultimately the decision rests with the individual patient (and family in many circumstances). In addition to the growing literature supporting the Shared Decision-Making Model, it appears, in point of fact, that it is a logical outgrowth of the rapid advancement of healthcare technologies. In my opinion, a maturation and evolution of the "position" of the patient is occurring in our era of cybermedicine, which is more adeptly aligned with the model of shared decision making.

2.2.2. Geometric Paradigms for the Interrelationships of the Models for the Physician–Patient Relationship

In the same vein as schematizing the models of clinical decision making, I will proceed with also schematizing the four models of the physician–patient relationship in the same manner. As a means of conceptualizing the intricacies of these four models, I will again propose a novel metaphorical geometric schematic paradigm (never previously introduced in the literature) consisting of a 3-dimensional tetrahedral triangular pyramid composed of four triangular-plane figure faces, six straight edges, and four vertices (Figure 4). This is the same geometric figure used in the schematization of the models of clinical decision making in Figures 2 and 3, although they involve a different subject matter. This geometric figure represents the summation and integration of the four models of the physician-patient relationship as a Principal paradigm. Each vertex represents one individual model of the physician–patient relationship, with the entire geometric figure consisting of and broken down into four separate metaphorical plane figure "triangulations" with the following reciprocal relationships:

- Sub-paradigm a: Shared Decision-Making Model—Counselor/Interpretive Model—Paternalistic Model (Figure 5a),
- Sub-paradigm b: Shared Decision-Making Model—Counselor/Interpretive Model—Consumerism/Informative Model (Figure 5b),
- Sub-paradigm c: Shared Decision-Making Model—Paternalistic Model/Consumerism/Informative Model (Figure 5c),
- Sub-paradigm d: Counselor/Interpretive Model—Paternalistic Model—Consumerism/Informative Model (Figure 5d).

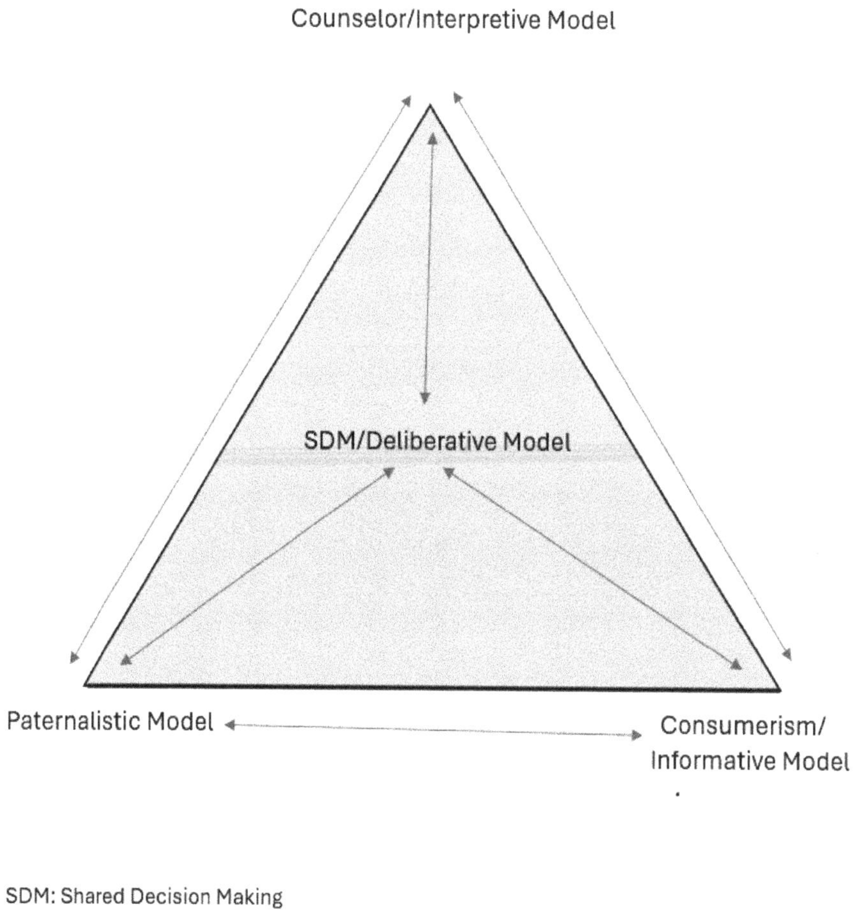

Figure 4. The Principal paradigm represented as a tetrahedral pyramid metaphorically demonstrating the summation and integration of the all the reciprocal relationships of the four models of the physician-patient relationship.

(a)

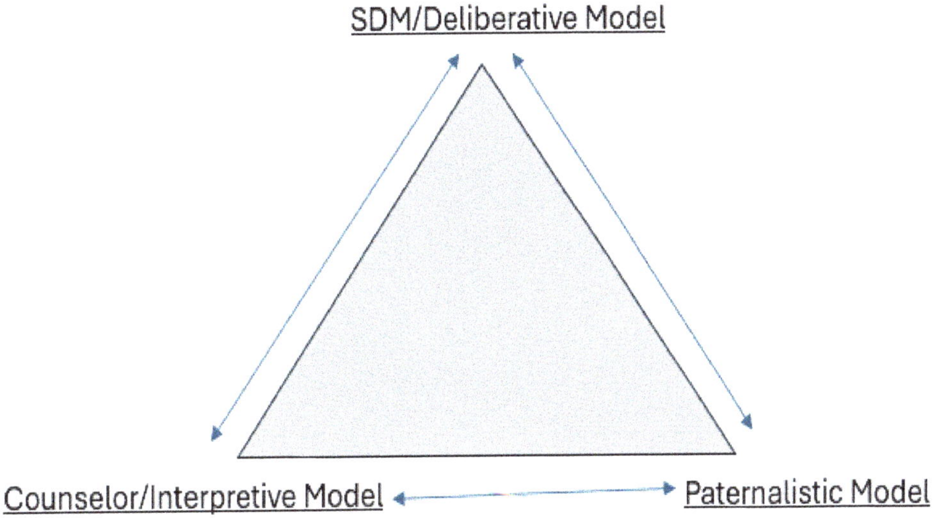

(b)

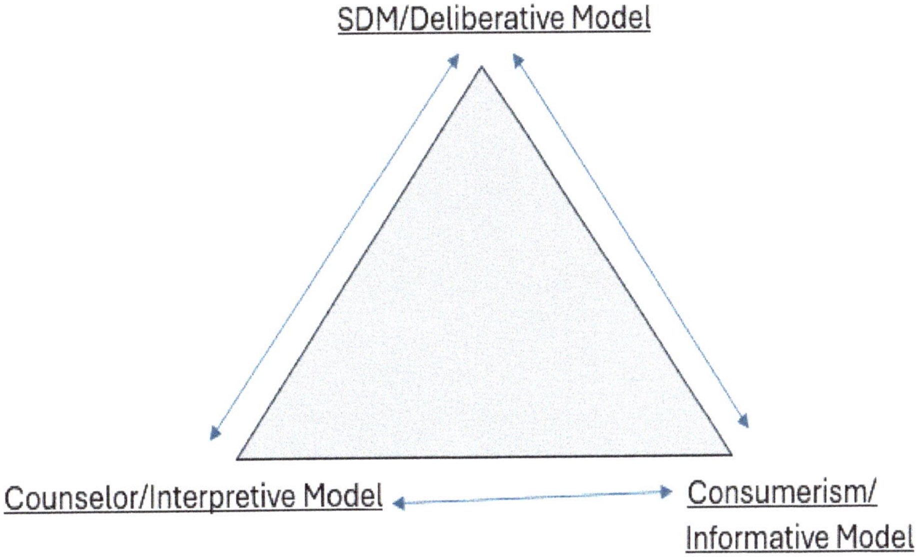

Figure 5. *Cont.*

(c)

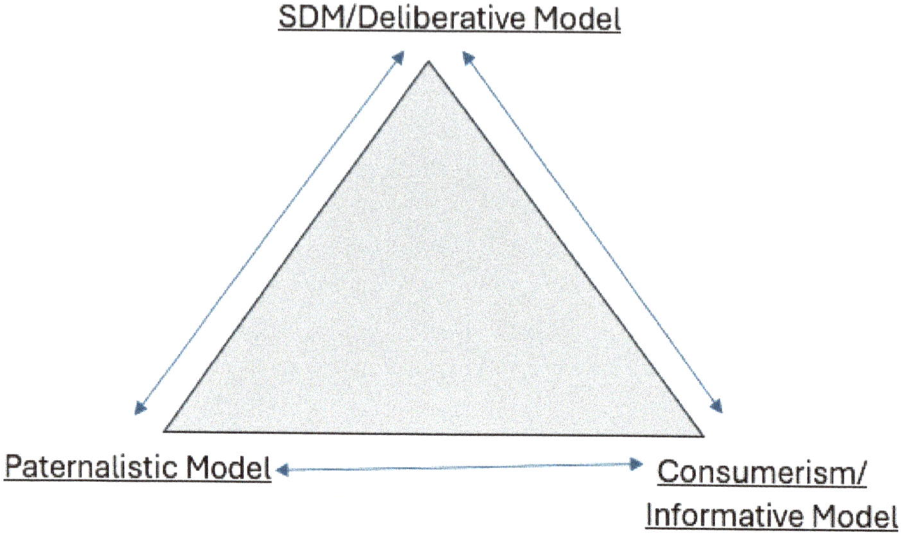

(d)

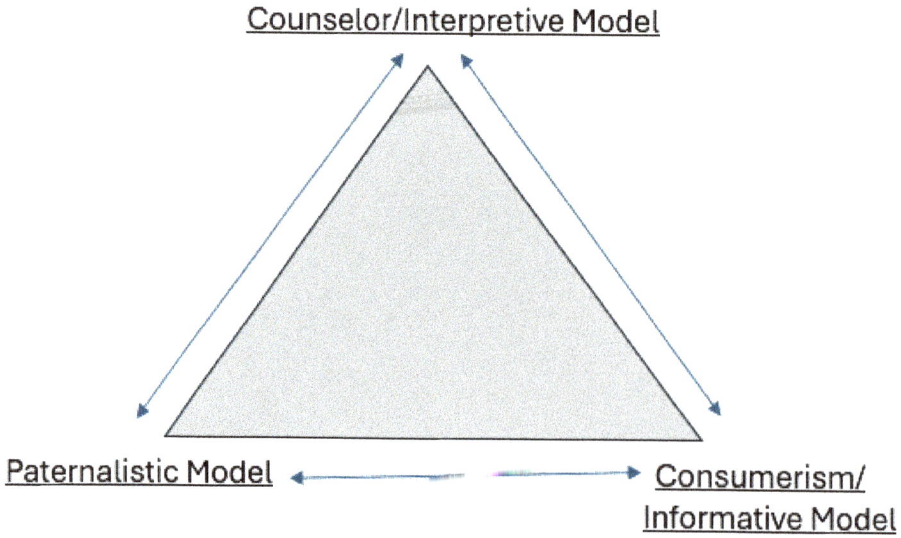

Figure 5. (**a**–**d**) The four separate triangular sub-paradigms which as a composite constitute the principal tetrahedral pyramid depicted in Figure 4. These plane figures metaphorically subtype all the interrelationships involved in the physician-patient relationships.

As with clinical decision making, the essence of the four separate "triangulations" of the physician–patient relationship is that no single model can be considered in isolation; rather, patient care involves a synthesis of elements from the multiple models. At a higher level, in order for the tetrahedral pyramid to take geometric form, each individual vertex must share a straight line with and thus be connected in a reciprocal fashion to each of the other three individual vertices. The mechanics of this novel paradigm follow those of the models of clinical decision making previously elaborated in Figures 2 and 3. The integration of the above results in a relative confluence of all four models of the physician–patient relationship, which is operative in the care of patients. That is, one individual model may take precedence during one period of time in the care of patients, although it does not exist alone, but rather as a convergence with the others to various degrees. Certain models may also contribute to a greater or lesser extent to the physician–patient relationship based on multiple factors: the nature and complexity of the disease processes, the preferences of the patient and the physician in the delivery and acceptance of care, the individual value systems of the physician and patient (as discussed above), social and cultural determinants, geographic and logistical issues, and patient "health literacy" (understanding of health-related issues), in addition to other considerations.

2.2.3. Clinical Examples of the Convergence of the Individual Models of the Physician Patient Relationship

Real-life examples of the intersection of the models of the physician–patient relationship are ubiquitous in the day-to-day practice of medicine. An example would include a patient followed for years with stable lung and kidney disease developing a rapidly progressive primary cancer of another organ system. The relationship has been built and based on years of mutual decision making, although benefits may ensue with the physician assisting in redefining the patient's own past system of values as a counselor/interpreter without his or her direct input. The patient may also wish to seek additional opinions (which may also be recommended by the physician) in a consumer-like fashion, although after this occurs, both parties again may partake in a collaborative relationship of shared decision making. Ultimately, the patient wishes to be guided and be "in the hands" of the original physician, viewed as a paternal figure. Another example is of a younger patient with a history of drug abuse (although abstinent for a number of years) presenting after a severe motor vehicle accident developing rhabdomyolysis (breakdown of muscle tissue) and ultimately multiorgan system failure. A shared decision-making relationship ensued in the Intensive Care Unit with the mutual collaboration of information and desired treatment plans with the family. The hospital course eventuated in the need and acceptance of a period of hemodialysis, although the patient also required revisiting his own set of values clarified by the physician (in a Counselor/Interpretive fashion) to include this individual's passion for life, exemplified by previous philanthropic activities and occupations. The patient also considered and valued the attending physician as an authoritarian figure in his continued and follow-up care. Such scenarios exemplify the real-life interrelations and interplay of the four separate models of the physician–patient relationship captured and schematized above by the paradigm of the metaphorical geometric tetrahedral pyramid and metaphorical triangulations.

2.3. The Variables of Trust, Empathy, and Communication: Hallmarks of Shared Decision Making

2.3.1. The Component of Trust

From a humanistic standpoint, devoid of deductive or inductive research, the essence of the physician–patient relationship is profoundly and poignantly captured by the modern-day Spanish infectious disease specialist, Dr. Teresa Hellin, in her analysis of the requisite tools for a physician to succeed in treating patients over twenty years ago:

> "To attend to those who suffer, a physician must possess not only the scientific knowledge and technical abilities, but also an understanding of human nature. The patient is a human being, at the same time worried and hopeful, who is searching for relief, help and trust. The importance of an intimate relationship between patient and physician can never be overstated because in most cases an accurate diagnosis, as well as an effective treatment, relies directly on the quality of this relationship". [20]

Trust by the patient has been shown to influence a number of clinical outcomes in a positive manner, as corroborated by the literature: emotional health, amelioration of symptoms, pain control, physiological parameters (including blood pressure control), and even mortality in certain groups [21–23]. Behavioral research in the early 2000s also strongly suggested that the trust of the patient in the physician is the bedrock of a privileged relationship and, coupled with the physician's positive attitude and approach, may be even more important to many patients than the medical issues themselves [24]. Conversely, well-performed studies also signify that the attitude and approach of the physician appear to be as important, or even more important to the patient, than any information being transmitted [25,26].

2.3.2. The Component of Empathy

An additional integral variable in the physician–patient "equation" is the key element of empathy demonstrated by the physician. Reviews investigating the subject of "empathic communication" in the acute hospital setting are based on relatively little research, although studies based on outpatient experience are numerous [27]. Intuitively, the expression of empathy in any type of human interaction will typically result in psychological benefits for both parties, particularly that of the physician and patient. In fact, research studies using qualitative assessment tools corroborate higher satisfaction [28] and determination of quality of care [29] among patients assessing their physicians as cognitively empathic. Furthermore, studies centering on empathy demonstrated by the physician are provocative in regard to subjective and objective (measurable) parameters of disease and infectious outcomes. As an example, a systematic review and meta-analysis of over 6000 patients revealed that greater practitioner empathy and communication of positive messages resulted in a modest reduction of pain (and other psychological outcomes) and a small benefit in physical outcomes, such as pulmonary function and length of hospital stay [30]. Moreover, in one report, levels of glycosylated hemoglobin (HbA1c) and low-density lipoprotein (LDL) among diabetic patients were found to be significantly improved in those who rated their physicians as more empathic [31]. Furthermore, a study of patients with the common cold revealed a shorter duration of illness and elevated levels of nasal wash Interleulin-8 and neutrophil counts among patients who rated their physicians as more empathic [32]. Although these reports suggest associations between empathy and medical outcomes, they cannot prove causality. Nonetheless, they certainly are compelling and are worthy of further research. The suggestions and implications of the above, therefore, are that empathy by the physician leads to improved clinical decision making, treatment plans, and patient compliance in the setting of a shared decision-making relationship.

2.3.3. The Component of Communication

In the spirit of the themes of confluences and reciprocities discussed throughout this perspective, the confidence of the patient in the physician can occur only through the art of communication between both parties. Communication is a learned skill affected by many factors, including verbal and non-verbal elements. Comparable to the ingredients of trust and empathy, communication between the physician and patient is multidimensional and complex in its behavioral, psychological, and cultural components. In tandem with the benefits of empathy, research supports effective communication as contributing to successful diagnoses and treatment of medical conditions [33]. Moreover, the most powerful diagnostic tool available to the physician is still age-old communication as the majority of information needed to make a diagnosis is often provided by the patient. Best practices and societal guidelines have now been published over the last decade, addressing communication as integral to the relationship between the physician and the patient [34,35]. Viewed from a different angle, communication can be construed as the cohesive factor linking both trust and empathy in the overall care of the patient in the context of shared decision making. The essential foundation of communication was undoubtedly implied by a passage written in the early 1990s by the therapist Deborah Rotter in ascribing great value to the patient's unique knowledge base (as the bearer of the disease process) as being just as important as the physician's medical knowledge such that "the medical visit is truly a meeting between experts" [36].

2.4. Neurobiological, Psychosocial, and Behavioral Components of Clinical Practice

2.4.1. Overview

Apart from the "mechanistic" analysis of clinical decision-making processes, the human elements provide their true underpinnings and foundation. A growing field of study is now exploring neuroscientific and neurobehavioral correlates involved in the physician–patient relationship and the ultimate results and outcomes of medical treatments. From a neurobiological point of view, a social–neural system has been proposed, which has evolved over the millennia (similar to our cellular–humoral immune system) as a defense and protective mechanism supporting the survival of man [37]. As such, and separate from the wonders of modern-day medical science, the mere "ritual" of the "therapeutic act" may result in responses equal to or even greater than the biological effects of the medications and procedures themselves [37]. These non-pharmacological (placebo) effects, in my opinion, may or may not be operative in physician–patient relationships or possibly in varying levels in tandem with the true pharmacologic treatments. However, the study of the activation and inactivation of neurochemicals and regions of the brain based on the physician's words, behaviors, and overall perception by the patient opens the door to an intriguing field of study to complement the "hardcore" physiological, biological, and medical sciences.

2.4.2. Specific Examples of Neuroscientific Findings

Although a "fledgling" scientific field, specific findings will be enumerated, which serve as springboards for ongoing research:

- The thickness of the left caudal anterior cingulate cortex was found to be inversely correlated with patients' trust in physicians using structural magnetic resonance imaging (MRI) [38]. Furthermore, using interactive functional near-infrared spectroscopy of both physicians and patients exhibiting a high level of trust in each other revealed increased inter-brain synchronization in the bilateral tempo-parietal junction and right inferior frontal gyrus [39].
- Functional MRI (fMRI) neuroimaging studies of physicians administering anesthesia to patients undergoing experimentally induced pain revealed the activation of the medial frontal brain regions [40]. More recent similar studies by the same group demonstrated the activation of additional brain regions of the physicians, including the right ventrolateral and dorsolateral prefrontal cortices [41].
- More intricate recent studies were conducted, consisting of interacting whole-brain mapping and fMRI of physicians administering anesthesia to patients during experi-

mentally induced acute and repetitive (chronic) pain stimuli. Significant brain-to-brain concordance with the dynamic coupling of brain nodes was demonstrated among physicians and patients (both of which with previously established rapport) [42].

- As per a systematic review of fMRI studies, the recently discovered mirror neuron system of specific areas of the brain appears to be important in establishing the basis for empathy: ventral premotor cortex, parietal and somatosensory areas, and limbic and paralimbic structures [43]. The mirror neuron system is a group of specialized neurons that fire when an individual is performing an activity, and it also fires in the same pattern when the same individual observes another person performing the same previous activity (as if the observer was performing the activity again). This neuronal system is also implicated in neurocognitive functions and neuropsychiatric disorders [44].
- The neuroendocrine system has also been implicated in correlates in the physician–patient relationship as manifested by fluctuations in the secretion of stress hormones (cortisol and epinephrine) as opposed to those secreted during "peaceful" activities (oxytocin) [45]. In fact, field-labeled socio-physiology is developing, which involves the associations between social behavior and physiology in multiple areas of medicine.

2.4.3. The Expanding Field of Placebo Research

A fascinating area of research involves that of placebo and nocebo effects, that is, the results of patients' positive and negative expectations, respectively, regarding a medication, procedure, or treatment [46]. The literature concerning this topic is vast, with multiple approaches proposed in its analysis and ongoing study. Neuroscientific evidence supports multiple complex brain systems and neurochemical mediators, which are actively being discovered as underlying the placebo effect [47–49]. A recent meta-analysis shows that parts of the thalamus, somatosensory cortex, and basal ganglia are key for the placebo effect to occur [50]. Psychosocial research posits that the placebo effect is based on and evoked by psychological processes, which are shaped by the contextual elements of social effects and the environment [51,52]. The effective application of the placebo effect in the contexts of clinical decision making and the physician–patient relationship has been advocated by multiple authors, although much remains to be learned regarding its neuroscientific basis [52,53]. In fact, the placebo effect is a compelling ingredient for the therapeutic milieu if harnessed properly. Interestingly, behavioral studies performed on physicians themselves demonstrated their liberal use of placebo techniques on their own patients, particularly if the former underwent tutorials regarding the benefits of placebo and if the patients themselves reported positive results from previous placebo treatments [54]. My perspective addresses this topic from another angle, that is, the grooming of a trusting, empathic, and communicative relationship in the setting of shared decision making is a powerful adjunct to the plan between physicians and patients based on medical science. The positive effect of each of these qualities in the activity of human interaction is intuitive and supported by many years of research. On the other hand, and in a broader neuroscientific sense, it can also be argued that trust, empathy, and communication may employ placebo neural pathways and patterns in the attainment of positive outcomes, although this requires further clarification and study.

2.5. The Essential Role of the Physician–Patient Relationship for the Effectuation of Advanced Clinical Decision Making

2.5.1. Interrelationships Between Paradigms of Clinical Decision Making and the Physician–Patient Relationship: The Secondary Analysis

In many ways, the models of physician–patient relationships parallel and are contingent on those of the clinical decision-making processes. I wish to posit a compelling argument that the bond between physicians and patients is the ultimate catalyst and effectuator for advanced clinical decision making to achieve fruition in optimal patient care. As asserted throughout this perspective, advanced clinical decision making and the physician–patient relationship are predicated on each other. The sub-relationships involving the individual models of clinical decision making and those of the physician–patient relationship are discussed separately above and schematized in Figures 2–5, respectively. Please indulge my proposition of novel higher "secondary and tertiary levels of analysis", again from a "bird's eye view" (Figure 4). The secondary level of analysis implies that the clinical decision-making models and processes cannot occur without the physician–patient relationship, and conversely, the latter cannot function without the former. Thus, the "domains" of clinical decision making and the physician–patient relationship do not represent a polarized dialectic with opposing forces and purposes, but rather a workable synergy and confluence required for optimal patient care. I would posit an imperative and, in effect, symbiotic interconnection of the two, depicted by an analogy from the field of astrophysics—a "harmonization" between all the "liaisons" and "sub-liaisons" within both domains. As a result, clinical decision making and the physician–patient relationship cannot exist without each other.

From a practical, pragmatic, and personal perspective, the existential aspects of a partnership between physicians and patients are manifested by mutual engagement in the framework of shared decision making in the analysis and execution by each party, as guided by the models of clinical decision making. The physician–patient relationship, therefore, has a large impact and influence on the models and processes of clinical decision making. Inversely, and in a similar fashion, the models/processes of clinical decision making will have a large impact and influence on the ensuing models and methods of interaction between physicians and patients. As schematized, the secondary analysis is, therefore, the determination from inductive reasoning that both domains of clinical decision making and the physician–patient relationship must interact with each other in order for each domain to function properly.

2.5.2. Clinical Examples of the Secondary Analysis

Real-life demonstrations of the proposed secondary analysis are rife in my practice. The models/processes contributing to clinical decision making (Participatory/Shared Decision Making, Evidence-Based, Rational, and Intuitive) will primarily affect the ensuing type of relationship between physicians and patients. Inversely, the type and character of the interaction between physicians and patients will primarily determine the model(s) that will be utilized in the decision-making process in the care of the patient. Therefore, clinical decision making will be affected based on the type of alliance between physicians and patients (Shared Decision making, Counselor/Interpretive, Consumerism/Informative, or Paternalism). In effect, the secondary analysis postulates that clinical decision making and the physician–patient relationship are tightly knit and thus reciprocally vitalized and energized by each other.

As cases in point, there are numerous examples of scenarios in which the models of clinical decision making will primarily affect the physician–patient relationship. With the advent of "cybermedicine", many patients are now conducting research on their own health issues via digital media and often proactively proceed with their own literature searches (complete with highlights and side notes). Typically, these patients are very interested in a collaborative interchange, including my ongoing opinions and feedback, without the intention of creating barriers to communication. As a result of these frequent occurrences, the clinical decision-making process that ensues is predominantly based on the Participatory/Shared Decision-Making Model and will most often lead to a relationship that is also predominantly based on shared decision making. On the other hand, another varying illustration would be a decision-making process based principally on evidence, which may lead primarily to a more consumerism/informative relationship between physicians and patients. In this case, the patient will often clarify their wishes for a decision-making process based primarily on up-to-date studies, trials, and societal guidelines without the desire for a true rapport or my personal input based on experience. Although this type of clinical decision-making model/process is not my preference, I will seek to incorporate some elements of the other models in formulating the decisions in the treatment of the patient and conduct the interactions in an informative fashion. However, a decision-making process based more on reason may result principally in a relationship between physicians and patients that is more counselor/interpretive in nature. In this case, assistance would be given to the patient in the clarification of their own thoughts and value systems (without my personal preferential input), which would then lead to the particular course of action. In sum, the above examples of my relationships with patients are shaped and take greater form and purpose predicated on the processes of decision making themselves.

The secondary analysis also consists of a reciprocation such that the type of operative physician–patient relationship primarily leads to and determines the model/process of clinical decision making. Correspondingly, multiple scenarios in clinical practice also shed light on this dynamic. As cases in point, if a shared decision-making relationship predominates, the model of clinical decision making in arriving at medical plans would most likely be based on that of Participatory/Shared Decision Making (although it may also include elements of the other three in various proportions). However, a consumerism/informative relationship may primarily result in an evidence-based and rational process of decision making. A counselor/interpretive alliance (although strong and collaborative) would likely and, in a similar fashion, primarily result in evidence-based and rational processes of clinical decision making. A Paternalistic Model has become quite rare in modern-day clinical medicine, although it may be appropriate in isolated situations. This may prevail when the physician is treating close family members or if a close relationship has been present for many years between the physician and the patient and family members. In these cases, the patient may not wish or be able to express their overriding preferences regarding the processes of arriving at decisions; therefore, the ensuing decision-making models may consist of a combination of evidence-based, rational, and possibly intuitive ones.

2.5.3. The Tertiary Analysis

The tertiary analysis in this construct reveals the critical nature of the physician–patient relationship as obligatory for the effectuation of advanced clinical decision making (Figure 6). In my opinion, the bond founded primarily upon shared decision making (although also including elements of the other models) gives the necessary energy and impetus for the process of clinical decision making to be translated into the treatment plan and overall care of the patient. The relationship is thus the metaphorical filter through which clinical decision making is distilled, crystallized, and activated in the care of patients. This tertiary analysis illustrates the critical importance of the physician–patient relationship for the analysis, interpretation, and ultimate translation of the models and precepts of clinical decision making. The conveyance of the information resulting from the decision-making process is afforded by the alliance of the physician and the patient, leading to its grasping, assimilation, and ultimate incorporation into the treatment plan. As highlighted in this perspective, both the processes of clinical decision making and the relationships between the physician and the patient are intertwined and actualize their constructs through each other. Moreover, in the simplest of terms, my perspective and opinion are that the pathway of decision making in the clinical arena is based on, and must "travel through", the existence of a strong bond between physician–patient based on mutual respect and collaboration.

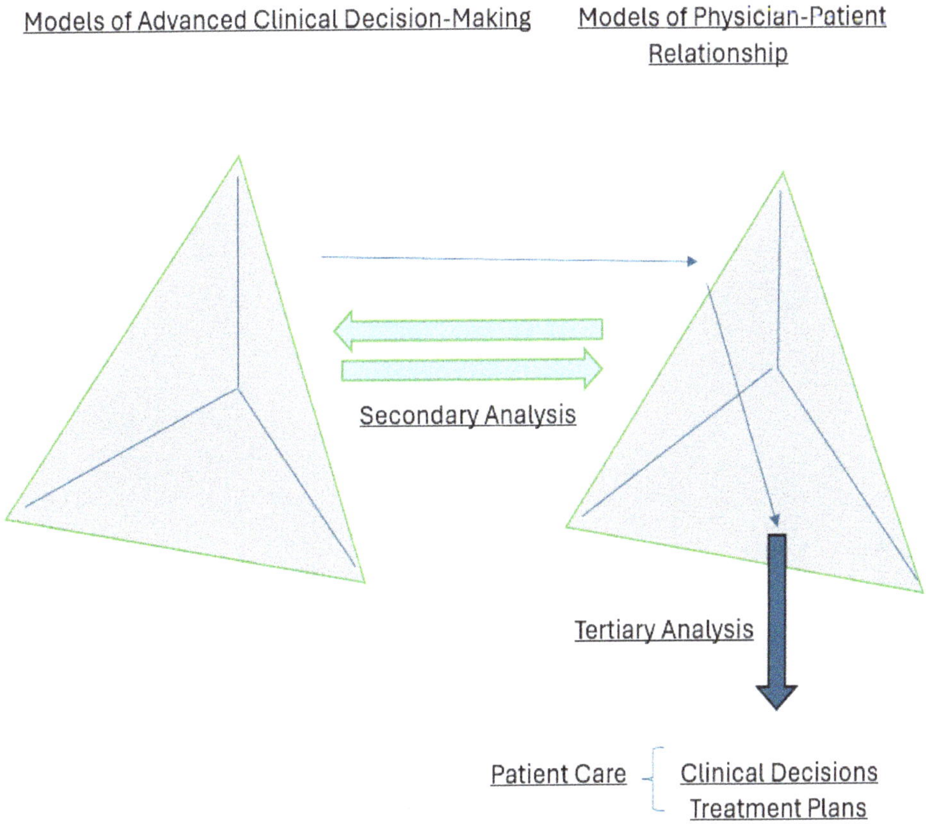

Figure 6. Interrelationships between Paradigms.

3. Conclusions

In summary, the complexities of advanced clinical decision making and the physician–patient relationship are interwoven amidst the multitude of interconnections and reciprocal relationships and sub-relationships detailed in this perspective. From my point of view, the resolute application of paradigms predominantly founded upon shared decision making within the domains of clinical decision making and the physician–patient relationship secures the most favorable results. Our modern-day digital era of mass-media "biomedicalization" is progressively impacting the terrain of healthcare, thus further necessitating a solid alliance between physicians and patients in the execution of the decision-making processes. The likelihood of successful medical outcomes is increasingly predicated on sound and robust practices within the clinical decision-making arena, filtered through robust collaborative interactions between the physician and the patient. These activities, including all their nuances and inherent challenges, will lead to the goal of optimal patient care in today's ever-complex medical and technological landscape. In conclusion, the practice of medicine is a delicate balance of art and science, which should be nurtured and groomed by trust, empathy, and communication between physicians and patients.

Funding: This research received no external funding.

Institutional Review Board Statement: Not applicable.

Informed Consent Statement: Not applicable.

Data Availability Statement: Not applicable.

Acknowledgments: The author wished to thank his cherished son and wife, Matthew and Laleh Musio, for the exceptional technical assistance and inspiration to complete this article.

Conflicts of Interest: There are no conflicts of interest.

References

1. Fiore, J.A.; Madison, A.J.; Poisal, J.A.; Cuckler, G.A.; Smith, S.D.; Sisko, A.M.; Keehan, S.P.; Rennie, K.E.; Gross, A.C. National health expenditure projections, 2023–2032: Payer trends diverge as pandemic-related polices fade. *Health Affairs* **2024**, *43*, 910–921.
2. Rodziewicz, T.L.; Houseman, B.; Hipskind, J.E. *Medical Error Reduction and Prevention*; StatPearls Publishing: Treasure Island, FL, USA, 2024. Available online: https://www.ncbi.nlm.nih.gov/books/NBK499956/ (accessed on 9 September 2024).
3. Kovacs, G.; Croskerry, P. Clinical decision making: An emergency medicine perspective. *Acad. Emerg. Med.* **1999**, *6*, 947–952. [CrossRef] [PubMed]
4. Trimble, M.; Hamilton, P. The thinking doctor: Clinical decision making in contemporary medicine. *Clin. Med.* **2016**, *16*, 343–346. [CrossRef] [PubMed]
5. Croskerry, P. A model for clinical decision-making in medicine. *Med. Sci. Educ.* **2017**, *27*, 9–13. [CrossRef]
6. Djulbegovic, B.; Elqayam, S.; Dale, W. Rational decision making in medicine: Implications for overuse and underuse. *J. Eval. Clin. Pract.* **2018**, *24*, 655–665. [CrossRef]
7. Bate, L.; Hutchinson, A.; Underhill, J.; Maskrey, N. How clinical decisions are made. *Br. J. Clin. Pharmacol.* **2012**, *74*, 614–620. [CrossRef]
8. Gaddis, G.M.; Greenwald, P.; Huckson, S. Toward improved implementation of evidence-based clinical algorithms: Clinical practice guidelines, clinical decision rules, and clinical pathways. *Acad. Emerg. Med.* **2007**, *14*, 1015–1022.
9. Harteis, C.; Morgenthaler, B.; Kugler, C.; Ittner, K.P.; Roth, G.; Graf, B. Professional competence and intuitive decision making: A simulation study in the domain of emergency medicine. *Vocat. Learn.* **2012**, *5*, 119–136. [CrossRef]
10. Thomas, E.; Bass, S.B.; Siminoff, L.A. Beyond rationality: Expanding the practice of shared decision making in modern medicine. *Soc. Sci. Med.* **2021**, *277*, 113900. [CrossRef]
11. Fraenkel, L.; McGraw, S. What are the essential elements to enable patient participation in medical decision making? *J. Gen. Intern. Med.* **2007**, *22*, 614–619. [CrossRef]
12. Frosch, D.; Kaplan, R.M. Shared decision making in clinical medicine: Past research and future directions. *Am. J. Prev. Med.* **1999**, *17*, 185–294. [CrossRef]
13. Bomhof-Roordink, H.; Gärtner, F.R.; Stiggelbout, A.M.; Pieterse, A.H. Key component of shared decision making models: A systemic review. *BMJ Open* **2019**, *9*, e031762. [CrossRef] [PubMed]
14. van Dam, H.A.; Van der Horst, F.; Van den Borne, B.; Ryckman, R.; Crebolder, H. Provider-patient interaction in diabetes care: Effects on patients' self-care and outcomes. *Patient Educ. Couns.* **2003**, *51*, 17–28. [CrossRef] [PubMed]
15. Ward, M.M.; Sundaramurthy, S.; Lotstein, D.; Bush, T.M.; Neuwelt, C.M.; Street, R.L., Jr. Participatory patient-physician communication and morbidity in patients with systemic lupus erythematosus. *Arthritis Rheum.* **2003**, *49*, 298–306. [CrossRef] [PubMed]
16. Parsons, T. Illness and the role of the physician—A sociological perspective. *Am. J. Orthopsychol.* **1951**, *21*, 452–460. [CrossRef]
17. Nelson, O. Doctor-patient relationship. In *The Wiley Blackwell Companion to Medical Sociology*; Cockerham, W.C., Ed.; John Wiley & Sons Ltd.: New York, NY, USA, 2021. [CrossRef]
18. Veatch, R.M. Models for ethical medicine in a revolutionary age. What physician-patient roles foster the most ethical relationship? *Hastings Cent. Rep.* **1972**, *2*, 5–7. [CrossRef]
19. Emanuel, E.; Emanuel, L. Four models of the physician-patient relationship. *JAMA* **1992**, *267*, 2221–2226. [CrossRef]
20. Hellin, T. The Physician-Patient Relationship: Recent Developments and Changes. *Haemophilia* **2002**, *8*, 450–454. [CrossRef]
21. Stewart, M. Effective Physician-Patient Communication and Health Outcomes: A Review. *Can. Med. Assoc. J.* **1995**, *152*, 1423–1433.
22. Lee, Y. Linking patients' trust in physicians to health outcomes. *Br. J. Hosp. Med.* **2013**, *69*, 28040. [CrossRef]
23. Schoenthaler, A.; Kalet, A.; Nicholson, J.; Lipkin, M., Jr. Does Improving Patient-Practitioner Communication Improve Clinical Outcomes in Patients with Cardiovascular Diseases? A Systemic Review of the Evidence. *Patient Educ. Counsel.* **2014**, *96*, 3–12. [CrossRef]
24. Lee, S.J.; Back, A.L.; Block, S.D.; Stewart, S.K. Enhancing physician-patient communication. *ASH Educ. Program* **2002**, *2002*, 464–483. [CrossRef] [PubMed]
25. Pearson, S.D.; Raeke, L.H. Patients' trust in physicians: Many theories, few measures, and little data. *J. Gen. Intern. Med.* **2000**, *15*, 509–513. [CrossRef] [PubMed]

26. Dang, B.N.; Westbrook, R.A.; Njue, S.M.; Giordano, T.P. Building trust and rapport early in the new doctor-patient relationship: A longitudinal qualitative study. *BMC Med. Educ.* **2017**, *17*, 32. [CrossRef] [PubMed]
27. Haribhai-Thompson, J.; McBride-Henry, K.; Hales, C.; Rook, H. Understanding of empathic communication in acute hospital settings: A scoping review. *BMJ Open* **2022**, *12*, e063775. [CrossRef] [PubMed]
28. Arshad, M.; Sriram, S.; Khan, S.; Gollapalli, P.K.; Albadrani, M. Mediating role of physician's empathy between physician's communication and patient's satisfaction. *J. Fam. Med. Prim. Care* **2024**, *13*, 1530–1534. [CrossRef]
29. Gerger, H.; Munder, T.; Kreuzer, N.; Locher, C.; Blease, C. Lay perspectives on empathy in patient-physician communication: An online experimental study. *Health Comm.* **2024**, *39*, 1246–1255. [CrossRef]
30. Howick, J.; Moscrop, A.; Mebius, A.; Fanshawe, T.R.; Lewith, G.; Bishop, F.L.; Mistiaen, P.; Roberts, N.W.; Dieninytė, E.; Hu, X.Y.; et al. Effects of empathic and positive communication in healthcare consultations: A systemic review and meta-analysis. *J. R. Soc. Med.* **2018**, *111*, 240–252. [CrossRef]
31. Hojat, M.; Louis, D.Z.; Markham, F.W.; Wender, R.; Rabinowitz, C.; Gonnella, J.S. Physicians' empathy and clinical outcomes for diabetic patients. *Acad. Med.* **2011**, *86*, 359–364. [CrossRef]
32. Rakel, D.; Barrett, B.; Zhang, Z.; Hoeft, T.; Chewning, B.; Marchand, L.; Scheder, J. Perception of empathy in the therapeutic encounter: Effects on the common cold. *Patient Educ. Couns.* **2011**, *85*, 390–397. [CrossRef]
33. Belasen, A.; Belasen, A.T. Doctor-patient communication: A review and a rationale for using an assessment framework. *J. Health Org. Manag.* **2018**, *32*, 891–907. [CrossRef]
34. American College of Obstetrics and Gynecologist. Effective Patient-Physician Communication. Committee Opinion (Committee on Patient Safety and Quality Improvement/Committee on Health Care for Underserved Women). Number 587. *Obs. Gynecol.* **2014**, *123*, 389–393. [CrossRef] [PubMed]
35. American Medical Association, Code of Medical Ethics. Chapter 1: Opinion Patient Physician Relationships. 2020. Available online: https://www.ama-assn.org/system/files/code-of-medical-ethics-chapter-1.pdf (accessed on 9 September 2024).
36. Rotter, D.; Hall, J. *Doctors Talking with Patients/Patients Talking with Doctors: Improving Communication in Medical Visits*; Greenwood Publishing Group (Auburn House Westport): Santa Barbara, CA, USA, 1992.
37. Benedetti, F. *The Patient's Brain: The Neuroscience Behind the Doctor-Patient Relationship*; Oxford University Press: New York, NY, USA, 2010.
38. Sadhu, M.; Jalalizadeh, B.; Fritz, A.; de Freitas Nicholson, T.; Garcia, R.; Lampley, S.; Rain, M.; Van Enkevort, E.; Brown, E.S. Trust in physicians and regional brain volumes: A population-based study. *Prim. Care Companion CNS Disord.* **2019**, *21*, 19m02461. [CrossRef] [PubMed]
39. Liu, Y.; Liu, Y.; Zhang, M.; Wang, P. Preserving trust in the doctor-patient interaction: Unveiling the interactive positive evolutionary process of doctor-patient trust though fNIRS evidence. *Res. Sq.* **2024**, *preprint*. [CrossRef]
40. Jensen, K.; Gollub, R.L.; Kong, J.; Lamm, C.; Kaptchuk, T.J.; Petrovic, P. Reward and empathy in the treating clinician: The neural correlates of successful doctor-patient interactions. *Transl. Psych.* **2020**, *10*, 17. [CrossRef]
41. Jensen, K.B.; Petrovic, P.; Kerr, C.E.; Kirsch, I.; Raicek, J.L.; Cheetham, A.; Spaeth, R.; Cook, A.; Gollub, R.L.; Kong, J.; et al. Sharing pain and relief: Neural correlates of physicians during treatment of patients. *Mol. Psych.* **2014**, *19*, 392–398. [CrossRef]
42. Ellingsen, D.M.; Isenburg, K.; Jung, C.; Lee, J.; Gerber, J.; Mawla, I.; Sclocco, R.; Jensen, K.B.; Edwards, R.R.; Kelley, J.M.; et al. Dynamic brain-to-brain concordance and behavioral mirroring as a mechanism of the patient-clinician interaction. *Sci. Adv.* **2020**, *6*, eacb1304. [CrossRef]
43. Derksen, F.; Bensing, J.; Lagro-Janssen, A. Effectiveness of empathy in general practice: A systemic review. *Br. J. Gen. Pract.* **2013**, *63*, e76–e84. [CrossRef]
44. Jeon, H.; Lee, S.H. From neurons to social beings: Short review of the mirror neuron system research and its socio-psychological and psychiatric implications. *Clin. Psychopharmacol. Neurosci.* **2018**, *16*, 18–31. [CrossRef]
45. Adler, H.M. The socio-physiology of caring in the doctor-patient relationship. *J. Gen. Intern. Med.* **2002**, *17*, 883–890. [CrossRef]
46. Colloca, L. The placebo effect on pain therapies. *Annu. Rev. Pharmacol. Toxicol.* **2019**, *59*, 191–211. [CrossRef]
47. Colloca, L.; Barsky, A.J. Placebo and nocebo effects. *N. Engl. J. Med.* **2020**, *382*, 554–559. [CrossRef] [PubMed]
48. Wager, T.D.; Atlas, L.Y. The neuroscience of placebo effects: Connecting context, learning and health. *Nat. Rev. Neurosci.* **2015**, *16*, 403–418. [CrossRef] [PubMed]
49. Benedetti, F. Placebo and the new physiology of the doctor-patient relationship. *Physiol. Rev.* **2013**, *93*, 1207–1246. [CrossRef] [PubMed]
50. Zunhammer, M.; Spisák, T.; Wager, T.D.; Bingel, U. Meta-analysis of neural systems underlying placebo analgesia from individual participant fMRI data. *Nat. Comm.* **2021**, *12*, 1391. [CrossRef]
51. Zion, S.; Crum, A.J. Mindsets matter: A new framework for harnessing the placebo effect in modern medicine. *Int. Rev. Neurobiol.* **2018**, *138*, 137–154.
52. Testa, M.; Rossettini, G. Enhance placebo, avoid nocebo: How contextual factors affect physiotherapy outcomes. *Manual. Ther.* **2016**, *24*, 65–74. [CrossRef]

53. Carlino, E.; Pollo, A.; Benedetti, F. The placebo in practice—How to use it in clinical routine. *Curr. Opin. Support Palliat. Care* **2012**, *6*, 220–225. [CrossRef]
54. Piedimonte, A.; Volpino, V.; Campaci, F.; Borghesi, F.; Guerra, G.; Carlino, E. Placebos in healthcare: A behavioral study on how treatment responsiveness affects therapy decisions in a simulated patient-physician interaction. *Clin. Pract.* **2024**, *14*, 2151–2165. [CrossRef]

MDPI AG
Grosspeteranlage 5
4052 Basel
Switzerland
Tel.: +41 61 683 77 34

Applied Sciences Editorial Office
E-mail: applsci@mdpi.com
www.mdpi.com/journal/applsci

www.ingramcontent.com/pod-product-compliance
Lightning Source LLC
Chambersburg PA
CBHW040835250926
51850CB00007BA/1319
* 9 7 8 3 7 2 5 8 6 0 5 3 1 *